The Fellows Manual
Techniques of Spine Surgery

The Fellows Manual
Techniques of Spine Surgery

Editors

Barrett S Boody MD
Assistant Professor
Department of Orthopedic Surgery
Orthopedic Spine Surgeon
Indiana Spine Group
Indiana University School of Medicine
Indianapolis, USA

Glenn S Russo MD MS
Clinical Assistant Professor
Connecticut Orthopedics
Frank H Netter School of Medicine
Quinnipiac University
Hamden, Connecticut, USA

Alexander R Vaccaro MD PhD MBA
Richard H Rothman Professor and Chairman
Department of Orthopedic Surgery
Professor of Neurosurgery
Thomas Jefferson University
Philadelphia, PA, USA

Greg Anderson MD
Professor
Department of Orthopedic and Neurological Surgery
Thomas Jefferson University
Philadelphia, PA, USA

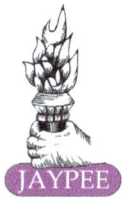

JAYPEE BROTHERS MEDICAL PUBLISHERS
The Health Sciences Publisher
New Delhi | London

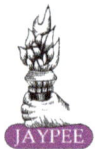 **Jaypee Brothers Medical Publishers (P) Ltd**

Headquarters
Jaypee Brothers Medical Publishers (P) Ltd
EMCA House, 23/23-B
Ansari Road, Daryaganj
New Delhi 110 002, India
Landline: +91-11-23272143, +91-11-23272703
+91-11-23282021, +91-11-23245672
Email: jaypee@jaypeebrothers.com

Corporate Office
Jaypee Brothers Medical Publishers (P) Ltd
4838/24, Ansari Road, Daryaganj
New Delhi 110 002, India
Phone: +91-11-43574357
Fax: +91-11-43574314
Email: jaypee@jaypeebrothers.com

Overseas Office
JP Medical Ltd
83 Victoria Street, London
SW1H 0HW (UK)
Phone: +44 20 3170 8910
Fax: +44 (0)20 3008 6180
Email: info@jpmedpub.com

Website: www.jaypeebrothers.com
Website: www.jaypeedigital.com

© 2023, Jaypee Brothers Medical Publishers

The views and opinions expressed in this book are solely those of the original contributor(s)/author(s) and do not necessarily represent those of editor(s) or publisher of the book.

All rights reserved. No part of this publication may be reproduced, stored or transmitted in any form or by any means, electronic, mechanical, photocopying, recording or otherwise, without the prior permission in writing of the publishers.

All brand names and product names used in this book are trade names, service marks, trademarks or registered trademarks of their respective owners. The publisher is not associated with any product or vendor mentioned in this book.

Medical knowledge and practice change constantly. This book is designed to provide accurate, authoritative information about the subject matter in question. However, readers are advised to check the most current information available on procedures included and check information from the manufacturer of each product to be administered, to verify the recommended dose, formula, method and duration of administration, adverse effects and contraindications. It is the responsibility of the practitioner to take all appropriate safety precautions. Neither the publisher nor the author(s)/editor(s) assume any liability for any injury and/or damage to persons or property arising from or related to use of material in this book.

This book is sold on the understanding that the publisher is not engaged in providing professional medical services. If such advice or services are required, the services of a competent medical professional should be sought.

Every effort has been made where necessary to contact holders of copyright to obtain permission to reproduce copyright material. If any have been inadvertently overlooked, the publisher will be pleased to make the necessary arrangements at the first opportunity.

Inquiries for bulk sales may be solicited at: jaypee@jaypeebrothers.com

The Fellows Manual: Techniques of Spine Surgery

First Edition: 2023

ISBN: 978-93-5465-539-5

Dedicated to

There are not enough words to properly thank those people in our lives who fill our lives with joy, so we attempt to capture our sentiment with brevity and sincerity.

The authors would like to dedicate this book to our families for their love and support during this lengthy endeavor. We are forever grateful to their patience and encouragement.

Contributors

Alan S Hilibrand	**Jacob Buchowski**	**Peter B Derman**
Alexander R Vaccaro	**Jacob Hoffmann**	**Peter G Whang**
Anthony Stefanelli	**Jael E Camacho**	**Peter R Swiatek**
Anthony Viola III	**James D Kang**	**Preetpaul S Bagi**
Aria Mahtabfar	**James D Lin**	**Rick C Sasso**
Ashley R Strickland	**James Harrop**	**R Matthew Wham**
Barrett S Boody	**Jason Savage**	**Rohan Gopinath**
Brett D Rosenthal	**Jeffrey Rihn**	**Ron Lehman**
Bruce V Darden	**John G Heller**	**Samuel Q Li**
Corey T Walker	**John R Dimar**	**Sean M Rider**
Daniel Franco	**Joon S Yoo**	**Sheeraz Quereshi**
Daniel Leas	**Joseph D Smucker**	**Sheila Kahwaty**
Daniel R Rubio	**Juan S Uribe**	**Shirvinda A Wijesekera**
David Casper	**Kern Singh**	**Sravisht Iyer**
David S Xu	**Lawrence Lenke**	**Srinivas Prasad**
Dil V Patel	**Leah Y Carreon**	**Steven C Ludwig**
Edward M DelSole	**Mark Kurd**	**Tom Mroz**
Fadi Al-Saiegh	**Matthew J Sabatino**	**Tyler Kreitz**
Glenn Gonzalez	**M Farooq Usmani**	**Vadim Goz**
Glenn S Russo	**Michael Yayac**	**Wellington K Hsu**
Greg Anderson	**Mostafa El Dafrawy**	**Yoji Ogura**
Han Jo Kim	**Munish C Gupta**	**Yoshihiro Katsuura**
Howard An	**Neel Anand**	

Message from Editors

*"Good judgment comes from experience,
And experience comes from bad judgment"*

While there are a number of textbooks that describe operative techniques, we felt that there may be an opportunity to capture the experience of our great teachers and present it in a manner that adds value to the reader and their patients. Our mission was to move past the well-established steps involved in performing a surgical procedure and to create a resource to help young surgeons capture the nuances of a well-performed procedure by diving into the "why" behind the "what" and the "how". Training with experienced surgeons in fellowship and residency, we participated in thousands of cases that went seamlessly and effortlessly. We would absorb the approaches and techniques of how a certain procedure was done but a certain surgeon and try to wrap our minds around the reasoning behind a certain retractor placement or tissue dissection. We then left training with a sense of ambition and confidence that our practice would soon resemble their practice.

Then, we began our practices. Sometimes, the seamless and effortless procedures seen in training didn't seem to go so seamlessly. The master surgeons' who smartly and adeptly placed retractors and assisted in the operating room were no longer there to help. We realized quickly that our mentor's techniques were not just a box to mark on a long checklist. Instead, the details and nuances of their work are the result of decades of lessons learned from successes and failures.

This book is meant for the surgeon who wants to dig deeper into a technique, learn a new technique, or even those who aspire to master the technique. But what makes this book different is that the authors for the techniques are not far removed from what it means to struggle and who firsthand understand the importance of the "why" something is done a certain way. For our chapters, we paired up fellows and early career surgeons with a senior master surgeon who has extensive experience in educating young surgeons. We sought to impart the wisdom of a career of experience written from a perspective of those to who was have targeted the book. Each author was given the instruction, "the reader knows how to perform this procedure, but we want to capture how to perform YOUR version of this procedure and WHY you do it the way you do."

We hope you enjoy and benefit from our efforts to compile a thoughtful technique guide to emphasize and extrapolate upon the core concepts and procedures of spine surgery.

Barrett S Boody
Glenn S Russo
Alexander R Vaccaro
Greg Anderson

Preface

Our book has sought to compile a technical and concept guide for the core practices of spine surgery. We have gathered master surgeons and young, talented surgeons to put into print some of the most important aspects of the procedures today's spinal surgeons perform on a daily basis. The result has been nearly 200 pages of lessons learned by dozens of expert surgeons. We believe that this text serves as a complement to the many other available texts on surgical techniques and builds upon the extensive information already available to young surgeons.

Barrett S Boody
Glenn S Russo
Alexander R Vaccaro
Greg Anderson

Acknowledgments

We further thank the chapter authors similarly for their dedication to providing excellent and concise material. This book would not have been possible were it not for the efforts of the authors who dedicated time and effort into thoughtfully writing their chapters.

Contents

SECTION 1 Cervical

1. Occipital Fusion 3
   Brett D Rosenthal, James D Kang

2. Posterior Cervical C1–2 Fusion 8
   Barrett S Boody, Glenn S Russo, Rick C Sasso

3. Posterior Cervical Decompression and Fusion 12
   Glenn S Russo, Barrett S Boody, Peter G Whang

4. Posterior Cervical Foraminotomy 17
   Yoshihiro Katsuura, Han Jo Kim

5. Posterior Cervical Laminoplasty 21
   John G Heller, R Matthew Wham

6. Anterior Cervical Discectomy and Fusion 28
   Anthony Viola III, Vadim Goz, Alan S Hilibrand

7. Anterior Cervical Corpectomy and Fusion 35
   David Casper, Jacob Hoffmann, Tom Mroz, Jason Savage

8. Anterior Cervical Discectomy and Disk Arthroplasty 39
   Bruce V Darden

9. Pearls of Upper Cervical Spine Trauma Management 42
   Daniel Leas, Barrett S Boody, Rick C Sasso

10. Technical Pearls in the Management of Subaxial Cervical Trauma 55
    Edward M DelSole, Michael Yayac, Alexander R Vaccaro

SECTION 2 Thoracolumbar

11. Thoracic Transpedicular Decompression and Costotransversectomy 65
    Preetpaul S Bagi, Glenn S Russo, Shirvinda A Wijesekera

12. Anterior Thoracic Discectomy/Corpectomy/Anterior Instrumentation 72
    Yoji Ogura, John R Dimar, Leah Y Carreon

13. Technical Pearls in the Management of Spinal Oncology 81
    Mostafa El Dafrawy, Jacob Buchowski

14. Percutaneous Thoracolumbar Pedicle Screw Fixation 91
    Barrett S Boody, Glenn S Russo, Greg Anderson

15. **Thoracolumbar Osteotomies: Posterior Column, Pedicle Subtraction, and Vertebral Column Resection** 96
    Daniel R Rubio, Sean M Rider, Munish C Gupta

16. **Thoracolumbar Instrumentation** 102
    Ron Lehman

17. **Sacral and Pelvic Instrumentation** 110
    Barrett S Boody, Glenn S Russo, Joseph D Smucker

18. **Transforaminal Lumbar Interbody Fusion** 115
    Barrett S Boody, Glenn S Russo, Jeffrey Rihn

19. **Technical Pearls in the Management of Adult Scoliosis** 118
    Lawrence Lenke, James D Lin

20. **Anterior Lumbar Interbody Fusion Technique** 123
    Barrett S Boody, Glenn S Russo, Mark Kurd

21. **Technical Pearls in the Surgical Management of Thoracic and Lumbar Trauma** 127
    Ashley R Strickland, Rohan Gopinath, Samuel Q Li, Jael E Camacho, M Farooq Usmani, Steven C Ludwig

22. **Open Microdiscectomy and Laminectomy** 137
    Tyler Kreitz, Howard An

SECTION 3 Miscellaneous

23. **Minimally Invasive Surgical Discectomy and Laminectomy** 145
    Sheeraz Quereshi

24. **Extraforaminal Approaches for Microdiscectomy and Foraminal Decompression in the Lumbar Spine** 149
    Barrett S Boody, Glenn S Russo, Rick C Sasso

25. **The Fellows Manual: Techniques of Spine Surgery Minimally Invasive Transforaminal Lumbar Interbody Fusion** 155
    Peter B Derman, Sravisht Iyer, Dil V Patel, Joon S Yoo, Kern Singh

26. **Lateral Lumbar Interbody Fusion** 160
    Corey T Walker, David S Xu, Juan S Uribe

27. **Ante-Psoas Interbody Fusion** 164
    Neel Anand, Sheila Kahwaty

28. **Navigation Techniques** 173
    Peter R Swiatek, Wellington K Hsu

29. **Technical Pearls in the Management of Spinal Cord Injury** 180
    Daniel Franco, Aria Mahtabfar, Glenn Gonzalez, James Harrop

30. **Dural Repair Strategies** 188
    Fadi Al-Saiegh, Anthony Stefanelli, Srinivas Prasad

31. **Minimally Invasive Sacroiliac Joint Fusion** 190
    Matthew J Sabatino, Glenn S Russo, Peter G Whang

Index 197

SECTION 1

Cervical

- **Occipital Fusion**
  Brett D Rosenthal, James D Kang

- **Posterior Cervical C1–2 Fusion**
  Barrett S Boody, Glenn S Russo, Rick C Sasso

- **Posterior Cervical Decompression and Fusion**
  Glenn S Russo, Barrett S Boody, Peter G Whang

- **Posterior Cervical Foraminotomy**
  Yoshihiro Katsuura, Han Jo Kim

- **Posterior Cervical Laminoplasty**
  John G Heller, R Matthew Wham

- **Anterior Cervical Discectomy and Fusion**
  Anthony Viola III, Vadim Goz, Alan S Hilibrand

- **Anterior Cervical Corpectomy and Fusion**
  David Casper, Jacob Hoffmann, Tom Mroz, Jason Savage

- **Anterior Cervical Discectomy and Disk Arthroplasty**
  Bruce V Darden

- **Pearls of Upper Cervical Spine Trauma Management**
  Daniel Leas, Barrett S Boody, Rick C Sasso

- **Technical Pearls in the Management of Subaxial Cervical Trauma**
  Edward M DelSole, Michael Yayac, Alexander R Vaccaro

CHAPTER 1

Occipital Fusion

Brett D Rosenthal, James D Kang

INTRODUCTION

Occipitocervical fusions may be required to treat various pathologic processes (e.g., traumatic, degenerative, inflammatory, infectious, neoplastic, or congenital).

INSTRUMENTS SUGGESTED

- Mayfield tongs
- Jackson table or a reversed standard operating room (OR) bed (to allow fluoroscopy clearance)
- Posterior cervical lateral mass screws
- Occipital plate
- Titanium or cobalt-chrome rods:
  - Hinged rods allow for easier insertion.
  - Titanium rods are typically strong enough and easier to contour.

NEUROMONITORING

- Recommend somatosensory evoked potentials (SSEPs)/motor evoked potentials (MEPs) intraoperatively.
- Can consider preflip testing in cases of acute or high instability (e.g., post-traumatic).
- Tell anesthesia staff to avoid paralytic so that neuromonitoring is not compromised during positioning and intraoperatively.

POSITIONING

- Maintain cervical spine precautions and perform log-roll technique during the flip. Keep cervical collar in place during the flip if surgery is being done for an acute injury.
- If using a reversed standard OR bed, gel rolls should be used to support the chest.
- Recommend using a Mayfield head positioner to allow for meticulous positioning of the head relative to the cervical spine.
- Prior to flipping, make sure a sheet is on the bed to allow for arms to be tucked at the patient's sides.
- Use heavy tape and/or a seat belt to further secure the patient to the bed.
- Maintain the bed in slight reverse Trendelenburg position.
- Keep the knees bent with adequate padding.
- The position of the head is critical to success in this operation. The patient will be permanently locked in this position.
  - Obtain radiographs after flipping to confirm an appropriate of head/neck.
    - Several landmarks to consider, including the following:
      - *Occipitocervical distance:* Distance from superior aspect of C2 spinous process to occipital protuberance: Mean is 21.5 mm in neutral position
      - *Occipitocervical angle:* Angle between McRae's line and superior endplate of C3: Mean is 44° in neutral position
      - *Mandible-cervical distance:* Distance from midpoint of mandibular angles to the anterior aspect of C2: Compare to preoperative neutral if available
  - Avoid excessive flexion or extension.
  - Chin position is a useful point of focus.
  - Confirm the nose, lips, and chin are pointing directly perpendicular to the axis of the body.

RADIOGRAPHY

- Lateral fluoroscopy or plain radiograph should be performed to assess alignment prior to prepping/draping.
- Adjust Mayfield position to achieve an acceptable alignment.

MEDICATION
- Provide preoperative antibiotics.
- *Consider initiation of tranexamic acid if clinically warranted:* The authors use tranexamic acid routinely unless if clinically contraindicated.

DRAPING
Be sure to have shaved the patient closely and widely to 1–2 cm above the external occipital protuberance: Postoperative dressings will not stick if hair is not shaved widely.

EXPOSURE
- *Cephalad extent:* Occipital inion
- *Caudal extent:* Based on preoperative plan for distal extension:
  - At minimum, exposure should be to C2.
  - Include two normal caudal levels in setting of acute trauma.
- Avoid high amplitude electrocautery to protect dura.
  - The authors typically use the 35 W setting.
- Incise the skin and use electrocautery to achieve hemostasis.
- Use electrocautery to identify the superficial fascia.
- Dissect down the midline raphe to spinous processes.
  - Raise large flaps to preserve vascularity.
  - Handle soft tissues gently.
- Remove all soft tissue from the midline while exposing out laterally to the lateral edge of the lateral masses.
- At C1–C2, take extra care to avoid the wide interspace.
- C1 dissection should be performed carefully.
  - To avoid iatrogenic risk to the vertebral arteries, be extremely careful when exposing beyond 1 cm from midline.
    - The authors recommend carefully using a small periosteal elevator and bipolar cautery to expose this region.
    - If possible, avoid monopolar electrocautery on the cephalad portion of the C1 ring beyond 1 cm from the midline.
    - Expose as much of the lateral C1 ring such that an adequate amount of bone is exposed for later decortication and grafting.
      - This is especially critical if a C1 laminectomy is planned.
  - Do not hesitate to take a radiograph to confirm the midline if in doubt.
- Preserve as much soft tissue attachment as possible to the caudal-most level's midline structures to minimize risk of iatrogenic instability.

INSTRUMENTATION
- We recommend an occipital plate with cervical rods/screws construct.
- Subaxial vertebrae can be instrumented using the standard lateral mass screw technique.
- C2 can be instrumented using pars or pedicle screw trajectories.
  - Laminar screw trajectory may be used as a salvage option as this makes rod contouring much more difficult and often requires offset connectors.
- C1 instrumentation may be performed in the typical fashion.
  - One technique is to burr the outer cortex and then cannulate the trajectory using a straight gear-shifter.
  - If needed, the head position can be temporarily flexed to allow easier access to C1.
  - We recommend the use of fluoroscopy in a lateral position to assist with achieving a correct trajectory.
  - Often C1 screws are not necessary, add time, and increase the difficulty of placing rods.
    - The authors usually do not include C1 screws so long as screw purchase is acceptable at the caudal levels.
- The occipital plate should be placed in the midline near the external occipital protuberance (thickest bone) **(Fig. 1)**.
  - Screws above the superior nuchal line risk injury to the transverse sinus **(Fig. 2)**
  - Optimal screw positions form an inverted triangle configuration.
    - ~20 mm lateral to the external occipital protuberance at the level of the superior nuchal line.
    - ~5 mm lateral from midline at ~20 mm inferior to superior nuchal line.
  - Three unicortical screws on each side may be used.
  - Bicortical screws are much stronger, but have increased risk.
    - When placing these, we recommend use of a hard-stop drill sleeve with adjustable lengths. Go up in 1–2 mm increments and check with a ball-tip probe between each pass until a soft endpoint is achieved.
    - Using this technique is safe, and bicortical screw purchase is always preferred in the occiput.
    - If cerebrospinal fluid (CSF) leaks from the screw hole, simply place the screw to stop the leak.
    - The authors prefer using bicortical screw fixation.
  - Keep in mind, revision scenarios may require larger diameter screws as a rescue option.

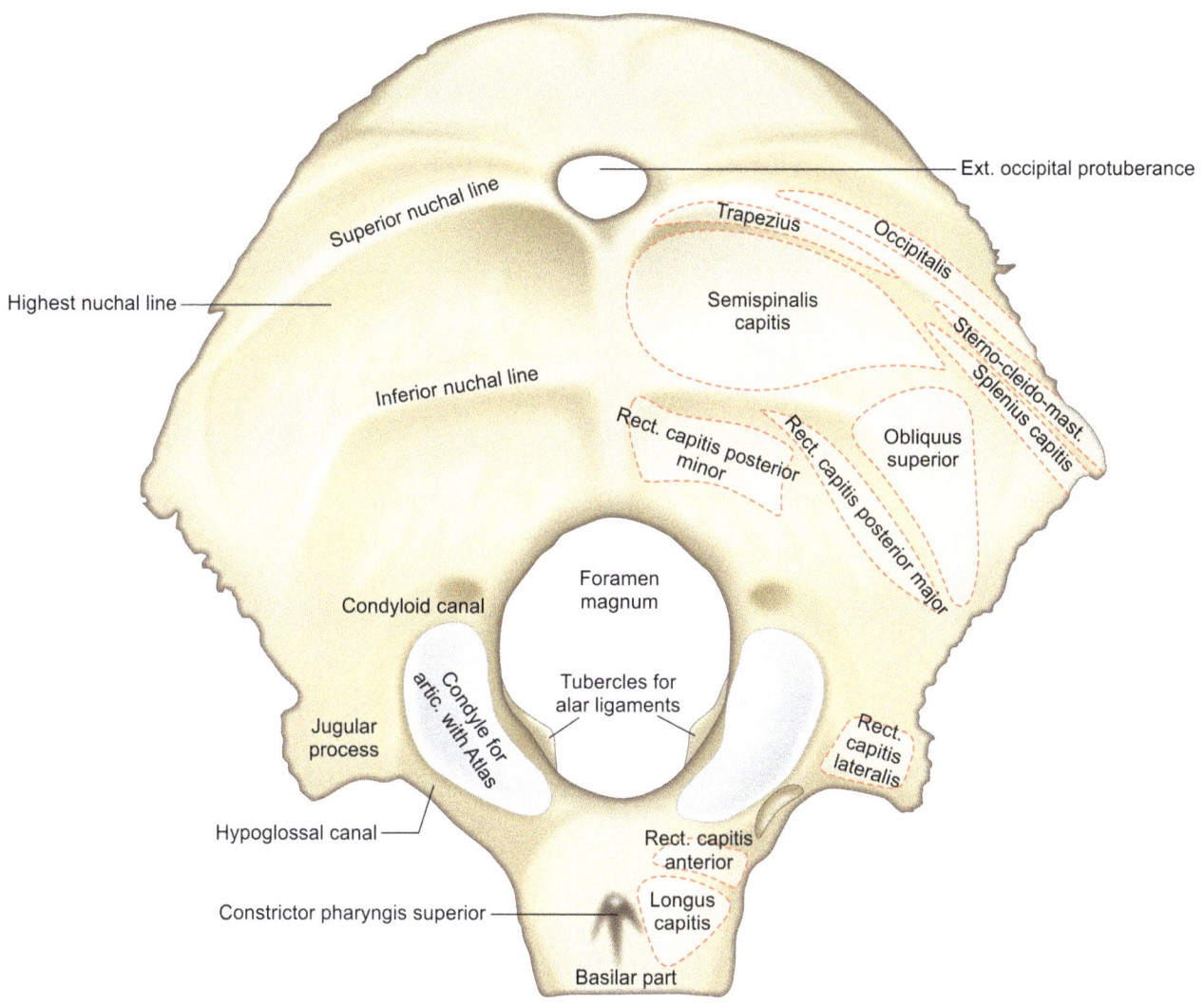

Fig. 1: Occipital bone (exterior surface).
Source: Anatomy of the Human Body (1918) – Henry Gray

DECOMPRESSION

If needed, a decompression of the occipitocervical junction can be performed using Kerrison rongeurs.
- If there is severe stenosis, avoid using a Kerrison and opt for either a side-cutting burr or a diamond tip burr to remove the central bone by making cuts on either side and then elevating the central bone using a curette.
- Always be cognizant of the location of the vertebral arteries when performing the decompression of the C1 arch.
- Take care to keep maintain adequate bone for a robust fusion to occur between the remaining surfaces.

FINAL INSTRUMENTATION/DECORTICATION

- After all screws and plate are in place, contour the rods and link all segmental fixation (**Figs. 3A to C**)
  - Instrumentation with a hinge built in is often easier to insert than prebent rods.
  - The authors recommend a hinged rod for this reason.
- Recheck position and alignment with fluoroscopy or plain radiographs.
  - Aim for neutral position:
    - If possible, use a neutral preoperative film as a guide.
    - In a trauma setting, refer to radiographic landmarks discussed above.
  - Avoid excessive flexion or extension:
    - This results in worsened ability to maintain horizontal gaze and swallow as one deviates further from neutral alignment.
    - Refer to radiographic parameters described above if in doubt.
  - Decorticate the occiput, remaining lamina, and lateral mass bone
- Pack autograft/allograft bone onto decorticated surfaces.
  - Consider iliac crest bone autograft for its robust fusion rates.
  - Depending on extent of decompression and remaining decorticated bone available for fusion,

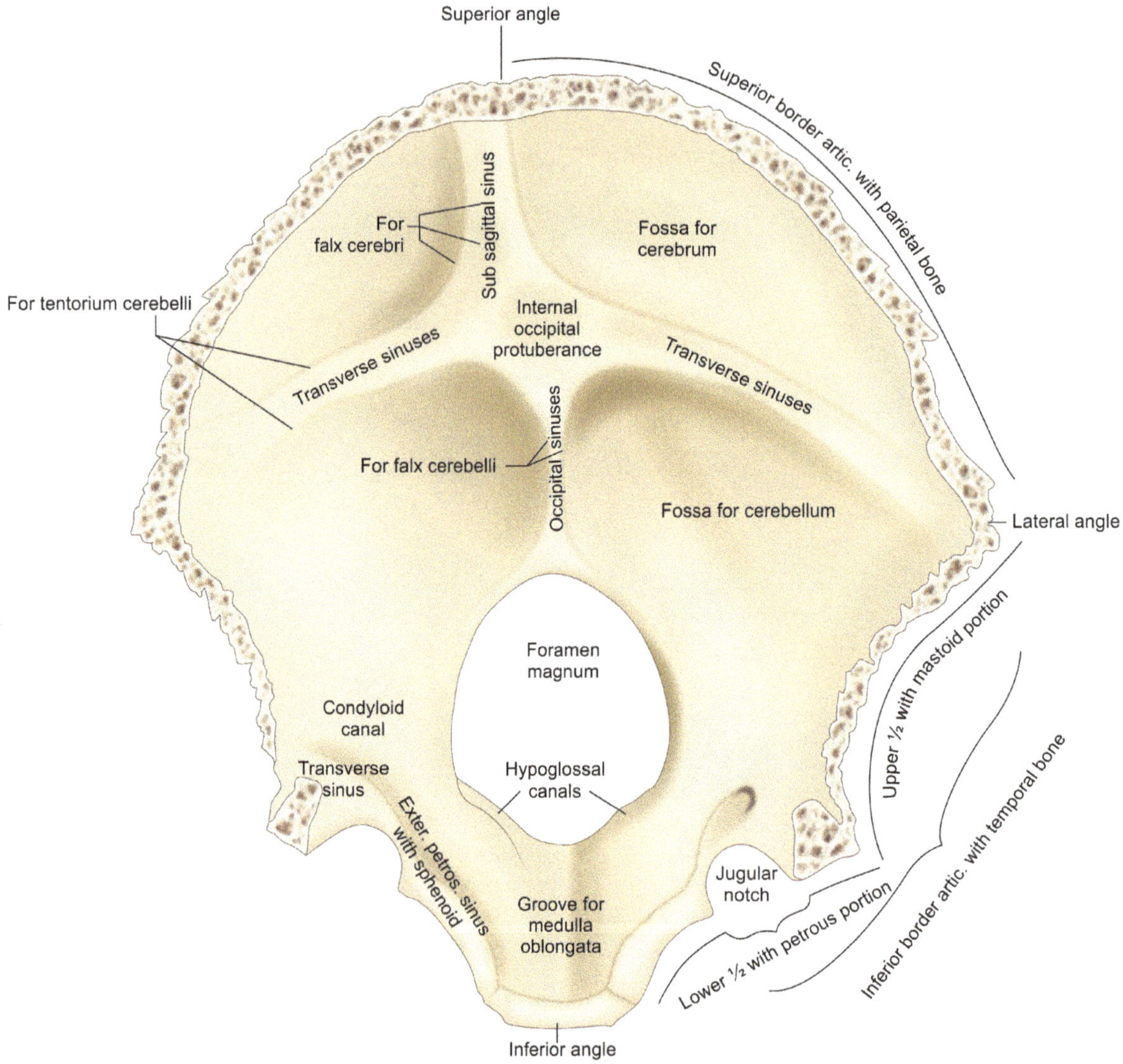

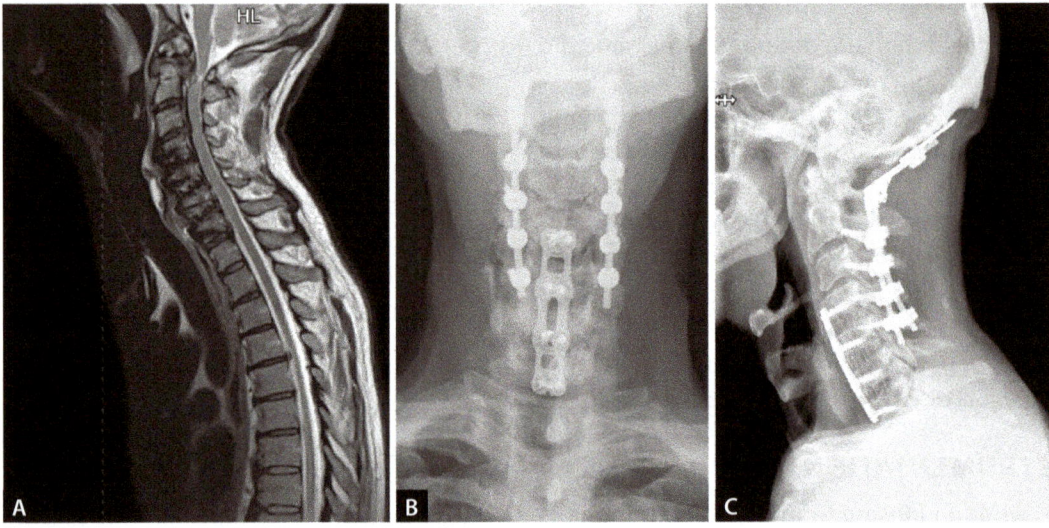

Fig. 2: Occipital bone (inner surface).
Source: Anatomy of the Human Body (1918) – Henry Gray

Figs. 3A to C: (A) Sagittal T2 image of a 64-year-old male patient with a remote history of os odontoideum/C2 nonunion status postprior C4–C7 anterior cervical discectomy and fusion from an outside hospital. C1–C2 stenosis is severe with associated cord signal changes; (B) Anteroposterior (AP) radiograph after C1–C2 decompression and occipitocervical fusion; (C) Lateral radiograph after C1–C2 decompression and occipitocervical fusion.

consider using structural corticocancellous iliac crest graft to span from the occiput caudally.
- The authors recommend using a heavy suture to tie the graft into place. The suture can be anchored to the rods and remaining bony structures.
- The authors use iliac crest bone graft routinely for occipitocervical fusions.

CLOSURE

- The authors routinely use antibiotic powder (e.g., vancomycin) in diabetic patients and patients with multiple comorbidities.
- The authors routinely place a subfascial drain.
- *Multilayer closure with interrupted figure-8 stitches:* Tight closure of the fascia is of utmost importance.

DRESSING

- Standard sterile dressings may be used.
- The authors routinely use an incisional negative pressure dressing in obese or diabetic patients.

IMMOBILIZATION

The authors recommend a cervical hard collar for immobilization for a minimum of 6 weeks: Appropriate fit of the cervical collar around the patient's mandible is critical to provide rotational stability.

CHAPTER 2

Posterior Cervical C1–2 Fusion

Barrett S Boody, Glenn S Russo, Rick C Sasso

■ INDICATIONS

- Commonly held indications for C1-2 posterior cervical fusions are for C1-2 instability and type 2 odontoid fractures. Etiologies for instability may be traumatic, oncologic, infectious, inflammatory/rheumatoid, or congenital. Instability is sometimes difficult to assess based upon computed tomography (CT) or magnetic resonance imaging (MRI) alone. When appropriate, upright plain radiographs can be useful to better understand upper cervical stability. With neurologic compromise, we would favor a more aggressive approach.
    - The posterior C1-2 fusion is our work-horse fixation choice for displaced type 2 odontoid fractures with risk factors for nonunion.
    - Anterior odontoid screws for type 2 odontoid fractures should be used only in carefully selected cases, including reducibility with positioning, adequate bone stock, and favorable fracture plane orthogonal to the screw trajectory are mandatory.
- Familiarity with C1 and/or C2 fixation is important as well as "bail-out" options for fixation with occipito-cervical instrumentation is needed before managing cervical deformity and trauma.
- Review preoperative imaging scans (MRI and CT) to plan hardware. Look for aberrant vertebral artery courses that complicate or contraindicate pedicle screw fixation.
    - Plan an appropriate length and trajectory for a C1 screw. Evaluate for the presence of a ponticulus posticus.
    - Specifically determine the most appropriate trajectory and length of a C2 pars or pedicle screw.
        - Also evaluated the C2 laminar dimensions to determine whether laminar screws would be possible.

■ ROOM SET-UP

- Our preferred positioning option is using an open Jackson with Mayfield head attachment. Arms are tucked at the sides using a drawsheet. Pad bony prominences and be aware of intravenous (IV) lines pressing against the skin. Posterior iliac crest can be prepped into the field for structural autograft if needed. Before placing the patient on the bed, raise the pins at the head of the open Jackson frame to start with more reverse Trendelenburg, as this often helps with positioning and access to the posterior cervical spine. Place a belt at the level of the buttocks and secure the belt to the frame above the hip pads to create a sling, preventing sliding of the patient caudad during reverse Trendelenburg or potentially "hanging" the patient from the Mayfield head holder.
    - Alternatively, you may use a standard operating room (OR) bed with the head board removed and the Mayfield attachment. This allows for more aggressive reverse Trendelenburg as the foot of the bed can be raised to prevent patient sliding. Make sure the sternal notch is above the end of the bed to prevent sliding of the head or jaw onto the bed during positioning.
    - We prefer the Mayfield head attachment as it gives more control of the head intraoperatively. This can be useful for reduction of instability or odontoid fractures if needed. Alternatively, bivector traction with a garner-well tongs or simply a foam or horseshoe style head-holder can be used as well, but limits positioning and reduction options if needed.
- Neuromonitoring
- Posterior cervical screws and instrumentation sets. For C1, partially threaded 3.5 mm screws may reduce C2 nerve root irritation from the exposed shank, however minimal data exists to support this theoretical claim. For C2 pedicle screws, common lengths will be approximately 18–30 mm depending on anatomy, technique, and how "proud" you

need the screw to be to line up with your C1 screw. Pars screws may be 14–20 mm in length. C2 laminar screws are approximately 22–30 mm in length and require offset connectors occasionally for rod placement.
- Graft options. We prefer using structural autograft from the iliac crest. Alternatively, structural iliac crest allograft may be used as well. We believe the structural autograft more strongly promotes fusion due to the presence of viable osteoblasts/progenitor cells as well as osteoinductive growth factors, but does increase the risk of complications due to graft harvest and time required in the case.
  - We commonly secure the structural graft with nonabsorbable suture, either #1 or #2 size.
  - Alternatively, the C1-2 joints can be decorticated and a site of potential fusion as well. Our graft preference for intra-articular fusion, local autograft, and/or bone graft extender (hydroxyapatite/tricalcium phosphate) soaked in bone morphogenetic protein (BMP).
- C-arm fluoroscopy for screw placement.

POSITIONING PEARLS

- If the odontoid fracture or instability appears displaced on upright X-rays, but is improved in reduction on supine imaging (CT or MRI), applying a rigid collar while supine and leaving in place during prone positioning can help prevent displacement. Also, take lateral X-rays before draping to ensure reduction. Manipulation for reduction is easier prior to draping. Oftentimes slight traction and extension or flexion is all that is required for reduction. More sophisticated intraoperative techniques of reduction can be employed if needed.
- We avoid military tuck positioning for exposure, as this can displace the fracture or C1-2 alignment. This may result in a longer initial incision, but minimizes the manipulation required to achieve or maintain reduction.

Exposure

- A standard midline longitudinal incision and approach is utilized. First identify the bulbous C2 spinous process and subperiosteally expose the C2 lamina. Continue lateral toward the inferior articular process of C2 and identify the medial aspect of the C2 pars using a nerve hook. This is commonly as wide as the dissection needs to be and serves as a reference of the width of the C1 posterior arch exposure. For placement of C2 pars screws, exposure caudad to the C2/3 joint is required.
  - Be careful using Bovie cautery cephalad to C2, as the O-C1 and C1-2 interspaces are only covered with thin connective tissue.
- Bluntly identify the midline of the C1 arch and expose the caudad half of the posterior C1 arch out to the widths of the C2 pedicles bilaterally using a Penfield 1 dissector or key elevator.
  - Avoid exposure of the cephalad half of the arch, as the vertebral artery can be in close proximity. In many patients, as you dissect from midline out laterally, you may encounter a groove in the cephalad boarder of the C1 ring that marks proximity to the vertebral artery.
- Next using a Penfield 4, identify the C1 lateral masses bilaterally.
  - These can be extremely vascular and require patience to expose and mobilize the C2 nerve root. An extensive venous plexus surrounds the C2 nerve roots. With mobilization of the C2 nerve, bleeding can be minimized. However, if the plexus is violated, the bleeding can be brisk, and in this area, can prompt concern for a vertebral artery injury. Do not use Bovie or bipolar in this area as it can tear vessels and cause additional bleeding. If significant bleeding is encountered, utilize thrombin soaked gel foam and tamponade. Allow an ample amount of time for coagulation to mature before resuming work in the area.
  - Use a nerve hook to identify the medial border of the C1 lateral mass.

INSTRUMENTATION (FIGS. 1 AND 2)

- We place the C1 lateral mass screws for two reasons:
  - C1 screws tend to be more difficult.
  - Depending on what type of C2 fixation, it can be in your way as you mobilize the C2 nerve.
- C1 lateral mass screw:
  - Use a Penfield 4 to gently retract the C2 nerve caudally. The tip of the Penfield 4 can be placed in the C1-2 joint to help hold the retracted position of the nerve root. Significant venous bleeding can be encountered and can be stopped with thrombin soaked gel foam as previously described. Patience with mobilizing the C2 nerve can significantly limit the bleeding encountered with C1 screw placement.
  - Identify the medial aspect of the C1 lateral mass again with the nerve hook and use a high-speed drill/burr to create the start point in the middle of the lateral mass.
  - Use the straight probe set to start a bony corridor. The trajectory of the C1 lateral mass is somewhat forgiving. Ideally aim approximately 10-15° medial. Use intraoperative fluoroscopy to determine the appropriate cephalad angulation, paralleling the path of the lateral mass and aiming for the caudal half of the anterior ring of C1 to avoid intrusion into the OC joint space.
  - The path is completed with a tap and probed to confirm the absence of breaches.

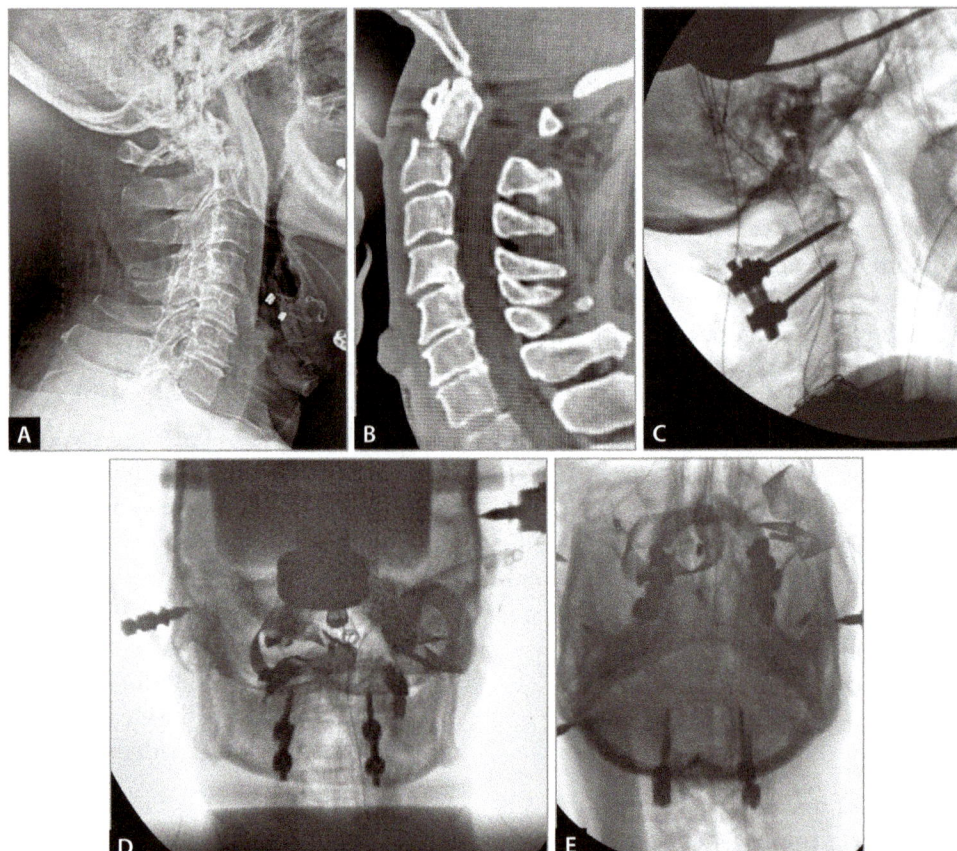

Figs. 1A to E: A 69-year-old male presented after a bicycling accident with neck pain as well as pain, paresthesias, and weakness in his hands. (A) Lateral X-ray and (B) mid-sagittal computed tomography (CT) demonstrate a type 2 odontoid fracture with posterior displacement as well as a fracture of the posterior C1 ring. (C through E) Intraoperative images of posterior C1–2 instrumentation. The lateral fluoroscopic Image C demonstrates interval fracture reduction and appropriate cephalad-caudad C1 and C2 screw trajectories. (D) A standard anteroposterior (AP) view but is of limited utility for intraoperative decision-making due to obliquity and overlap of bony anatomy. (E) The Waters view, adding 45° of cephalad Ferguson tilt to the standard AP projection in order to view the C1 vertebra from a "top-down" perspective; similar to a pelvic inlet view, this allows for improved understanding of the C1 the medial-lateral screw trajectory.

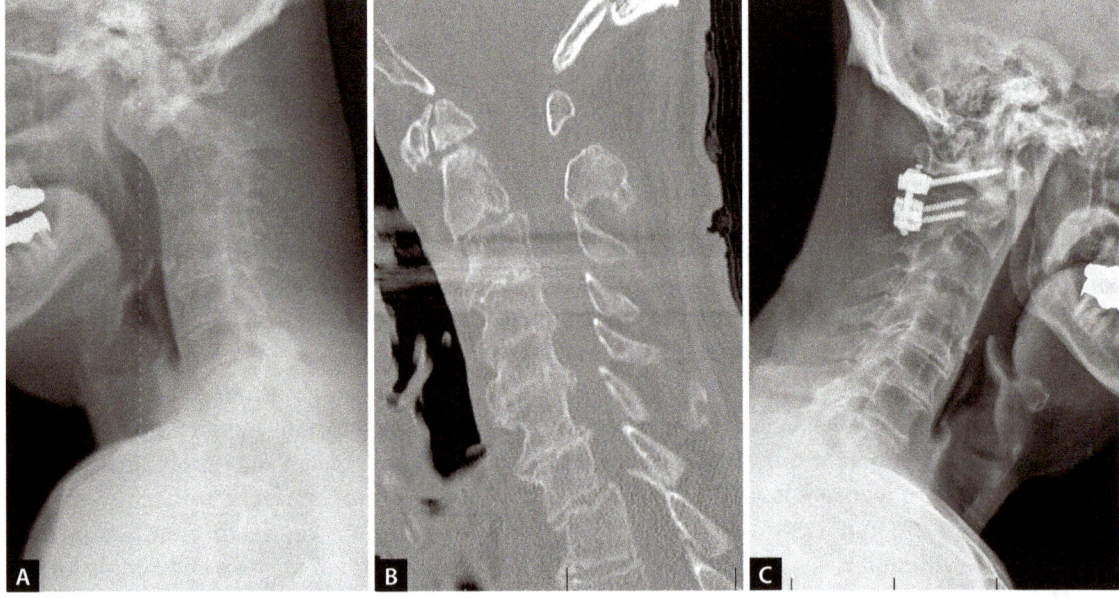

Figs. 2A to C: An 80-year-old male reported a distant fall with progressively worsening cervical deformity and neck pain. He noted significant difficulty maintaining horizontal gaze. Neurological examination demonstrated intact motor and sensory function. (A) A kyphotic alignment of a chronic type 2 odontoid fracture; (B) A mid-sagittal computed tomography (CT) scan with reduction of the chronic odontoid nonunion with supine positioning; (C) 6-month follow-up with posterior C1–2 instrumentation and improved C1–2 alignment.

- Measure the screw length using the ball tip probe, from the bottom of the C1 tapped path to a point that lines up with your C2 screw. This significantly helps with rod placement by having equal depth of the screw tulips.
- *C2 instrumentation:* Take care to ensure true lateral C-arm imaging as suboptimal images can result in errant screw placement.
  - A note on "pedicle screws" versus "pars screws": While these are two distinct techniques described in the literature, in our practice, we essentially try to identify the longest corridor of bone for screw placement. Sometimes, this trajectory is a blend between the more traditional paths of the classically defined pedicle or pars screws.
  - *Pedicle screws:*
    - The start point is identified after confirmation of the medial and superior borders of the pedicle with the nerve hook. Cephalad/caudad starting location is typically along the superior border of the lamina. Medial/lateral start point will depend on angulation of the pedicle (as determined by preoperative imaging and intraoperative referencing).
    - Use a burr to create the start point.
    - Next, we utilize a freehand drill with a depth stop, typically at 16-18 mm to start. Lateral fluoroscopy can be helpful to determine cranial/caudal orientation. After the initial advancement, use a straight probe to confirm trajectory and intrapedicular location.
      - Erring medial is preferred to lateral breaches, as the canal is capacious at C2 and laterally the vertebral artery is in close proximity.
    - After determining the proper trajectory, exchange the drill for a tap and we will advance the rest of the way. Confirm trajectory again with a ball tip probe.
    - Finish with pedicle screw placement under fluoroscopic guidance.
  - *Pars screws:*
    - Although it is an option for C2 fixation, it is the authors' preference to avoid pars screws due to risk of vertebral artery injury and inferior biomechanical properties compared to laminar and pedicle screw fixation. Pars screws can be utilized for bail-out options if the lamina and pedicle are suboptimal for screw placement.
    - The start point is slightly (1-2 mm) medial and cephalad (1-2 mm) of the midpoint at the C2-3 joint. The hand drill is set to 14-18 mm depending on preoperative measurements of the pars. Using fluoroscopic imaging, the hand drill is advanced roughly in line cephalad with the dorsal cortex of the C2 pars, but slight ventral angulation can be helpful to avoid dorsal cortical breakout. The trajectory can be neutral medial/lateral or with a few degrees of medial angulation to prevent inadvertent vertebral artery injury.
    - The trajectory is confirmed with a ball tip probe, appropriately undertapped, confirmed again with ball tip probe, and finished with screw placement.
    - For pars screws, due to the cephalad angulation needed, extra soft tissue dissection caudally will assist with proper screw trajectory.
  - *Laminar screws:*
    - Use a burr at the inflection point of the lamina to the spinous process at C2 to create a start point. Use visual cues of the contralateral lamina to determine how high or low on the spinous process to create your start point. Additionally, stagger the start points more cephalad on one side and more caudal on the other to avoid overlapping trajectories. Use a straight probe/awl to follow the dorsal plane of the contralateral lamina, with care taken to err dorsally to avoid spinal canal intrusion. Use a ball tip probe to confirm trajectory, appropriately undertap the trajectory, probe the pathway again, and place the screw.

ROD PLACEMENT AND FUSION

- Place rods bilaterally and provisionally tighten endcaps. Take anteroposterior (AP) and lateral images to confirm reduction of the C1-2 articulation and/or odontoid. Next, final tighten the end caps and irrigate the wound.
- Decorticate the caudal C1 arch and C2 lamina and spinous processes and place the structural bone graft over the C1-2 interspace. Using a rongeur, a small resection of the caudal midline aspect of the graft (making an upside-down U-shaped graft) can help seat the graft and accommodate the C2 spinous process and maximize bony contact. Any remaining graft can be morselized and placed in the interspace.
- A nonabsorbable suture can be threaded beneath the bilateral rods and tied over the dorsal surface of the graft to buttress it into position.

CLOSURE

- A standard layered closure is performed next.
- A drain can be placed if there is concern for hematoma. It is the authors' practice to avoid drain placement for posterior C1-2 fusions.

POSTOPERATIVE CARE

- Commonly the patient is admitted overnight for pain control and monitoring.
- A soft collar can be provided for comfort postoperatively.
- The patient is permitted to mobilize as tolerated. No formal restrictions are commonly needed.

Posterior Cervical Decompression and Fusion

Glenn S Russo, Barrett S Boody, Peter G Whang

■ INTRODUCTION

- Posterior cervical decompression and instrumented fusion is an essential tool for the able spine surgeon. There are a wide variety of indications necessitating this intervention. These include, but are not limited to, acute or chronic instability including fractures and ligamentous injury; decompression in the setting of tumor, infection, or diffuse spondylosis; stabilization for nonunion or failed cervical arthroplasty; and deformity correction.
- Each construct needs to be uniquely tailored for the specific patient and pathology. A variety of constructs may be utilized using a combination of lateral mass and, if needed, pedicle screw instrumentation.
  - Inclusion of levels involves a complex decision-making process. The major considerations are the levels of stenosis and sagittal alignment.
    - Unlike the lumbar spine, decompression is generally performed by removal of the entire lamina versus an interspace partial laminectomy. Therefore, since stenosis is commonly located at the interspaces, we typically perform a complete laminectomy of the level cephalad and caudad to decompress the stenotic level (i.e., for C3-4 stenosis, a C3 and C4 laminectomy would be performed), although in some cases, a partial laminectomy may be performed depending upon the location of the stenosis.
    - Instrumentation is performed at all levels undergoing laminectomy. Consideration of extending the construct cephalad or caudad can be made for cases in which there is kyphotic alignment (which may require more robust fixation to hold lordotic posture) or for fractures (which may benefit from improved stability).
  - One construct that is commonly used in our practice is a C3-6 laminectomy and a C3-T1 instrumented fusion with lateral mass screws placed from C3 to 5 and pedicle screws at C7-T1. One reason for including T1 in the construct is because there is some evidence suggesting that extension to this level may be associated with a lower revision rate.[1]

■ INSTRUMENTS

- Regular table with Mayfield head holder
- Fluoroscopy/navigation
- Neuromonitoring
- Weitlaner, Cerebellar, and Gelpi Retractors
- 1.7 mm burr
- 3 mm side-cutting burr
- 2 mm Kerrison
- Nerve hook
- Towel clips.

■ SETUP

- As with many procedures, the setup is a critical early step in achieving a successful outcome. In particular, the setup for a posterior cervical procedure can greatly influence the complexity of this procedure.
- May be prudent to obtain baseline neuromonitoring potential with the patient in the supine position, especially those with severe stenosis.
- The patient is positioned in a prone position on a regular table with the head secured in tongs with a Mayfield extension.
  - The regular table can either be rotated so that the foot of the bed is on the same side as anesthesia, whereas certain tables may allow for the translation of the top relative to the base. The goal is to ensure that the post for the table is far enough down by the patient's lower body so that the fluoroscope may be moved freely and adequate imaging of the cervical spine may be obtained.

- Two large gel rolls are placed on the regular table which should be aligned with the long axis of the table.
  - The gel rolls tend to separate or slide laterally when the patient is placed on top, so the authors tend to move the rolls a little more medially that one might expect in order to compensate for this anticipated movement.
  - The rolls and table pad should be right at the edge of the table to help protect the patient from any exposed metal on the table and avoid pressure breakdown during the course of the surgery.
  - A long draw sheet is placed over the rolls before positioning the patient.
- The patient is positioned in the prone position and the Mayfield head holder is secured.
  - Pay special attention to the patient's chin and forehead to ensure that they are free of any pressure with adequate space between the operating room (OR) bed and chin. When placed in the reverse Trendelenburg position, the patient can slide caudad and potentially cause contact of the head with the OR table.
- Pad all lines and intravenous (IV) sites with gauze to ensure that there is no excess pressure applied to the skin. Wrap the arms with gel sheets or pad them with foam.
- Wrap the draw sheet around the patient with the arms at the side.
  - Use 3-inch silk tape wrapped around the patient multiple times at the levels of the shoulders, just above the elbow, and mid-forearms. Support the wrists and hands with padding as needed.
  - Make sure that IV and arterial lines are functioning after the patient is secured.
- Bend the knees into a flexed position by either breaking the bed or supporting them with a stack of blankets.
- Place a safety strap at the level of the buttocks and tether it to the table around the level of the patient's waist as a sling so that it will provide support when the patient is moved into a reverse Trendelenburg position.
- Incline the table into a reverse Trendelenburg position until the neck is roughly parallel with the ground. Make sure to recheck the patient's chin and ensure that the patient is stable on the table.
- Gentle traction may be applied by wrapping tape around each shoulder and fastening it to the bed. It may be beneficial to obtain motor readings throughout this process to reduce the risk of an iatrogenic upper extremity nerve injury.
  - Improper positioning can result in neuromonitoring changes which will need to be addressed before commencing surgery.
  - Excessive neck extension can worsen cervical stenosis and may not be well tolerated in patients with a spinal cord injury or severe myelopathy.
  - Excessive shoulder traction can cause a brachial plexopathy (unilateral or even bilateral).
  - Inadequate padding of the elbows and hands can result in an ulnar or median neuropathy, respectively.
  - Placing the table in too much reverse Trendelenburg can result in "hanging" of the patient who can slide caudad and is held in place only by the Mayfield attachment which can result in similar global changes in neurologic function as excessive cervical extension.
  - Failure to address any changes in neuromonitoring at this stage may potentially give rise to a catastrophic neurologic injury. Global reductions in motors should first be treated with neck flexion and decreasing the degree of reverse Trendelenburg. In addition, ensure that the blood pressure is at an appropriate goal [85 mm Hg mean arterial pressure (MAP)]. If motors return to baseline within a few minutes, it may be reasonable to proceed but continue to be cautious of any changes in position. If motors continue to be globally diminished, the patient should be returned to the supine position and it may be necessary to consider aborting a posterior approach in which case performing an anterior decompression and stabilization operation may be indicated, either instead or before a posterior procedure.
- Shave the back of the head as needed and prewash with a chlorhexidine scrub brush. The authors utilize a universal drape.

APPROACH

- A midline incision is drawn over the posterior cervical spine. The vertebra prominens (C7) and spinous process of C2 can usually be palpated to help orient the surgeon. The incision should extend from the approximate area of C2–T2. Levels may also be confirmed using lateral fluoroscopy.
- The skin and paraspinal muscles are injected with a local anesthetic with epinephrine.
- After incision of the skin, the dissection is continued through the soft tissues making sure to work through the midline raphe.
- Self-retaining retractors may be used to apply tension to the adipose tissue in order to better visualize the midline tissue plane.
- At the level of the fascia, the vertebra prominens and C2 spinous can usually be palpated but in thick or muscular necks, the spinous processes of the remaining subaxial spine may not always be appreciated. A fascial incision is made distal to C2 to the spinous process of C7. Ensure that ligamentous attachments between C7 and T1 are preserved.
- Once the muscle is exposed, the bifid spinous processes of the subaxial spine can then usually be palpated.

- Dissect through the posterior cervical musculature, primarily bluntly in the midline with use of the Bovie electrocautery as needed.
- Identify the tips of the bifid spinous processes and perform a subperiosteal dissection down the laminae, extending it laterally to expose the lateral masses in their entirety, making sure to preserve the C2-3 facet joint capsule. Identify the T1 transverse process for use as a caudad landmark.
  - A common error is to not fully expose the lateral aspect of the lateral mass. This may lead to the medial placement of the lateral mass screws which can place the vertebral artery and nerve roots at risk for injury.

■ DECOMPRESSION AND INSTRUMENTATION

- *C7 and T1 pedicle screw placement:*
  - C7 pedicles are first identified via palpation through a laminotomy. A 3 mm side-cutting burr is used to create a laminotomy at C6-7. A 2 mm Kerrison rongeur is used to extend the laminotomy laterally so that a fine nerve hook can be used to palpate the C7 pedicle. With a clear understanding of location of the pedicle, a 1.7 mm burr is used to create a tract, taking care to ensure a bony floor can be palpated with the burr. If any difficulties are encountered identifying the bony anatomy, a small straight probe and ball-tip can be used to cannulate the pedicle. The bony corridor is tapped and the pedicle screw is placed; in most instances, a 3.5 × 18 mm screw is adequate.
    - For those inexperienced with the insertion of C7 pedicle screws, we recommend making sure that the laminotomy is flush with the medial wall of the C7 pedicle. It is common for the inexperienced surgeon to incorrectly identify the location of the medial and cephalad pedicle boundaries and a malpositioned C7 pedicle screw will complicate the T1 screw placement.
  - The starting point of the T1 pedicle is located by extending a line caudally from the C7 screw, moving one burr width medial, and making sure it is on the superior ridge of the T1 transverse process. The pedicle is cannulated and tapped in the same fashion as previously described. A 4.0 mm diameter screw can usually be placed safely but there is often sufficient room for larger implants; similarly, screws 25 mm in length or longer are generally able to be accommodated.
- *Lateral mass cannulation:*
  - It may be preferable to cannulate the lateral masses prior to decompression to minimize the passage of instruments over the exposed spinal cord.
  - The starting point is made a burr width inferior and medial to the midpoint of the lateral mass of the C3, C4, and C5 bilaterally. Be mindful of the placement of the starting points so that they are in line with one another, which will facilitate rod placement.
    - Before creating the tracts for lateral mass screws, it is important to confirm the medial and lateral aspects of the facet as well as the joint space above and below. Without properly identifying these landmarks, it may be difficult to correctly locate the proper starting point.
    - A common mistake is to employ insufficient cephalad angulation so it is important to maximize your cephalad angulation as much as possible. While we have frequently observed screws that are oriented too caudally, we personally have never seen nor placed a lateral mass screw with too much cephalad angulation.
    - To achieve the correct lateral angulation, visualize in your mind the anterolateral corner of the facet complex which may serve as a target. Starting too far laterally may lead to a breach of the lateral wall which may increase the risk fracture and the path may not be salvageable.
  - A 3.0 mm tap is used in preparation for a 3.5 mm screw. The tap is oriented along the facet with a cephalad and lateral trajectory to avoid the exiting nerve root and vertebral artery, respectively. This may be achieved by aligning the shaft of the driver so that it contacts the spinous process of the caudal vertebra medially.
- *Laminectomy:*
  - In our practice, a laminectomy is commonly performed from C3 to C6 or C7. However, the levels of the decompression are determined on a case-by-case basis depending on the specific pathology.
  - The goal is to remove the lamina as one continuous unit with minimal risk to the spinal cord.
  - A Leksell rongeur is used to remove the interspinous ligaments at the cephalad and caudad extent of the laminectomy.
  - Using a 3 mm burr, a trough is made at the spinolaminar line. The goal is to have a final laminectomy width of approximately 15 mm based on data suggesting that a wider laminectomy could predispose one to a C5 nerve palsy.[2]
    - The lamina is triangularly-shaped in cross-section with its base along the caudal aspect.
    - It is important to remember that the lamina is only 2-3 mm in width so if you are burring a trough deeper than this point, you are likely too far lateral and in the facet joint.
  - The authors preferred technique is to first score the trough by thinning the lamina at each level. This helps orient the trough and also allows for a more

controlled osteotomy when using the burr at the lamina-ligamentum interface.
- The burr is then used in a side cutting fashion in a caudad-to-cephalad direction to cleave the lamina throughout the trough.
    - A nerve hook can be used to help determine if there any residual bony bridges.
    - Sometimes there may be an "overhang" of tissue along the medial aspect of the trough that can limit visualization which can be taken down with the burr as well.
- After the trough has been completed bilaterally, towel clips are applied to each of the spinous processes so that an assistant may apply gentle upward pressure which may reduce the risk of an iatrogenic cord injury. The 2 mm Kerrison rongeur is also used to free any remaining soft tissue tethering the lamina.
    - Use the Kerrison to bite toward the edges of the laminae to increase the width of the bony troughs of the laminectomy as well as the ligamentum flavum present at the interspaces above and below the laminectomy which will help to free the laminar segments.
- Peel back the lamina working in a caudal-to-cephalad direction, ensuring that there is no excessive traction applied to the cord from dural adhesions which should be released in advance.
    - Use a nerve hook and a Woodson elevator to free the lamina from any dural adhesions.
    - Be patient with removal of the laminae and instruct the assistant to only apply gentle upward pressure with the towel clips. Excessive traction on incompletely freed laminar segments can cause a spinal cord injury.
- Remove the lamina as a single unit if possible which may be utilized as autograft.
- *Lateral mass instrumentation:*
    - Lateral mass screws are placed bilaterally at the appropriate levels; a typical screw size is 3.5 × 12 mm.
        - Avoid "hubbing" the screws because if the head of the screw impacts the facet, there is an increased risk of either stripping the screw or fracturing the facet so having the screw slightly proud may be preferable which will also increase the mobility of the screw head which will facilitate rod placement.
        - If a screw path becomes stripped, it may be possible to safely place a larger screw (i.e., greater diameter and longer length). If there is still no purchase, the screw should be removed on this side. However, if the compromised screw is at the upper instrumented level, it may be necessary to extend the fusion cephalad.
    - At this point, the Mayfield head holder may be adjusted to extend the neck and impart more lordosis.
- Once the cervical spine is in an acceptable position, appropriately sized rods can be placed and secured within the screw heads.

ALTERNATE WORKFLOW

When a first assistant is not available, an alternate workflow that minimizes switching sides and works well for the authors is as follows:
- For instance, if a surgeon is standing on the patient's left, C7 and T1 screws may be placed on the left side, followed by cannulation of the right C3–C5 lateral masses and then creation of the left laminectomy trough.
- The surgeon then moves to the patient's right for insertion of the right C7 and T1 screws, cannulation of the left C3–C5 lateral masses, and completion of the right-sided trough. From this position, the lamina can then be removed and the lateral mass screws placed bilaterally.

CLOSURE

- After copious irrigation, hemostasis is achieved and a deep subfascial drain is placed to minimize the risk of developing an epidural hematoma.
- 1 g of vancomycin powder is applied within the wound for antibiotic prophylaxis.
- The incision is approximated in a layered fashion with separate closure of the muscles and fascia.
    - The muscle layer is not a tension holding layer so the goal is apposition to obliterate "dead space" and the tissue should not be "strangled" during closure.
    - The fascial closure must be meticulous and watertight. We use #1 pop-off Vicryl sutures in a "figure of 8" fashion with generous bites of tissue. In addition to placing all of the sutures before tying them which allows for increased density of sutures, we also secure the margins of the fascia first and close the middle last.
- The subcutaneous tissues are closed with absorbable suture and the skin is closed with a running-locked 3-0 nylon suture.
    - Returning the head to a "military tuck" position by adjusting the Mayfield tongs may facilitate skin closure by reducing the redundant skin folds that may be encountered with neck extension.
- Of all spine surgery procedures, closure of posterior cervical wounds is perhaps the most critical. Consequently, an inadequate closure can result in potentially disastrous wound complications.
- A sterile, occlusive dressing is applied to cover the incision.
- A hard cervical collar is placed and the Mayfield head holder is removed before transferring the patient to the supine position.

POSTOPERATIVE CARE

- The head of the bed is kept at or above 45° for 3 days or while the patient is hospitalized.
- Consider observing the patient in the intensive care unit initially after surgery, especially for those with a spinal cord injury or significant preoperative neurologic deficits secondary to stenosis so that the MAP may be maintained at a minimum of 85 mm Hg postoperatively.
- Frequent neurological examinations must be performed to monitor for postoperative neurological decline secondary to hematoma or a nerve root palsy.
- The drain may be removed after two consecutive values of 30 cc or less during an 8-hour shift.
- Muscle spasms are a significant contributor to postoperative pain and should be addressed as part of a multimodal pain regimen.
- The patient is seen at 2, 6, and 12 weeks following surgery.
- The hard collar is generally used for 12 weeks.

REFERENCES

1. Schroeder GD, Kepler CK, Kurd MF, Mead L, Millhouse PW, Kumar P, et al. Is it necessary to extend a multilevel posterior cervical decompression and fusion to the upper thoracic spine? Spine (Phila Pa 1976). 2016;41(23):1845-9.
2. Radcliff KE, Limthongkul W, Kepler CK, Sidhu GD, Anderson DG, Rihn JA, et al. Cervical laminectomy width and spinal cord drift are risk factors for postoperative C5 palsy. J Spinal Disord Tech. 2014;27(2):86-92.

CHAPTER 4

Posterior Cervical Foraminotomy

Yoshihiro Katsuura, Han Jo Kim

INTRODUCTION

The posterior cervical foraminotomy is a motion-sparing procedure used to decompress the cervical nerve roots in the setting of radiculopathy. The primary goal of the operation is the removal of the medial half of the facet complex (composed of superior and inferior articular process) to relieve pressure from the cervical nerve root. The most common indication for this procedure is to treat compression from a lateral soft disk herniation or less commonly, from posterior osteophytes originating mainly from the superior articular process of the facet complex.[1] The posterior foraminotomy is advantageous as it may minimize the complications of adjacent segment disease resulting from decreased segmental motion with fusion procedures.[2] Furthermore, posterior approaches do not violate the retropharyngeal space, leaving the esophagus and recurrent laryngeal nerve untouched and thus have less dysphagia and airway complications. Finally, the posterior foraminotomy is advantageous over anterior cervical discectomy and fusion (ACDF) procedures as there is no possibility of pseudoarthrosis. However, as it is true with most posterior cervical procedures, careful attention must be made to preserve soft tissues to avoid postoperative kyphosis.[3] Moreover, bilateral radiculopathy or myelopathy type symptoms are better addressed with other approaches such as ACDF, laminectomy plus fusion, or laminoplasty. Nonetheless, cervical foraminotomy can be a powerful adjunct to any larger posterior cervical procedure to relieve radiculopathy in the setting of myelopathy or prevent C5 palsy. Studies in the past have failed to show superiority of posterior foraminotomy over ACDF, however, in certain indications, it can be advantageous.[4] The prime example is a patient with myeloradiculopathy resulting from multilevel compression which requires a posterior decompression.

ANATOMY

- *The cervical foramen has four boundaries:* The pedicles (superior and inferior), the superior articular facet of the facet complex and lamina (posterior), and the posterolateral aspect of the uncovertebral joint and intervertebral disk (anterior).[5]
- The overall shape of the foramen resembles a funnel, with the medial entrance being narrow, and the lateral exit being wide.[5] It may be divided into three zones: Medial (pedicle zone where most compression occurs, and corresponds to entrance of the cervical foramina), middle (posterior to vertebral artery), and lateral zone (lateral to the vertebral artery).[6]
- *Nerve root structure:* A single cervical nerve root is composed of bundles of ventral and dorsal rootlets (typically 14-23 bundles) which emerge from the spinal cord one segment higher than the nerve root. The dorsal bundles form the dorsal root ganglion and combine with the ventral bundles to form the spinal nerve root lateral to the foramen.[5]
- *Anatomic relations between the nerve root and disk:* The relationship between the nerve root and the disk varies depending on cervical level.
  - *C4-5 nerve roots:* Disk is proximal to or at the level of the nerve root take off (shoulder position).
  - *C6-7 nerve roots:* Disk is caudal to nerve root take off (axillary position).
  - *C8 nerve root:* Disk is caudal and does not directly contact the nerve root.[5]
- Most nerve roots may be fully decompressed with removal of the medial ½ of the facet complex to the level of the pedicle. The exception to this is the C8 nerve root which may require a larger resection as the result of the longer width of the medial portion of the cervical foramina and morphology of the superior articular process of T1.[5,6]

SUGGESTED INSTRUMENTS

- Jackson table with bivector traction set up
- Neuromonitoring
- McCullough retractor set
- High-speed burr 3 mm diamond tip
- Cervical Kerrison rongeurs
- Codman microcurette set
- Micropituitary
- Cervical nerve hook
- Cervical ball hook
- Paralysis is not typically used as it will interfere with motor evoked potentials (MEPs).

APPROACH

- *Position:*
  - After induction of general anesthesia, Gardner-Wells tongs are placed 1 cm superior to the pinna and in-line with the external auditory canal.
  - The patient is then placed prone on a Jackson table with the head secured to bivector traction.[7]
  - 15 lbs of weight is attached to the flexion rope, keeping the extension rope free. The extension rope is generally not critical for this procedure and keeping the head in the flexed position is beneficial for exposure (nonetheless, we always set up the extension rope in case of possible conversion to a fusion procedure). The flexed position allows the cervical facet joints to maximally displace which facilitates removal of the medial facet joint complex. It also elongates and flattens the posterior soft tissues of the neck allowing for easier dissection. It is important to position the body in reverse Trendelenburg in order to prevent venous pooling to the head.
  - The patient's arms are well padded around the cubital and carpal tunnels and tucked using a figure of 8 sheet **(Fig. 1)**.

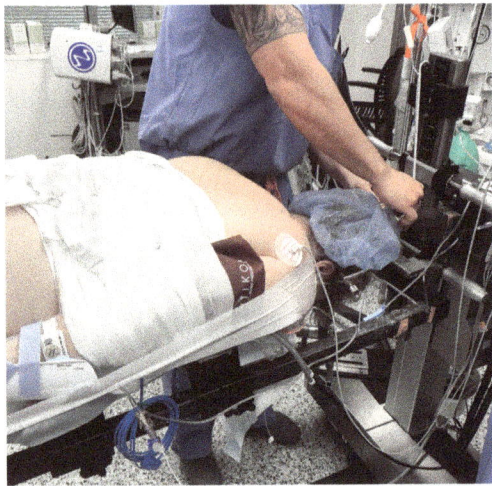

Fig. 1: *Preoperative draping for posterior cervical procedure:* The arms are padded and tucked in a figure of 8 position and the head is attached to the bivector traction device.

- *Fluoroscopy:*
  - We find that the tendency is to make the incision too proximal, which can result in unnecessary restriction by soft tissues. This prevents the surgeon from sliding the Kerrison cranially under the facet joint. Thus the incision should be places slightly caudal to allow a trajectory which is perpendicular to the facet and lamina.
  - Thus, fluoroscopy is brought in to confirm the levels with a metallic marker on the skin or a spinal needle. A 2–3 cm incision is all that is necessary for a single level, and will typically be more distal than first thought because of the flexed posture of the neck. If soft tissues prevent adequate visualization by X-ray, we recommend using a computed tomography (CT) navigation system which will allow correct identification of levels.

- *Draping:* Skin is then prepped with iodine-based scrub solution or other sterilizing agent and the patient is draped in a sterile fashion.

- *Approach:*
  - A careful midline incision is made through the epidermis of the skin, completing the dermal incision with electrocautery. We do not complete the final 2 mm of dermal incision at the proximal and distal ends of the incision in order to optimize the cosmetic appearance of the incision after healing and to prevent tearing of the epidermis.
  - The fat is carefully dissected with electrocautery until the fascia is encountered. For a unilateral foraminotomy, the dissection through the fascia should only be performed on a single side.
  - Meticulous periosteal dissection is then carried out lateral to the spinous process across the lamina making all attempts to avoid the synovial capsule of the facet joint and the interlaminar space is isolated. The synovial capsule and facet joint should be identified using a blunt instrument (such as a cervical nerve hook) to palpate and define the lateral border of the facet through the soft tissue. This step gives an understanding of the dimensions of the joint complex and how much dissection and resection can take place safely. Usually, you can identify the spinous processes of the levels above and below the foraminotomy site and partially elevate the muscles.
  - A McCullough retractor of the depth appropriate for the soft tissue thickness is selected and placed to expose the medial aspect of the facet joint. If the incision is too small to utilize the full size blade of the McCullough, it is possible to instead utilize the spike blades, which are thinner and when positioned correctly, can provide adequate visualization.

Decompression

- Once again, we ensure that the neck is in the position of maximal flexion to best expose the cranial border of the superior articular facet once resection is begun.
- An outline of the proposed resection should be made with electrocautery to denude the bone of joint capsule covering the facet to be removed. Again, a blunt instrument can be used to palpate the unexposed lateral border of the facet to determine the extent of resection.
- The cranial and caudal lamina at the medial aspect of the facet joint (interlaminar V) must be identified before starting the bony resection.
- High-speed side cutting burr is then used to remove the inferior articular facet in a medial to lateral and then superior to inferior fashion to uncover the superior articular facet. This resection is not >5 mm lateral (<50% of the facet joint). This creates a resection in the shape of an inverted L making a window to visualize the superior articular facet. Although the inferior articular facet is generally not the source of compression, it must be removed to gain access to the superior articular facet.
- The medial facet resection must be limited to ≤50% (on average 5.9 mm) of the total width of the facet to prevent segmental hypermobility and destabilization of the joint **(Fig. 2)**.[8]
- Attention is now turned to the visible portion of the superior articular facet. The high-speed burr is once again utilized to resect the portion of the facet which is visible in a medial to lateral and cranial to caudal fashion, starting from the lateral portion that is visualized. Again, a window is created by removal of superior articular facet in the shape of an L.
- The ligamentum flavum may be partially resected but should be kept mostly intact to preserve stability of the segment.
- With the ligament removed, the surgeon is now able to palpate the pedicle (the medial border of which can typically be palpated with 2–3 mm of bony exposure). The surgeon must not exceed 5 mm of lateral resection until you can be sure where the lateral edge of the pedicle is located.
- As we burr down, the cancellous bone becomes visible which is the sign that the far cortex is approaching. As this is the bone closest to the underlying nerve root, care should be taken not to exceed the depth of the far cortex. At this point, the trough may be completed with a cervical Kerrison.
- Once the L-shaped trough is completed, a Codman 1B microcurette is used to excise the bone fragment of the medial superior articular facet fragment. This is performed by slipping the curette ventral to the fragment and applying a gentle a dorsolateral force. This will disrupt any remaining cortical attachments. If the fragment is adherent to soft tissue, a micropituitary may be used to remove the bone.
- Any sharp bone edges are then carefully smoothed with a 1 mm Kerrison rongeur.
- A cervical nerve hook is then used to assess the foraminotomy by palpating the medial and lateral margins of the pedicle to ensure full decompression (decompression should reach the lateral border of the pedicle). The cranial border is assessed for any remnant of bone from the superior articular facet resection. If bone is left, it may cause residual symptoms **(Fig. 3)**.
- In cases of soft disk herniation, the nerve should be gently mobilized with a cervical hook or ball tipped probe to identify any extruded fragments. If the fragment

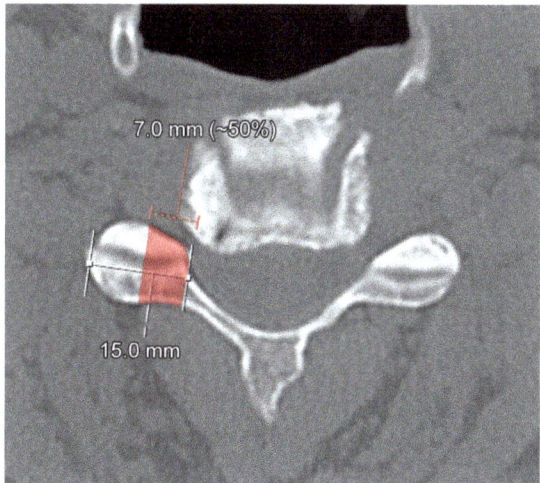

Fig. 2: Cross-sectional demonstration of facet complex which may be safely resected (red outline).

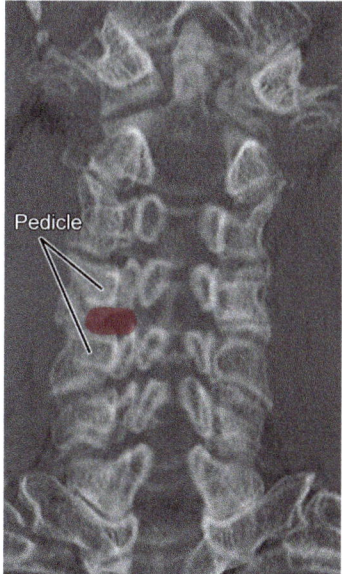

Fig. 3: Computed tomography overlay image demonstrating coronal anatomy and orientation of resection (red oval) in relation to cervical pedicles.

is contained within annulus, a small annulotomy may be made to carefully express the fragment.
- Hemostasis is achieved using bone wax for bony surfaces and a combination of bipolar electrocautery, thrombin, and gelatin hemostatic matrix for epidural vessels.
- The wound is then irrigated with copious normal saline to remove any bone fragments or dust, and closed in layers.

REFERENCES

1. Jagannathan J, Sherman JH, Szabo T, Shaffrey CI, Jane Sr JA. The posterior cervical foraminotomy in the treatment of cervical disc/osteophyte disease: a single-surgeon experience with a minimum of 5 years' clinical and radiographic follow-up: Clinical article. J Neurosurg Spine. 2009;10(4):347-56.
2. Hilibrand AS, Carlson GD, Palumbo MA, Jones PK, Bohlman HH. Radiculopathy and myelopathy at segments adjacent to the site of a previous anterior cervical arthrodesis. J Bone Jt Surg. 1999;81(4):519-28.
3. Albert TJ, Vacarro A. Postlaminectomy kyphosis. Spine. 1998;23(24):2738-45.
4. Herkowitz HN, Kurz LT, Overholt DP. Surgical management of cervical soft disc herniation. A comparison between the anterior and posterior approach. Spine. 1990;15(10):1026-30.
5. Tanaka N, Fujimoto Y, An HS, Ikuta Y, Yasuda M. The anatomic relation among the nerve roots, intervertebral foramina, and intervertebral discs of the cervical spine. Spine. 2000;25(3):286-91.
6. Ebraheim NA, An HS, Xu R, Ahmad M, Yeasting RA. The quantitative anatomy of the cervical nerve root groove and the intervertebral foramen. Spine. 1996;21(14):1619-23.
7. Karikari IO, Bumpass DB, Gum J, Sugrue P, Chapman TM, Elsamadicy AA, et al. Use of bivector traction for stabilization of the head and maintenance of optimal cervical alignment in posterior cervical fusions. Glob Spine J. 2017;7(3):227-9.
8. Zdeblick TA, Zou D, Warden KE, McCabe R, Kunz D, Vanderby R. Cervical stability after foraminotomy. A biomechanical in vitro analysis. J Bone Joint Surg Am. 1992;74(1):22-7.

CHAPTER 5

Posterior Cervical Laminoplasty

John G Heller, R Matthew Wham

■ INTRODUCTION

In the properly selected patient, laminoplasty has been shown to have equal efficacy versus anterior procedures and posterior laminectomy with fusion in the treatment of multilevel cervical myelopathy. The procedure reliably arrests the progression of the myelopathy, and leads to significant clinical improvement in a majority of patients.[1-3] Laminoplasty does so with less morbidity while preserving segmental spinal motion, and reduced risk of adjacent level disease.[4-13]

■ INSTRUMENTS SUGGESTED

- Mayfield tongs, operating table with Mayfield attachment
- Intraoperative neuromonitoring (suggested but not required)
- 3.0 and 4.0 mm burrs of choice
- Kerrison rongeurs
- Angled curettes (1 and 2 mm)
- Laminoplasty plate/screws device of choice
- Intra-arterial catheter for continuous blood pressure monitoring to ensure maintenance of mean arterial pressure.

■ APPROACH

Pearls

- Discuss with anesthesia preoperatively the steps to be taken to ensure maintenance of adequate mean arterial pressure. Significant hypotension risks a spinal cord infarction. Having an intra-arterial pressure monitor in place prior to induction with vasopressors immediately available is wise, especially when the spinal cord compression is severe.
- The standard midline posterior cervical approach is utilized. The lateral extent of the exposure should be limited to the midpoint of the lateral masses. This will facilitate proper identification of the lamina-lateral mass junction where troughs are to be placed.
- Care is taken to preserve the muscular attachments to C2 as much as possible.
- Partially exposing one level above and below will facilitate removal of ligamentum flavum in the interlaminar spaces cephalad and caudal to the sites of laminoplasty. It will also allow for dome laminectomies where indicated, or partial laminectomies where necessary to facilitate adequate laminar excursion of the levels to be decompressed.
- *Localization:*
  - The spinous processes of C2 and C7 are most prominent and serve as palpable landmarks with which to localize the incision.
  - Radiographic confirmation of the surgical levels is strongly advised to avoid wrong-level surgery.
- *Table and positioning:*
  - Position in the patient prone on a table with a Mayfield attachment. The cervical spine should be in a slightly flexed position in order to minimize "shingling" of adjacent lamina.
  - Asking the patient to demonstrate their position of comfortable maximum forward flexion prior to surgery will be helpful for intraoperative positioning.
  - A cross-table radiograph can assist in confirming adequate neck positioning and can also be utilized for localization.
  - Place the operating room table in the reverse Trendelenburg position in order to ensure that the operating field will be parallel to the floor and to help reduce venous pressure.
- The arms are padded and tucked at the patient's side **(Figs. 1 and 2)**.
  - *Draping:* Prepare a surgical field adequate to ensure that the base of the occiput and the upper thoracic spine are accessible, if necessary.

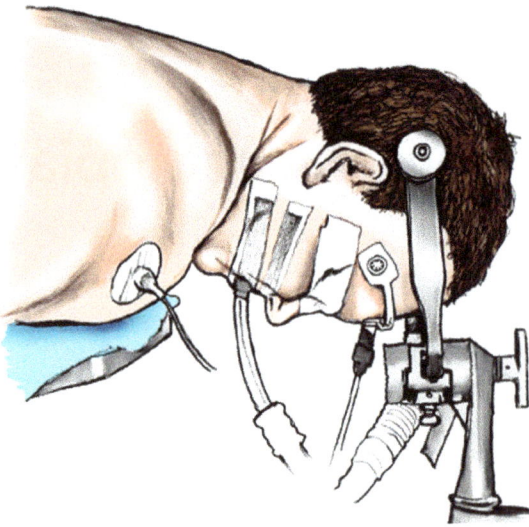

Fig. 1: *Patient positioning.* Position the patient in relative cervical flexion in order to minimize the "shingling" effect of adjacent lamina.
Courtesy: Dr Heller JG

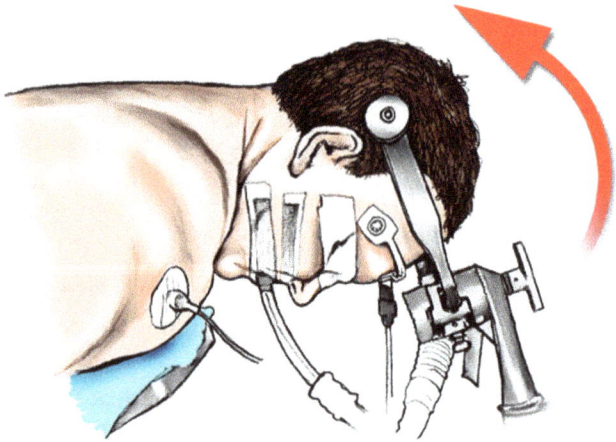

Fig. 2: *Table positioning.* After flexing the patient's cervical spine, place the operative table in reverse Trendelenburg position in order to maintain an operative field that is parallel to the floor and reduced epidural venous pressure.
Courtesy: Dr Heller JG

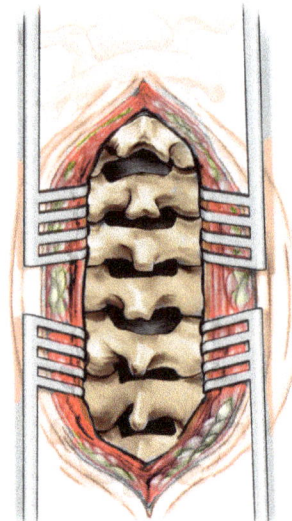

Fig. 3: *Midline exposure to the cervical spine.* After bilateral subperiosteal exposure, two self-retaining cerebellar retractors are placed to maintain exposure. The lateral extent of exposure is less than that for a posterior cervical fusion, and ought to be just lateral enough to accurately identify the lamina-lateral mass junction.
Courtesy: Dr Heller JG

- *Exposure:*
  - Begin the midline posterior cervical approach. The levels above and below the proposed laminoplasty should also be partially exposed. Take care to maintain a midline approach through the relatively avascular midline raphe in order to obtain adequate hemostasis. Optionally, infiltrating the dermis 0.25% Marcaine with epinephrine will assist with hemostasis and minimize dermal cautery and necrosis. Upon reaching the spinous processes, proceed with subperiosteal exposure past the laminae to the medial portion of the lateral masses. The lateral extent of the exposure is significantly less than for a laminectomy and fusion procedure. Release the insertion of the extensor muscle tendons at their point of insertion onto the inferior margins of the spinous processes and laminae. This will reduce bleeding and muscle necrosis.
  - Muscular bleeding should be controlled with a combination of mono- and bipolar electrocautery. Some osseous bleeding points should be sealed with bone wax. After adequately exposing one side of the posterior elements, pack this area with a sponge and proceed with similar exposure on the contralateral side. Ensure that the posterior elements are adequately cleared of soft tissue, including the interspinales muscles, so that appropriate landmarks can be identified.
  - During the exposure, secure a suitable instrument to one of the more cranial spinous processes and obtain a cross table lateral radiograph in order to confirm the anatomic level. These levels should be marked with indelible ink and referenced throughout the case.
  - The author recommends removing the spinous processes of the laminoplasty levels to improve visualization and facilitate closing the incision.
- *Retractor placement:*
  - During and after completion of the posterior cervical exposure, a pair of angled self-retaining cerebellar retractors will be adequate to maintain visualization. They ought to be repositioned from time to time to both facilitate exposure where the surgeon is working, and to reduce muscle ischemia.
  - At the time of closure, look carefully for occult bleeding points where the retractor blades were **(Fig. 3)**.

DECOMPRESSION

- The spinous processes of the working levels should be removed at their base using a rongeur. Seal bleeding points with bone wax.
- For an open door laminoplasty, first identify the side to be opened. Criteria to help guide this choice include:
  - The side with the greater degree of spinal cord compression
  - The side on which one might be adding supplemental foraminotomies to decompress certain nerve roots
  - The hand dominance of the surgeon. If none of the other factors apply, a right-handed surgeon will generally feel more comfortable with the ergonomics of making the opening trough on the patient's left, while standing on the patient's left.
- Start with the "open door" side using the burr of the surgeon's choice. The authors prefer either a 4.0 millimeter round burr, or a so-called "match stick" tip for this initial step **(Figs. 4 and 5)**.
  - Identify the lamina-lateral mass junction by correlating the preoperative axial images and the intraoperative bone landmarks.
  - Descending from cranial to caudal, remove the dorsal cortex and cancellous bone until the ventral cortical bone is reached. Seal the bleeding bone surfaces with bone wax as you go to enhance visibility.
  - Using either the same burr or changing to a 3.0 mm diamond burr, thin the ventral cortex until it becomes a translucent blue. Depending on the surgeon's experience and comfort, the rest of the bone may be removed with the same burr tip, or by using a 1 or 2 mm Kerrison rongeur. Ensure complete separation of the lamina-lateral mass junction at each of the laminoplasty levels.
  - An angled curette, nerve hook, or periosteal elevator can be used to confirm the separation by placing into the epidural space and underneath the lamina, applying a dorsally-directed force. The most common source of incomplete detachment is a bridge of bone at the upper end of the lamina concealed by overlapping bone from the lamina above **(Fig. 6)**.
  - If epidural bleeding is encountered at this stage, one should be cautious about using bipolar cautery for fear of harming a nerve root. The spinal canal stenosis causes epidural venous hypertension, thus increased bleeding. It may be wisest to use powdered gelfoam and thrombin with a 0.5 × 0.5 inch cottonoid to check the bleeding. Once the laminoplasty is opened, the venous pressure is reduced and the bleeding is easier and safer to control.
- Next, begin making the "hinge side" trough. The placement of the trough is the same as for the "open"

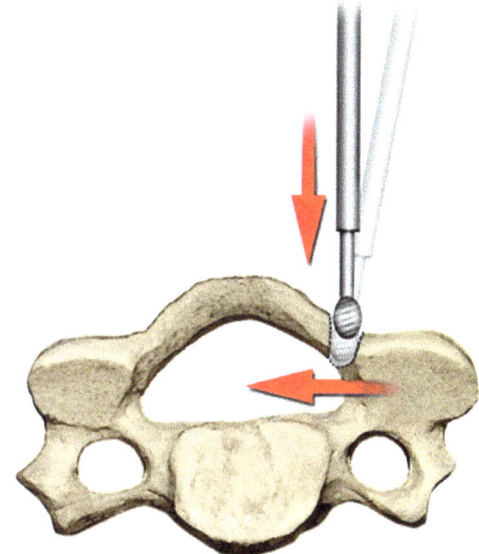

Fig. 4: *Burring technique.* When creating troughs, identify the lamina-lateral mass junction by correlating the local anatomy with the preoperative axial images. Then begin by removing the dorsal cortex and the cancellous layer to the inner cortex. The authors prefer a 4.0 mm burr for this purpose, as the burr should be directed ventrally to a depth no >4 mm. Any additional burring is directed medially as one removes the remaining inner cortical bone for the "open" side. On the hinge side, one must carefully thin the inner cortex only so far as to create a hinge that will deform plastically.
Courtesy: Dr Heller JG

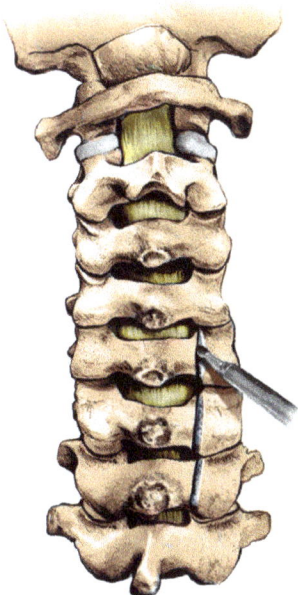

Fig. 5: *Opening side.* Begin with trough creation on the "open door" side. Proceed in a stepwise fashion, level-by-level, until the dorsal cortex and cancellous bone are removed. Seal bleeding bone with wax as needed to maintain clear visibility.
Courtesy: Dr Heller JG

side. Remove the dorsal cortex and cancellous bone of the laminae as before.
- To avoid issues with "healing" of the bone hinge, osseous bleeding points on the hinge side ought to

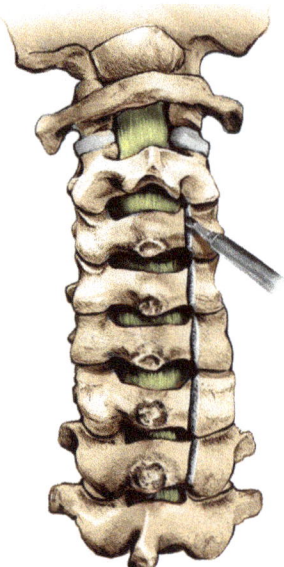

Fig. 6: *Completion of the opening side.* Complete the "open" side trough by thinning and removing the ventral cortices at each level. Confirm that the separation is complete at each level before moving on to the "hinge" side trough.
Courtesy: Dr Heller JG

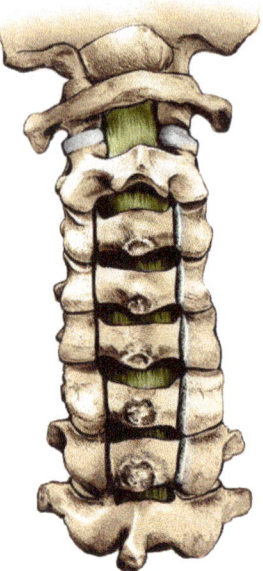

Fig. 7: *The "hinge" trough.* This is symmetrically located opposite the "open" side. After removing the dorsal cortex and cancellous bone, carefully remove just enough of the ventral cortex to render a slightly stiff hinge.
Courtesy: Dr Heller JG

be controlled with powdered gelfoam and thrombin rather than with bone wax, if possible. Sometimes the bleeding is brisk enough that only bone wax will be effective.
- Level by level, proceed with thinning the ventral cortex until the hinge is rendered slightly flexible. The stiffness of the hinge is assessed by applying an upward force at the edge of the lamina on the "open" side with the instrument of choice, such as a nerve hook or angled curette. Avoid removing too much bone and creating a floppy hinge and the risk of displacement when the laminoplasty is opened **(Figs. 7 and 8)**.
- Once the hinges have been fashioned, begin by removing the ligamentum flavum bilaterally at the interspaces above and below those laminae that are to be opened.
  - A straight, narrow rongeur can be utilized to initiate the removal in the midline until the median raphe is identified. Kerrison rongeurs (2.0 or 3.0 mm) are used to complete the removal of the ligamentum flavum on both sides.
  - If one is careful to place the Kerrison between the ligamentum flavum and the epidural veins, bleeding can be minimized during this step **(Fig. 9)**.
- The laminoplasty is now ready to be opened and the spinal cord decompressed. The exact technique and instruments used may vary with surgeon preference. The authors recommend that the assistant standing on the "hinge" side use a nerve hook placed under the cut edge of the "open" side to apply a gentle upward force, while the primary surgeon applies a similar force with

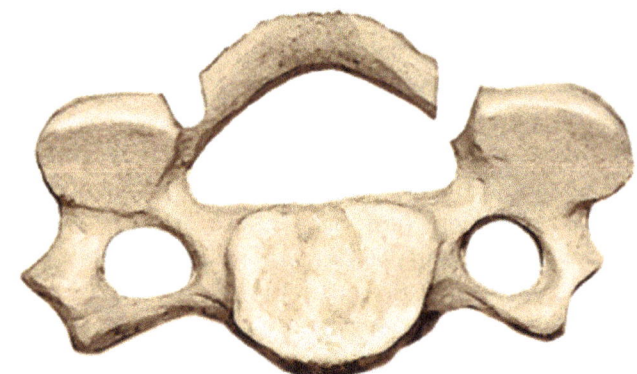

Fig. 8: *An axial schematic of completed troughs bilaterally.* Note that only a thin section of ventral cortex remains on the hinge side. If anything, the angle of the troughs is directed slightly medially in order to aim into the canal rather than the lateral masses.
Courtesy: Dr Heller JG

an angled curette. Once the lamina is displaced a few millimeters, the assistant maintains the position with the nerve hook. The surgeon then shifts to the next level to apply a similar opening maneuver. Then the assistant releases the nerve hook at the initial levels and replaces it at the level where the surgeon is now holding the lamina with the curette. This sequence of steps is repeated ascending and descending until the laminoplasty is fairly open **(Fig. 10)**.
- As the laminoplasty is opened in this fashion, the epidural veins and remaining capsular tissue and ligamentum flavum at each level will be revealed. The capsular tissues and flavum may be divided with a Kerrison rongeur. The epidural veins need to be coagulated and divided, which

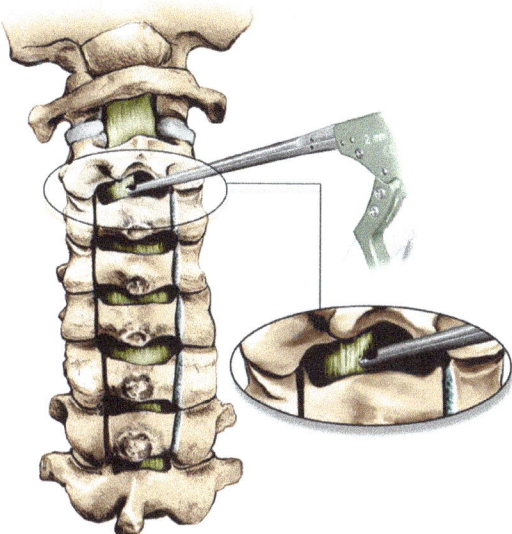

Fig. 9: *Removing ligamentum flavum.* After creation of the troughs, the ligamentum flavum is removed at the cranial and caudal ends of the laminoplasty to allow opening. If possible, the Kerrison rongeur is used in the plane between the ligamentum flavum and the epidural veins in order to minimize bleeding.
Courtesy: Dr Heller JG

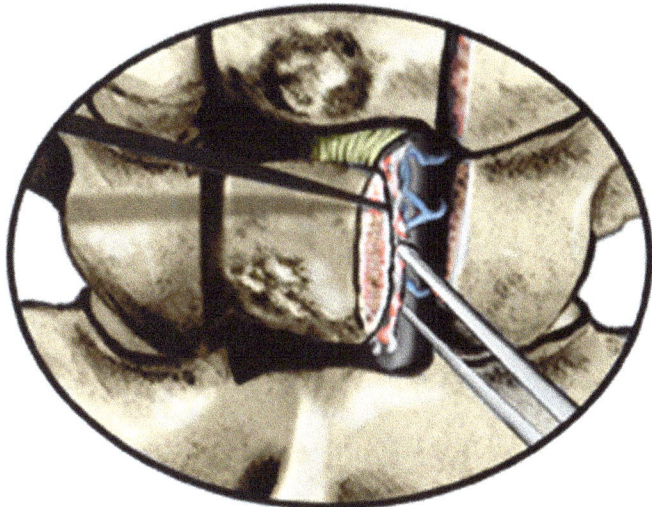

Fig. 11: *Hemostasis.* While opening the laminoplasty, epidural veins will be revealed and must be addressed as necessary with bipolar electrocautery. Coagulating the veins as far dorsally as possible will reduce bleeding. Remaining capsular tissue must also be divided to permit full opening of the laminae.
Courtesy: Dr Heller JG

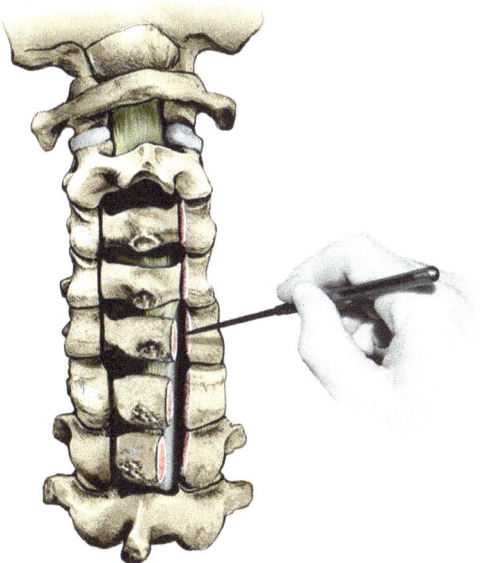

Fig. 10: *Opening the laminoplasty.* The assistant should use a nerve hook under the "open" side of the laminoplasty to apply a gentle upward force while the primary surgeon applies a similar force with an angled curette. The assistant then holds the lamina open while the surgeon proceeds to open the lamina cranial to this. This is done in a stepwise fashion until all laminae have been opened and demonstrated adequate excursion.
Courtesy: Dr Heller JG

is most effectively done with bipolar cautery. The more dorsal one coagulates the veins and the more effective one will be in preventing bleeding. Once this has been accomplished at each level, the steps described above are used again to complete the opening of the laminoplasty until the dura has expanded to its full extent. It is wise to use an angled dural elevator to check for any epidural adhesions before fully opening the laminae (**Fig. 11**).

- If brisk venous bleeding is encountered, control it with tamponade via a patty until the laminoplasty is fully opened and the venous pressure is reduced. It will then be easier and safer to identify and control the active bleeding point.

INSTRUMENTATION

After ensuring adequate excursion at each level, begin securing the laminae in place level by level.

- Have an assistant utilize a nerve hook or angled curette to hold the lamina open. This curette should be placed on the cephalad portion of the lamina to ensure that the plate can be placed at its center.
- Select a plate of appropriate size such that once in place, the assistant may release pressure and the lamina will remain open with the instrumentation well-seated before placing screws. Use an Adson clamp or plate holder to place the laminar side of the plate first, after which the lateral mass aspect of the plate can be rotated into proper position. The plate should be in the center of the lamina and lateral mass, in a craniocaudal direction. It should not interfere with the facet joint above when the patient fully extends their cervical spine postop (**Fig. 12**).
- While holding the plate in position, drill the hole for the first lateral mass screw and insert it. Then place the second lateral mass screw before finally drilling and inserting a single laminar screw. Using an appropriate type of clamp to provide a counter-torque force on the lamina can avoid accidental hinge fracture or displacement while inserting the laminar screw.

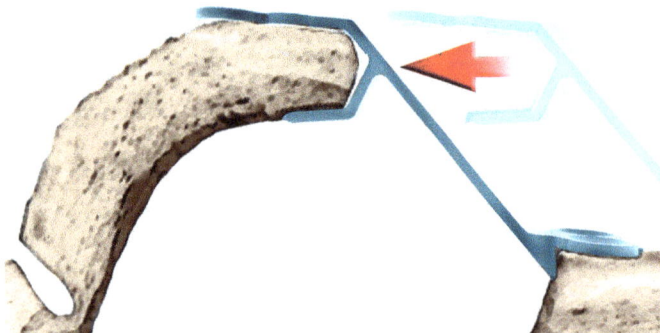

Fig. 12: *Plate insertion.* While an assistant holds the lamina open with a nerve hook or angled curette, slide the laminar portion of the plate into position before rotating the lateral portion of the plate into position. Ensure that the plate fits the lamina well and that no "toggling" is present.
Courtesy: Dr Heller JG

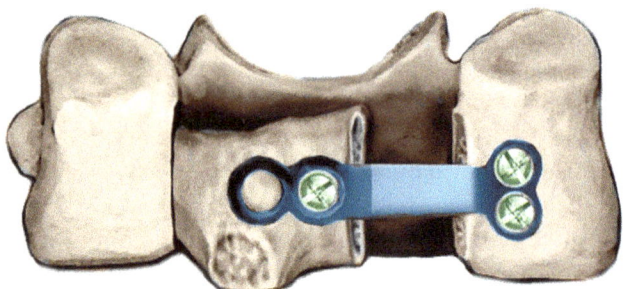

Fig. 13: *Plate positioning.* Each plate should be at the center of the lamina and lateral mass. It should not interfere with the supra-adjacent facet joint in maximum extension.
Courtesy: Dr Heller JG

- Depending on the patient's local anatomy, one should select the type of plate which allows a pair of screws to be used in securing the lateral mass portion of the plate. Some companies offer both vertical and transverse screw orientations on their plates to facilitate this choice.
    - Proceed by repeating the above process at each level to be instrumented **(Figs. 13 to 15)**.

■ CLOSURE

- First ensure meticulous hemostasis. Bipolar cautery is recommended for muscle bleeding points to minimize necrosis. Look carefully where the retractors blades where placed. Vancomycin powder may be utilized to minimize infection risk. A subfascial drain is strongly recommended.
- When closing posterior cervical incisions, ensure that both the muscle layer and fascial layers are closed as separate layers. Closing the muscle layer first, in figure-of-8 fashion with #1 Vicryl will minimize dead space and thus risk of postoperative seroma or hematoma. Next, proceed with fascial layer closure with closely spaced #1 Vicryl in figure-of-8 fashion. Subcutaneous layer sutures are used when necessary. Finally, 2-0 Vicryl

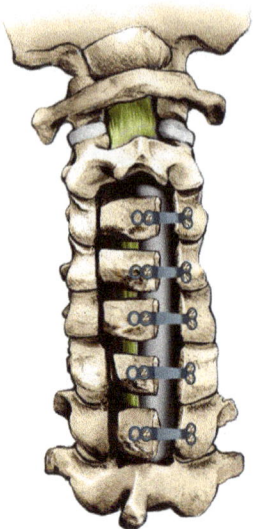

Fig. 14: *Completed instrumentation.* The laminoplasty has been properly secured with sufficient opening to allow full expansion of the dura. Note that a pair of screws has been inserted through the plate into each lateral mass while only a single screw is needed to secure the laminar side.
Courtesy: Dr Heller JG

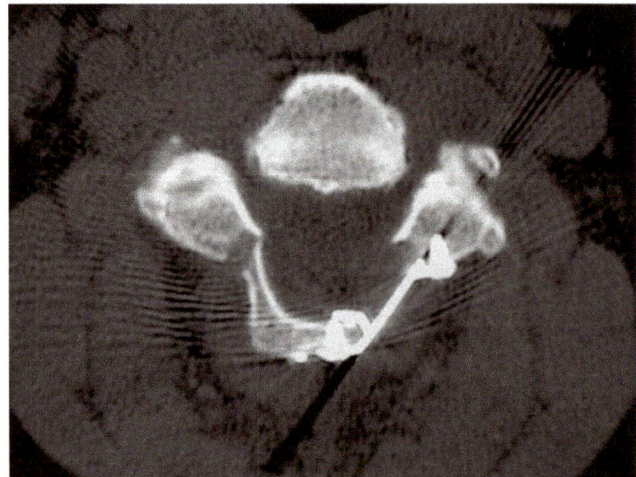

Fig. 15: *Postoperative axial computed tomography image.* Note the final position of bilateral troughs and instrumentation. This image is also illustrative of the amount of decompression possible with laminoplasty.
Courtesy: Dr Heller JG

is used for interrupted deep dermal layer closure and the skin is closed with a running subcuticular 3-0 monocryl.

■ POSTOPERATIVE CARE AND REHABILITATION

- Laminoplasty is intended as a motion-sparing operation. As such it is important to encourage early active range of motion of the cervical spine. Postoperative bracing is not necessary, and in fact should be discouraged. The use of a soft cervical collar for 1–2 weeks could be at the

surgeon's discretion. But it should not discourage active range of motion exercise.
- Patients should avoid any strenuous or repetitive upper extremity activity during the first 6 weeks of recovery to protect the midline tissue repair.
- Active resisted neck/shoulder/upper extremity exercises with elastic bands are initiated under the supervision of a physical therapist 6 weeks after surgery.

REFERENCES

1. Bartels R, van Tulder M, Moojen W, Arts M, Peul W. Laminoplasty and laminectomy for cervical spondylotic myelopathy: a systematic review. Eur Spine J. 2015;24(Suppl 2):S160-7.
2. Ratliff J, Cooper P. Cervical laminoplasty: a critical review. J Neurosurg Spine. 2003;98(3):230-8.
3. Zhu B, Xu Y, Liu X, Liu Z, Dang G. Anterior approach versus posterior approach for the treatment of multilevel cervical spondylotic myelopathy: a systematic review and meta-analysis. Eur Spine J. 2013;22:1583-93.
4. Rhee JM, Register B, Hamasaki T, Franklin B. Plate-only open door laminoplasty maintains stable spinal canal expansion with high rates of hinge union and no plate failures. Spine. 2011;36(1):9-14.
5. Yoon S, Hashimoto R, Raich A, Shaffrey C, Rhee J, Riew K. Outcomes after laminoplasty compared with laminectomy and fusion in patients with cervical myelopathy: a systematic review. Spine (Phila Pa 1976). 2013;38(22 Suppl 1):S183-94.
6. Highsmith J, Dhall S, Haid RJ, Rodts GJ, Mummaneni P. Treatment of cervical stenotic myelopathy: a cost and outcome comparison of laminoplasty versus laminectomy and lateral mass fusion. J Neurosurg Spine. 2011;14(5):619-25.
7. Heller J, Edwards CI, Murakami H, Rodts G. Laminoplasty versus laminectomy and fusion for multilevel cervical myelopathy: an independent matched-cohort analysis. Spine (Phila Pa 1976). 2001;26(12):1330-6.
8. Park A, Heller J. Cervical laminoplasty: use of a novel titanium plate to maintain canal expansion-surgical technique. J Spinal Disord Tech. 2004;17(4):265-71.
9. Steinmetz M, Resnick D. Cervical laminoplasty. Spine J. 2006;6(6 Suppl):S274-81.
10. Patel C, Cunningham B, Herkowitz H. Techniques in cervical laminoplasty. Spine J. 2002;2(6):450-5.
11. Lee DG, Lee SH, Park SJ, Kim ES, Chung SS, Lee CS, et al. Comparison of surgical outcomes after cervical laminoplasty: open-door technique versus French-door technique. J Spinal Disord Tech. 2013;26(6):E198-203.
12. Chiba K, Ogawa Y, Ishii K, Takaishi H, Nakamura M, Maruiwa H, et al. Long-term results of expansive open-door laminoplasty for cervical myelopathy–average 14-year follow-up study. Spine (Phila Pa 1976). 2006;31(26):2998-3005.
13. Okada M, Minamide A, Endo T, Yoshida M, Kawakami M, Ando M, et al. A prospective randomized study of clinical outcomes in patients with cervical compressive myelopathy treated with open-door or French-door laminoplasty. Spine (Phila Pa 1976). 2009;34(11):1119-26.

CHAPTER 6

Anterior Cervical Discectomy and Fusion

Anthony Viola III, Vadim Goz, Alan S Hilibrand

INTRODUCTION

Anterior cervical discectomy and fusion (ACDF) is a proven treatment to address symptomatic cervical radiculopathy or myelopathy secondary to disk degeneration. It is a safe approach that is soft tissue friendly, avoids damage to the neural elements, and provides excellent exposure to allow decompression and correction kyphosis if present in the cervical spine.

PREOPERATIVE PLANNING

- The preoperative magnetic resonance imaging (MRI) must be carefully evaluated for specific site of compression.
    - For central disk herniations, the authors recommend decompression until the medial wall of the pedicle can be palpated with a nerve hook.
    - For compression from lateral disk herniations, it is recommended that decompression is carried lateral until the lateral aspect of the pedicle can be palpated with a nerve hook.
    - Studies have shown that the length of nerve root between the take off of the root and the vertebral artery is approximately 6 mm in the V2 segment of the vertebral artery.
- Vertebral artery location must be noted on the MRI as anomalous vertebral artery anatomy may predispose to vertebral artery injury during the procedure.
- Measure the vertebral body length in order to estimate the appropriate length of the Caspar pins and screws to use during surgery and for the final construct, respectively.

SURGICAL ANATOMY

- Exposure requires sound understanding of the involved anatomy.
- Anatomical surface landmarks are utilized to estimate the level of the incision: The hyoid bone is at approximately C3, thyroid cartilage is at C4–C5, cricoid cartilage and carotid tubercle estimate C6 (**Fig. 1**).
- The sternocleidomastoid (SCM) divides the neck into two triangles, referred to as the anterior and posterior triangles.
- The borders of the anterior triangle are the anterior edge of the SCM, inferior border of the mandible, and the midline of the neck.
- The ACDF approach accesses the ventral spine via the interval between the SCM and the strap muscles, in the anterior triangle of the neck (**Fig. 2**).
- The anterior approach traverses three distinct fascial layers:
    - The deep cervical fascia, deep to platysma, envelopes the SCM muscle anteriorly and the trapezius muscle posteriorly. It continues as a circumferential single layer throughout the rest of the neck.
        - The external jugular vein and the communicating vein reside superficial or "on top of" the deep cervical fascia.

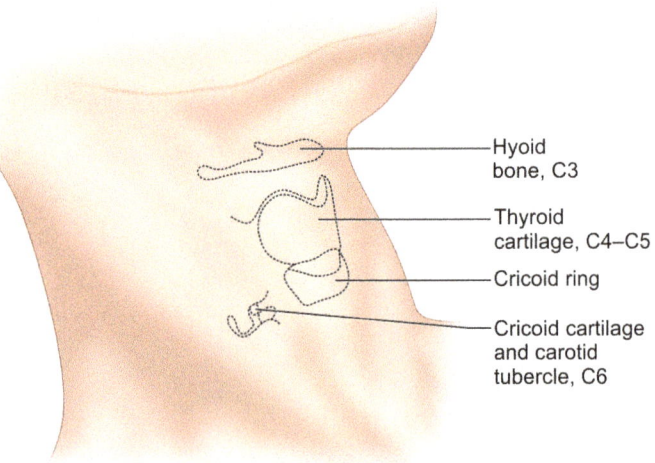

Fig. 1: Anterior cervical landmarks.

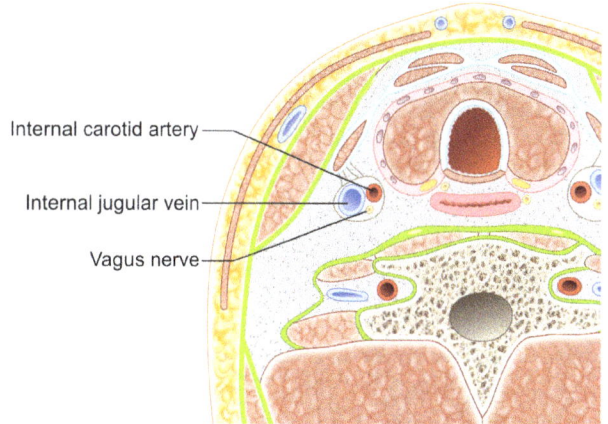

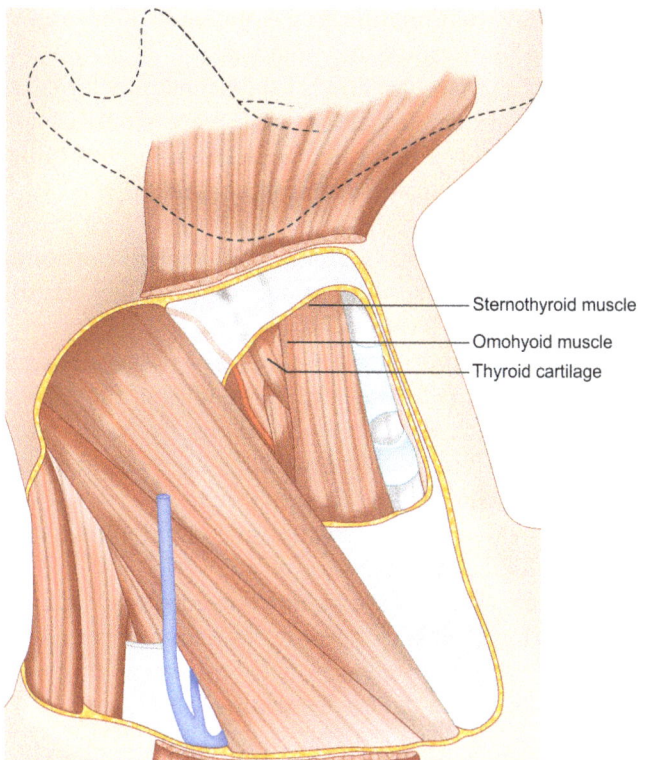

Fig. 2: Once the platysma is reflected, the anterior cervical triangle is visualized. The boundaries of the triangle are the medial border of the sternocleidomastoid, the midline of the neck, and the inferior border of the mandible.

- The pretracheal fascia is deep to the deep cervical fascia and connects the strap muscles to the carotid sheath.
- The prevertebral fascia lies directly on longus colli muscles. The cervical sympathetic plexus runs superficial (ventral) to the prevertebral fascia, on the lateral aspect of the longus colli muscles.
- While performing the anterior approach to the cervical spine, the surgeon should be aware of a number of anatomic structures.
  - Three veins reside in the anterior triangle of the neck immediately beneath the platysma: (1) External jugular vein, (2) anterior jugular vein, and the (3) communicating vein.
    - The external jugular vein runs from the angle of the mandible toward the middle of the clavicle, crossing the SCM from medial to lateral as it courses distally. The external jugular is typically lateral to the field of dissection, but may be encountered with more cranial incisions.
    - The anterior jugular vein is rarely encountered as it is a midline structure residing medial to the exposure.
    - The communicating vein courses over the medial aspect of the SCM and can be a useful marker for the interval between the SCM and strap muscles.

Fig. 3: The carotid sheath is noted above by the black line. The carotid sheath contains in the internal jugular vein, internal carotid artery, and the vagus nerve.

- *The carotid sheath:*
  - Immediately lateral to the dissection plane
  - Contains the internal carotid artery, internal jugular vein, vagus nerve, and the lymphatic plexus **(Fig. 3)**
- *The recurrent laryngeal nerve (RLN):*
  - Branch of the vagus nerve
  - On the right, the RLN loops under the subclavian artery at the level of T1-3 and then courses superiorly toward the larynx. The right RLN has a more oblique course and may still be lateral to the tracheoesophageal groove at C7 and thus lies within the field of dissection.
  - On the left side, the RLN loops around the aorta at approximately T3-6. The left RLN is typically in the tracheoesophageal groove throughout the extent of the cervical spine.
- *The superior and inferior thyroid arteries:*
  - Two paired arteries that cross the interval between the SCM and strap muscles.
  - The superior thyroid arteries are accompanied by the superior laryngeal nerves and can be found crossing the surgical interval at the level of hyoid bone or approximately C3.
  - The inferior thyroid arteries are accompanied by the RLNs and can cross the surgical field between C5 and C7.
- *The hypoglossal nerve:*
  - Can be encountered in high ACDF exposures
  - The nerve courses next to the carotid sheath until it crosses medially at the level of the mandible to innervate the tongue.
- *The ansa cervicalis:*
  - Composed of nerve fibers from the C1 to C3 nerve roots
  - Forms a loop that lies superficial to the carotid sheath and innervates the strap muscles

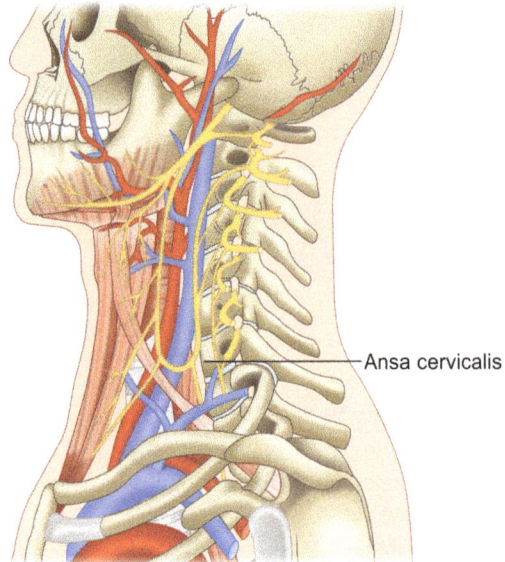

Fig. 4: Ansa cervicalis.

- Branches of the ansa cervicalis can be seen in a careful exposure within the surgical interval used for an ACDF as nerve fibers course across the interval to innervate the strap muscles **(Fig. 4)**.
  - *The vertebral artery:*
    - Runs within the foramen transversarium typically between C2 and C6. The vertebral artery runs approximately half way in terms of ventral to dorsal depth relative to the vertebral body. At the level of the foramen, the vertebral artery is just ventral to the exiting nerve root.
    - The vertebral artery is immediately adjacent to the uncovertebral joint.

OPERATIVE TECHNIQUE

- *Table:* Position the patient supine on a regular surgical operating room (OR) table.
- *Positioning:*
  - An inflatable pressure infusion bag is placed horizontally underneath the shoulders, centered at the level of the scapula.
  - The shoulders are pulled distally and taped down to help with visualization of the cervical spine on lateral radiographs.
  - The head is placed on a small circular foam headrest. The pressure bag is inflated until approximately 10–15° of neck extension is obtained.
  - At this point the patient is prepped and draped.
  - Use a 1010 to square off the ear lobe to make sure chin is in the field, allowing estimation of midline.
  - Drape with four towels, Ioban strips, and a thyroid drape.
- *Neuromonitoring:*
  - The authors routinely use neuromonitoring for ACDF cases.
  - Baseline neuromonitoring is obtained after intubation prior to taping the shoulders.
  - Preintubation baseline is established only for cases with cervical instability or severe stenosis and myelopathy where there is concern for cord injury with neck extension during intubation.
- *Localization:*
  - The location of the incision is based on the anatomic landmarks described above, with a focus on the inferior most level.
    - For example, if a C4–C7 ACDF is planned, the incision will be closer to the level of the cricoid cartilage, as the C6–C7 level is typically more difficult to visualize than the C4–C5 level due to the lordosis of the cervical spine.
  - A left-sided approach is routinely used unless prior left-sided approach was utilized.
  - In the revision setting where a left-sided approach was used for the index procedure, the authors recommend obtaining a laryngoscopy, if both vocal cords are mobile, than a right-sided approach is utilized.
- *Incision:*
  - The incision extends from midline to the medial border of the SCM.
  - An electrocautery is used to dissect through the dermis.
  - A Raytec sponge is used to clearly define the platysma.
  - Dissection is carried out with a pair of Metzenbaum scissors and Gerald forceps. The Metzenbaum scissors are used to carefully dissect deep to the platysma.
    - This is often easiest to do in a medial-to-lateral fashion, elevating the platysma off of the contents below, and allowing it to be safely transected with an electrocautery without injuring tissue deep to the muscle. If a 3 or 4 level procedure is planned, more inferior exposure is often needed and a "T" is developed in the platysma by transecting the inferior flap in a longitudinal manner.
  - The superior and inferior aspects of the platysma are elevated with curved Metzenbaum scissors in order to minimize the tension on the soft tissue throughout the procedure.
  - Utilize bipolar as needed for bleeding control.
  - The deep cervical fascia which envelopes the platysma is a thin layer and is bluntly transected early in the dissection.
  - The interval between the SCM and strap muscles is now located. The communicating vein is a useful landmark for this interval and typically has to be mobilized either laterally or medially. The Metzenbaum scissors are used to gently dissect within this interval which contains loose areolar tissue that spreads easily.

- It is important to note that the interval of interest migrates laterally as one moves cranially due to the oblique course of the SCM **(Fig. 5)**.
- *Deep fascial incision:*
  - As the dissection is carried deeper between the SCM and strap muscles, the first thick fascial layer encountered is the pretracheal fascia.
  - At this point, the pulse of the internal carotid artery is palpated to ensure that the dissection remains medial to the carotid sheath.
  - The pretracheal fascia is either bluntly separated via finger dissection or gently incised with Metzenbaum scissors and the dissection is carried deeper until the vertebral bodies and disks can be palpated.
  - Again, it is confirmed that the carotid sheath is lateral by palpating the pulse of the internal carotid artery.
  - Handheld cloward or appendiceal retractors are placed within the interval.
  - The prevertebral fascia is bluntly dissected off of the vertebral bodies and disks using two Kittners **(Fig. 6)**.
- *Neurovascular structures:*
  - A number of neurovascular structures may be encountered within the interval between the SCM and strap muscles. Depending on the level of the dissection, these include the superior and inferior thyroid arteries, the superior and RLNs, the hypoglossal nerve, and the ansa cervicalis.
  - Vessels encountered in the dissection are carefully ligated with a bipolar electrocautery. The ansa cervicalis can be ligated as well if it is in the field of the dissection without postoperative morbidity.
  - The authors take care to preserve the laryngeal nerves in order to minimize risk of postoperative hoarseness, however these at times do need to be ligated if directly in the field.
  - The omohyoid may also be in the field, especially at the C5–C7 levels. The muscle is isolated using a right angle forceps and divided using an electrocautery with the division being closer to the lateral edge of the interval.
    - This prevents remnants of the muscle from obscuring the dissection.
- *Exposure:*
  - Hand-held Cloward retractor is used in the interval, allowing a good view of longus colli and prevertebral fascia.
  - Once the prevertebral fascia is cleared off of the vertebral disks and bodies, a hemostat is clamped on the soft tissue over the disk, and a lateral radiograph is taken to confirm the operative level.
  - With careful direct visualization, the hemostat is taken off and the disk is marked with the electrocautery. Next the longus colli is elevated off of the disks and vertebral bodies of the operative levels

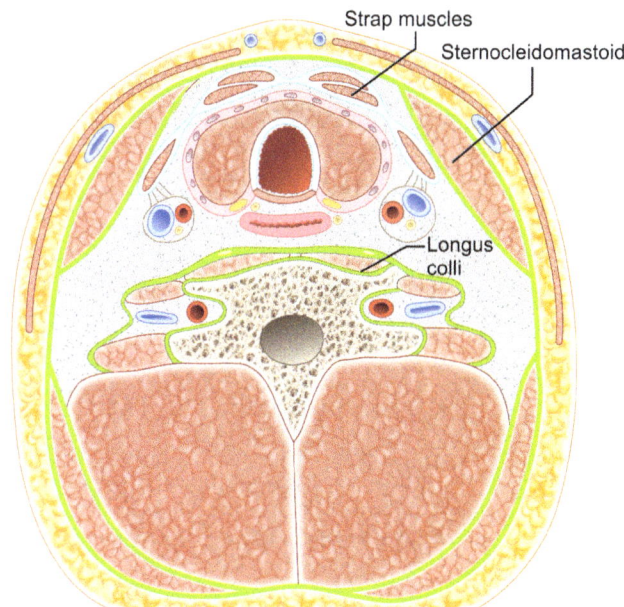

Fig. 5: Key muscles to anterior approach.

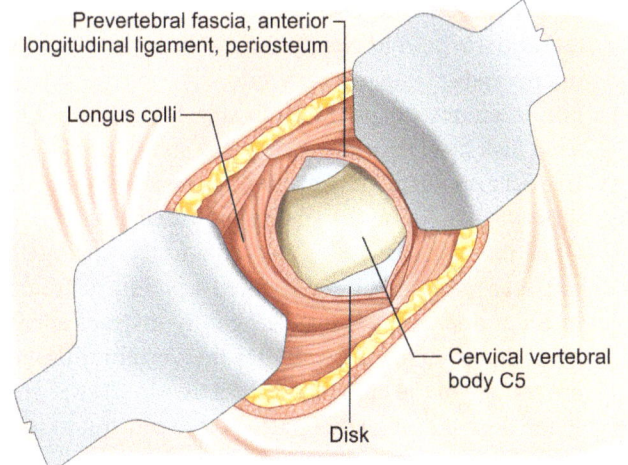

Fig. 6: Deep dissection.

using the bipolar electrocautery. It is important to do so in a subperiosteal manner moving from medial to lateral. The sympathetic chain resides on the longus colli.
  - Subperiosteal dissection minimizes damage to this structure.
- Self-retaining retractors are inserted at the operative level. If the operation is a single- or two-level ACDF, then one or both of the disks are exposed respectively.
- *Discectomy:*
  - For a two-level procedure, an annulotomy is performed with a 15 blade scalpel of both disks ensuring that the annulotomy extends laterally to the uncovertebral joints.
  - Appendiceal retractors are used to isolate the disk for annulotomy, protecting the soft tissue as a blade is used to start the annulotomy **(Fig. 7)**.

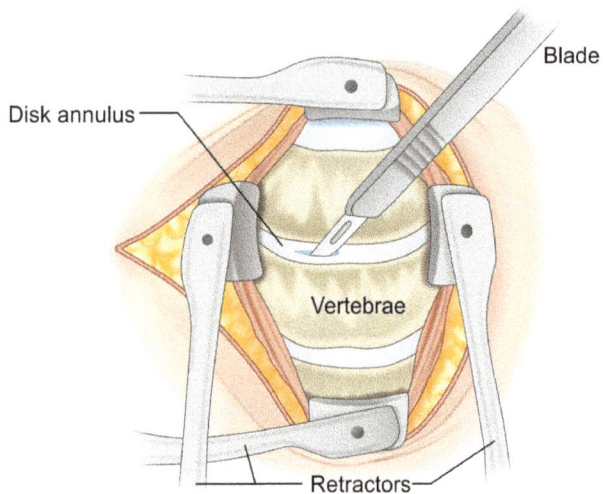

Fig. 7: Annulotomy.

- For a three- or four-level procedure, an annulotomy is performed working from the inferior level up.
- The disk material is then cleared away using pituitary and Kerrison rongeurs and Karlin curettes, close attention is paid to clearly define the upslope of the uncovertebral joint on each side.
- For efficiency purposes, each step is performed on each disk in a factory assembly line style workflow.
- Use a 3 mm Kerrison to clean the lateral aspect of the disk space defining the upslope of the uncus.
- Once the disk material is cleared and the upslope of the uncovertebral joints is defined, a paddle distractor or a cervical cobb is used to gently distract across each disk space, ensuring that the vertebral bodies are mobile in the cranial-caudal axis.
- Place floseal and a large patty before moving to next level.
- In a two-level ACDF, the Caspar pins are next inserted into the superior most and inferior most vertebral bodies.
- In a three-level and four-level ACDF, the retractors are moved to expose the bottom two levels first, Caspar pins are placed across bottom two levels.
  - Typically 14 mm Caspar pins are used, however if the vertebral bodies are particularly small as measured on preoperative measurement, then 12 mm pins may be used.
- Careful attention is paid to the Caspar pins being in the center of the vertebral body both in the cephalad-caudad direction and medial-lateral. Gentle distraction is applied across both disk spaces.
- At this point, the rest of the procedure is performed under the microscope. The inferior level(s) are addressed first.
- A round AM8 burr is used to fashion the disk space into a rectangular prism shape. The superior endplate is domed with a large inferior overhang anteriorly. The cranial aspect of the dome can be palpated with a Woodson or tip of a Kerrison in order to gain an appreciation for the most cephalad extent of the disk space. The anterior overhang of the superior end plate is burred down to the level of the high point of the dome, this helps with adequate visualization of the disk space. Next the anterior portion of the dome is burred down until the anterior half of disk space is flat. This trajectory is taken posteriorly to the level of the posterior longitudinal ligament (PLL).
- It is important that all of the disk material is cleared and the cortical bone is burred to expose bleeding bone while maintaining endplate integrity.
  - Cancellous bone will cause bleeding, and burring through the cortical bone of the endplate negatively impacts the structural integrity and predisposes to graft subsidence.
- The superior endplate of the level below is usually fairly flat throughout the majority of the disk space. The upslope of the uncovertebral joint can be gently leveled with a burr in order to widen the flat aspect of the disk space and accommodate a wider graft.
  - The vertebral artery is just lateral to the uncovertebral joint approximately halfway in the disk space in an anterior to posterior direction.
- The posterior most aspect of the disk space is now flattened as well in order to complete the posterior aspect of the rectangular prism.
  - There will often be superior and inferior bony projections of the caudad and cephalad vertebra respectably that need to be burred down.
- The PLL is then taken down. A nerve hook is used to get plane under PLL and a 2 mm Koros rotating rongeur to clear PLL laterally to the uncus. Decompression of the disk space is then completed.
  - The decompression is deemed to be lateral enough when the surgeon is able to palpate the medial aspect of the pedicle with a nerve hook. If foraminal stenosis is present on preoperative MRI, then decompression is continued until the nerve hook can palpate the lateral aspect of the pedicle.
- A rasp is used as the final instrument to prepare the disk space and a graft, typically machined fibular allograft is inserted into the disk space **(Fig. 8)**.
- Disk prep and grafting for multi-level ACDF (vertebra are numbered in ascending order with 1 indicating superior most vertebral body, i.e., in C5–C6 ACDF C5 = vertebra 1 and C6 = vertebra 2)
  - Two-level ACDF:
    - Annulotomy of inferior disk, followed by annulotomy of superior disk

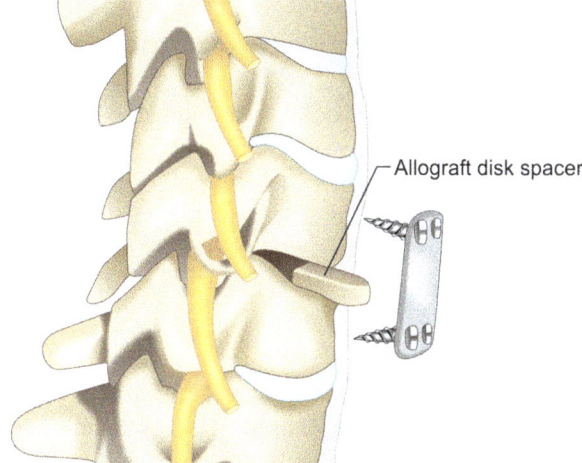

Fig. 8: Allograft disk.

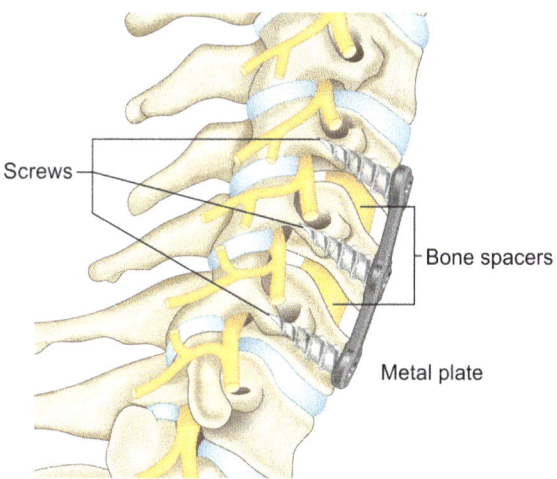

Fig. 9: Fusion.

- Caspar pins placed vertebra 1 and 3, distraction
- Prepare endplates of inferior level, then superior level
- Insert inferior graft, insert superior graft
• Three-level ACDF:
- *Annulotomy and preliminary preparation of superior level:* Remove only gross disk material with curettes and pituitary
- Move retractor to middle and inferior level
- Annulotomy inferior level, annulotomy middle level
- Preliminary disk prep of inferior level, then middle level
- Gently paddle distract both levels
- Caspar pins in vertebra 2 and 4, distract
- Endplate prep of inferior most then middle level
- Graft inferior level, graft middle level
• Four-level ACDF:
- Preliminary discectomy of top two levels
- Set retractors to bottom two levels
- Preliminary discectomy of bottom two levels
- Caspar pins into vertebra 3 and 5, distract
- Bring in microscope, decompress bottom two levels
- Graft bottom two levels
- Move Caspar pins to vertebral bodies 1 and 3
- Decompress top two levels
- Graft second level from the top
■ *Plating:*
• Drill holes in the inferior aspect of the superior vertebra
• Graft top level
• *Place plate:* Plate should span from the very bottom of the superior most vertebra to top edge of the inferior most vertebra.
• Provisional fixation (screw not all the way down to allow leigh way) in top level
• Ensure that the plate is directly midline, checking alignment outside of the microscope relative to the sternum.
• Drill/place screws in bottom most level
• *Proceed superiorly drilling and tightening screws into plate:* As a general rule of thumb, men and women tend to measure about 16 mm and 14 mm, respectively, for the superior-most and inferior-most screws. The middle screws are variable **(Fig. 9).**
■ *Closing:*
• Irrigation with normal saline is utilized.
• Additional graft is then placed on the side of the allograft.
• Floseal is used at each level to slow bleeding.
• A penrose drain is placed.
• The incision is closed with multiple layers of Vicryl followed by prolene, steri strips and mastisol.

POSTOPERATIVE PROTOCOL

■ *Hospitalization:*
• The practice of the authors is for all patients undergoing ACDF to be observed for 23 hours.
  ♦ A 23-hour observation period allows the surgeon to assess for any development of postoperative neurological deficits or airway obstruction.
• Under certain circumstances, patients may be discharged home prior to this, including:
  ♦ Strong patient preference for discharge home
  ♦ One- or two-level procedures
• All ACDF patients leave the OR with a Philadelphia cervical collar on.
• Postoperative day 1:
  ♦ Drain is discontinued.
  ♦ Dressing is changed.

- Postoperative cervical collar is discontinued and replaced:
  - Soft collar for one- or two-level ACDF (except in cases of surgery for adjacent segment disease). This is continued for 2 weeks postoperatively and allowing earlier return to work and driving.
  - Hard collar for three- or four-level ACDF, and for those having surgery for adjacent segment disease. This is continued for 3-4 weeks postoperatively and prior to allowing work and driving.
- Physical therapy is not routinely ordered during hospitalization or postoperatively on discharge unless the patient complains of ongoing mechanical neck pain for more than 1 month following surgery.

- *Follow-up:*
  - The first follow-up visit is typically made at 2-4 weeks.
    - Anteroposterior (AP) and lateral radiographs are obtained at this visit.
  - The patient is then seen in the office postoperatively at:
    - 2-3 months
    - 4-6 months
    - 1 year
    - 2 years
  - Flexion/extension lateral radiographs are ordered at all postoperative visits after the initial follow-up.
  - Less than 1 millimeter of motion at each fused level is considered a solid fusion.

CHAPTER 7

Anterior Cervical Corpectomy and Fusion

David Casper, Jacob Hoffmann, Tom Mroz, Jason Savage

■ INDICATIONS

- Cervical spondylotic myelopathy
- Multilevel cervical spinal cord compression with preexisting kyphosis
- Cervical osteomyelitis recalcitrant to intravenous (IV) antibiotics or compressive epidural abscess
- Cervical neoplasm
- Cervical disk herniation with migrated fragments posterior to the vertebral body (retrovertebral stenosis)
- Vertebral burst fracture with neurologic deficit
- Unstable flexion-distraction injuries (tear-drop type fractures) with or without neurologic injury.

■ INSTRUMENTS

- Regular table [Flat Jackson or regular (AMSCO) bed. Prefer Flat Jackson if Gardner-Wells tongs (GWTs) traction needed to help restore alignment]
- Consider GWTs and weight to provide cervical traction
- Pressure bag or bump (behind scapula)
- Vein retractor, appendiceal retractor, and handheld Cloward retractor
- Electrocautery (monopolar and bipolar)
- Self-retaining retraction system with optional weights
- Caspar pin distractor
- Microscope
- High-speed burr
- Micro Kerrison rongeur
- Curettes
- Nerve hook
- Interbody graft [prefer fibular strut allograft, other options include stackable polyetheretherketone (PEEK) cage, expandable cage, structural autograft]
- Sagittal saw to "fashion" bone graft.

■ NEUROMONITORING

- The use of neuromonitoring is often beneficial and should be considered when performing a cervical corpectomy. Neuromonitoring is particularly helpful in the setting of trauma/instability and/or deformity correction. Neck extension and shoulder traction during positioning can lead to brachial plexus palsy or spinal cord injury. Therefore, checking pre- and postpositioning motor evoked potentials (MEPs) and somatosensory evoked potentials (SSEPs) ensures that the patient's neck has not been over extended and that too much traction has not been placed on the upper extremities.
- MEPs are also recommended intraoperatively, as changes in spinal cord perfusion, spinal cord injury, or root injury can be addressed at the time of surgery. Mean arterial pressures can be elevated, grafts can be repositioned, and cord or root compression can be evaluated when an alert is triggered. Examples of points in the procedure when MEPs prove valuable include endplate distraction, discectomy, foraminal decompression, corpectomy, graft placement, and postfinal hardware placement.

■ POSITIONING

- The patient is positioned in a supine position on a regular table with arms at the side, tucked with a sheet. GWTs are often used with 10 pounds of cervical traction to provide better distraction during the corpectomy and assist in alignment/lordosis restoration. An inflatable pressure bag or bump is placed beneath the patient at the interscapular level and a gel donut is placed beneath the head.
- Using the pressure bag or bump, the neck is placed in slight extension to improve access to the cervical spine.

- Caution should be taken so as to not overextend the patient's neck in cases of myelopathy or spinal cord compression.
- Tape is then placed bilaterally on the shoulders, and in line traction is used to tape the shoulders down to the foot of the bed. This traction helps to provide adequate localization of the cervical spine during intraoperative lateral radiographs.
- The surgical site is preliminarily draped lateral to the sternocleidomastoid (SCM) muscles, just caudal to the sternal notch, and along the anterior aspect of the mandible.
- Sterile preparation of the site is then preformed, and the incision is often marked/localized with intraoperative fluoroscopy.

■ APPROACH

- A right- or left-sided Smith-Robinson approach is utilized based on surgeon preference.
- A transverse incision achieves excellent visualization of 1–4 cervical levels; however, if exposure of more than four levels is required, an oblique incision (in-line with the SCM) should be considered.
- Using surface landmarks, a transverse incision is preferentially placed in a skin crease. However, if skin creases are not within adequate location to the desired surgical level, a crease should not be utilized.
- The incision is centered over the interval between the SCM and strap muscles, and often begins at the medial aspect of the SCM. This ensures adequate space for decreasing tension during retraction, and crossing the midline produces a more cosmetic result due to symmetry of the incision.
- Once the incision is made, generous flaps are elevated anterior to the platysma. The platysma is then undermined with Metzenbaum scissors and divided using electrocautery.
- Using a vein retractor, the lateral edge of the incision is tensioned, which helps to identify a cleft in the tissue that marks the interval between the SCM laterally and the strap muscles/tracheoesophageal structures medially. This interval is developed in both the cephalad and caudal directions starting superficial and working deep. The superficial layer of the deep cervical fascia (investing the SCM) is released along the medial edge of the SCM as far cranial and caudal as possible. Proper release of adhesions within this interval allows for adequate exposure to several vertebral levels.
- The interval is then further developed using blunt dissection, ensuring the carotid sheath is lateral. Often at the fifth and sixth vertebral bodies, the omohyoid is encountered. If impeding on visualization or dissection, the omohyoid may be divided using a right angle forceps to circumferentially expose and elevate the muscle, followed by electrocautery for transection of the omohyoid muscle.
- Once the spine is bluntly palpated through this interval, a finger should be run cephalad and caudal along the spine so as to elevate the esophagus prior to retractor placement. By freeing the esophagus, focal retractor pressure on a small area of the esophageal musculature is also avoided.
- Using an appendiceal or handheld Cloward retractor, the midline viscera and lateral vasculature are retracted and any further deep cervical fascia at the cephalad or caudal aspects of the surgical field is released.
- The prevertebral fascia is then bluntly dissected with two peanuts, or Metzenbaum scissors may be utilized to dissect this layer. Care must be taken to ensure that the esophagus surrounding tissue is retracted medially during the exposure of the anterior vertebral bodies.
- Once adequate visualization of disk space and vertebral body is achieved, a marking film is acquired. A Caspar pin can be placed into the vertebral body or a tonsil clamp can be placed over the anterior longitudinal ligament (ALL) to serve as a marker for localization with a lateral radiograph. Utilization of a spinal needle in the disk space should be avoided, as this can cause iatrogenic injury to a disk not included within the fusion.
- After localization is achieved, subperiosteal dissection of the longus colli and ALL is performed. Developing this muscular flap allows for placement of a self-retaining retractor and also serves to minimize injury to the sympathetic chain.
- The longus colli muscles are elevated bilaterally to the level of the apex of the uncovertebral joint. This should be done in a medial to lateral fashion to avoid injury to the sympathetic chain and/or vertebral arteries. A "flap" of longus colli should be developed on the medial aspect of the muscle and the retractor blades should be placed underneath the flaps.

■ DISCECTOMY

- Once the bilateral uncovertebral joints are exposed and subperiosteal dissection has been carried out over the vertebral body planned for corpectomy, discectomy at the level above and below is performed.
- A self-retaining, expandable retractor is first placed, and weights are hung off either side of the retractor using umbilical tape. Typically, two pounds are placed on the side retracting the midline structures, and one pound is placed on the side of the carotid sheath. Once the retractor blades are placed, the cuff of the endotracheal tube is deflated and reinflated to reduce pressure on the esophagus.

- An annulotomy of the disks is then performed using a 15-blade scalpel, and disk fragments are removed using a pituitary rongeur.
- The anterior osteophyte along the caudal aspect of the cephalad vertebral body is then removed. This is performed with either a high-speed burr or micro Kerrison rongeur. Care should be taken to preserve any bone that can later serve as autograft.
- The disk material and endplate cartilage are removed with a series of curettes, Kerrisons, pituitary rongeurs, and/or high-speed burr. The disk and endplate cartilage is removed from uncinate to uncinate in an anterior to posterior fashion.
- Once preliminary discectomy is complete, Caspar pins are placed in the vertebral bodies above and below the level of the corpectomy.
- The Caspar pin distractor is then placed, and distraction over the two disk spaces is achieved to provide visualization to the posterior annulus, posterior osteophytes, and posterior longitudinal ligament (PLL).
- A microscope may be utilized to achieve optimal visualization. Using the microscope, it is apparent that the discectomy progresses at each level until the PLL is encountered. The PLL is typically preserved until after the corpectomy is completed. It is particularly important to maintain your "orientation" when using the microscope, as this prevents an "oblique" corpectomy and minimizes the risk of inadvertent injury to surrounding structures, including the vertebral artery (VA).
- Bilateral foraminotomies are performed using a 1 mm Kerrison rongeur, and a nerve hook may be passed into the neuroforamen to confirm adequate decompression.

CORPECTOMY

- It is imperative to review the course of the carotid artery (CA) and VA from preoperative imaging. Approximately 2% of patients have an "aberrant" CA or VA, and it is critical to identify these abnormalities prior to surgery to avoid potentially catastrophic complications. The CA may be retropharyngeal and in the "path" of the standard anterior exposure, and the VA may be outside of the transverse foramen and within the vertebral body.
- Complete discectomy of the cranial and caudal extent of the planned resection allows for knowledge of the depth and identification of the lateral borders (uncovertebral joints) of the planned corpectomy.
- The uncovertebral joints are used to center the resection, as the medial border of the unciform processes dictate the lateral borders of the corpectomy.
- The planned resection is then marked with a high-speed burr or electrocautery. Avoiding using the burr "outside" or superficial to the disk space as inadvertent injury to surrounding tissue may occur. It is also critical to maintain the width of the corpectomy from anterior/posterior. A small ruler can be cut to the desired width of the corpectomy for reference throughout the case.
- Lateral troughs are initially made with a high-speed burr to "outline" the extent/width of the corpectomy. This is typically done just medial to the uncovertebral joints. Ventral corpectomy is then started with a Leksell rongeur. This can be used for approximately two-third of the ventral vertebral body. This bone is saved and used for locally obtained autograft in the fusion part of the procedure.
- In the setting of trauma, be cautious to "pull out" fragments of bone with a rongeur as a fragment may be attached to the transverse foramen.
- As the spinal canal is approached, use of a high-speed burr to remove the posterior portion of the vertebral body makes for a more controlled decompression.
- The posterior cortex is thinned, and remaining bone should be removed using a high-speed burr, 1-mm or 2-mm Kerrisons, or angled curettes.
- If the PLL was not taken down during the prior discectomies, a nerve hook can now be utilized to develop a plane in between the PLL and underlying dura. This is accomplished by either sweeping under the cephalad vertebral body and "popping" through the PLL, followed by rotating the nerve hook caudal and pulling anterior traction to create a defect in the PLL, or by orienting the nerve hook 30° to the PLL and applying a controlled posterior force in the midline in order to develop a plane in the PLL. Once a plane is developed posterior to the PLL, a 2-mm Kerrison rongeur is used to finish the resection of the remainder of the ligament.
- In situations of ossification of the posterior longitudinal ligament (OPLL), where the dura is extremely adhered to the ossified ligament, the PLL can be left intact and an anterior floating technique can be utilized when the corpectomy is performed. In this situation, first thin the OPLL mass, flush with the normal PLL (if you leave it bulky, the graft may not allow it to float back adequately), then a circumferential sub-PLL resection around the fragment confirmed with a nerve hook. Once the decompression is complete, the spinal cord will drift away from the small bone island left adherent to the dura.
- Care should be taken not to violate the endplates of the cranial and caudal limits of the corpectomy, as this could increase the risk of interbody subsidence. If subsidence occurs, consider posterior fixation to prevent further collapse/subsidence, deformity, and/or nonunion.
- Meticulous hemostasis from epidural bleeding is obtained with bipolar cautery, cottonoid, and hemostatic agents throughout the decompression.

GRAFT PLACEMENT AND INSTRUMENTATION

- Fusion after corpectomy may occur using a tricortical graft and plate, mesh cage, or expandable cage devices.
- *Tricortical graft:*
  - Harvested tricortical iliac crest autograft or allograft may be used. Locally obtained autograft from the corpectomy site can be placed in the structural allograft (fibula, radius, etc.).
  - The structural graft is then inserted into the defect.
  - The graft must match the length of the defect in order for it to share the axial load with the plate. In the setting of trauma or tumor, be careful not to "overdistract" with a large graft. The graft size is often measured using a cut ruler or caliper.
  - A small ridge of bone is left on the posterior aspect of the caudal and cephalad vertebral bodies to avoid translation of the graft into the canal.
  - After the graft is inserted, the Caspar pins are removed. A snug fit of the graft within the defect should be noted in order to avoid graft kick out or translation.
- *Mesh cage or expandable cage application:*
  - Corpectomy defect is measured with a caliper.
  - The largest diameter mesh cage (that fits into the corpectomy defect) is selected and cut to appropriate length.
  - The cage is tightly packed with locally obtained autograft bone and/or allograft.
  - Endplate rings can be added in patients with poor bone quality. In order to accommodate nonparallel endplates, variable angulation endplate rings can be added.
  - Under lateral fluoroscopic guidance, the cage is inserted and tapped into its final position and the Caspar pins are removed. An expandable cage can then be opened to ensure adequate fit.
- *Application of plate:*
  - Remove anterior osteophytes with high-speed burr or Leksell rongeur to ensure plate sits flush against the vertebral bodies.
  - An appropriate length plate should be selected to ensure that screws are not placed near the mobile disks above and below.
  - Ideally, the plate would extend as little as possible above and below the endplates of the corpectomy.
  - The plate is contoured to accommodate the patient's lordosis.
  - Temporary pins can be placed while anteroposterior (AP) and lateral views confirm appropriate plate positioning.
  - Lengths and trajectory of the screws can be templated based on preoperative measurement of the vertebral body depth.
  - Set the stop guide of the drill to appropriate length. Two screw paths are drilled in each vertebra aiming slightly medial and away from the corpectomy.
  - Screws are applied but not fully tightened until all screws have been inserted.
  - The cranial most screws are first tightened to ensure the plate sits flush with the vertebral body. This can potentially prevent any impingement of the plate onto the pharynx.
  - Final imaging verifies appropriate instrumentation placement.
  - Posterior fixation should be considered with multi-level corpectomies, and/or in the setting of significant instability (bilateral facet fracture dislocation, tumor involving multiple vertebral bodies, etc.).

CLOSURE

- The incision should be copiously irrigated, and meticulous hemostasis is achieved using bipolar electrocautery, hemostatic agents, and bone wax.
- In corpectomy cases, a deep drain is placed and either brought through the incision, in line with the incision, or through a separate incision just caudal.
- 3-0 Vicryl is used to close the platysmal and superficial cervical fascial layer, followed by 4-0 Vicryl on the dermal layer, and lastly 4-0 running absorbable suture on the skin.
- Steri strips or skin glue is then utilized, followed by a sterile dressing and foam tape.
- Postoperative day 1, the dressing and drain are removed.

AFTERCARE

- Overnight intubation should be considered for patients requiring extensive dissection or extended operative time that are at risk for retropharyngeal hematoma or edema.
- The patient should be positioned with the head of the bed >45° overnight.
- Local and/or IV steroids may be used in an attempt to minimize postoperative dysphagia.
- The use of a cervical collar is at the discretion of the operative surgeon.

CHAPTER 8

Anterior Cervical Discectomy and Disk Arthroplasty

Bruce V Darden

INTRODUCTION

Cervical disk arthroplasty (CDA) following anterior cervical discectomy offers an alternative to anterior cervical discectomy and fusion (ACDF). CDA allows continued motion at the affected vertebral segment, theoretically diminishing stresses on the adjacent disks, thereby diminishing adjacent segment degeneration. Clinical studies are starting to provide evidence that CDA may positively affect adjacent segment disease. However, not every patient undergoing ACDF is a candidate for CDA.[1] **Box 1** lists generally accepted indications and contraindications for CDA, based on the Food and Drug Administration (FDA) Investigational Device Exemption studies. Barbagallo et al. report an algorithm for when CDA is appropriate for cervical pathology.[2]

BOX 1: Indications and contraindications for cervical disk arthroplasty (CDA).

Indications:
- 1–2 level symptomatic cervical disk disease (radiculopathy and/or myelopathy) between C3 and C7 in a skeletally mature patient
- Disk herniation, osteophyte formation, and/or disk height on imaging studies
- Functional deficit and/or neurologic deficit in a pattern consistent with findings on imaging studies
- Failure of nonoperative treatments for at least 6 weeks in the absence of progressive neurologic deficits

Contraindications:
- Allergy to any component of desired CDA
- Active local or systemic infection
- Osteoporosis with T score < –2.5
- Moderate to advanced spondylosis, bridging osteophytes
- Disk collapse >50% of normal height
- Absence of motion at implantation levels
- Advanced facet arthropathy
- Cervical instability: >3 mm of translation on flexion/extension radiographs and/or >11° of angulation of disk space compared to adjacent levels
- Significant kyphotic deformity
- Retrovertebral pathology ossification of the posterior longitudinal ligament

Source: Adapted from ProDisc-C FDA IDE study protocol

INSTRUMENTS SUGGESTED

- Radiolucent bed [Mayfield head holder cannot be used unless radiolucent-prevents—anteroposterior (AP) visualization]
- Gel head pad
- Roll for neck/shoulders
- Fluoroscopy—the caudal vertebra at the affected disk must be visualized or will have to convert to ACDF
- Soft tissue anterior approach retractors should be radiolucent
- Caspar disk retractors (some CDA prosthesis sets provide these)
- Standard ACDF instruments.

CHOICE OF IMPLANT

- Keeled implants may have higher rates of heterotopic ossification (HO).
- ProDisc-C CDA (Centinel Spine, West Chester, PA) more constrained prosthesis; Bryan disk (Medtronic, Minneapolis, MN) less constrained. There are no strict criteria for how much constraint is optimal. A less constrained prosthesis restores the mobile instantaneous center of rotation. A more constrained prosthesis limits shear strain to the facet joints, theoretically delaying facet degeneration if this is a concern.
- Mobi-C (Zimmer Biomet, Warsaw, IN) and Prestige LP (Medtronic, Minneapolis, MN) have FDA clearance for two-level use.
- Use of keeled implants at more than one contiguous level carries a risk of vertebral body fracture, especially in smaller individuals.

- Hybrid procedures (combination of CDA, ACDF) have in multiple studies been shown to be safe and effective, but currently are off-label through the FDA.

APPROACH

- Standard ACDF approach (Smith-Robinson) is used.
- Shoulders are taped to allow fluoroscopic visualization of target level **(Fig. 1)**.
- Initial AP/lateral fluoroscopy prior to incision to establish optimal C-arm position. The aim of positioning is to recreate typical upright lordosis. Mayo table is not used at head of the bed so C-arm can be moved cephalad when not in use.
- Draping—standard for ACDF, allowing room for C-arm cephalad. Lateral C-arm drape is used for sterility.
- Exposure—meticulous hemostasis is critical to minimize the risk of HO. Exposure of the longus colli muscles should be limited for the same reason.
  - Self-retaining retractors are then placed, the approach level marked, and confirmed by radiography.
- Confirmation of the midline in the AP plane is obtained prior to placing Caspar-type retaining/distracting pins. The midline of the cephalad and caudal vertebrae are confirmed by AP fluoroscopy. The pins can then be placed in the midline, which simplifies the centering of the prosthesis placement. They should be as far from the disk as possible, parallel to affected disk in the lateral plane, to allow adequate room for endplate preparation.
- *Decompression:*
  - Should be tailored to the pathology. Discectomy is typically done to the medial uncovertebral joint. A portion of the medial joint may be resected to remove an extruded fragment. If bony foraminal stenosis is the problem and a significant amount of the joint must be removed, consider fusion.

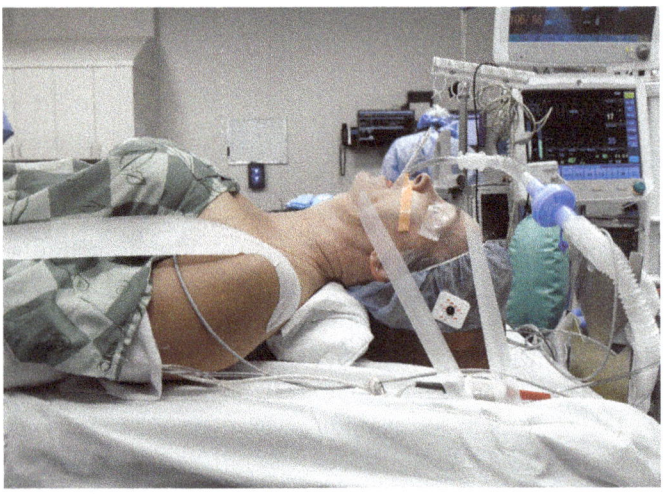

Fig. 1: Photography of intraoperative positioning for cervical disk arthroplasty.
Courtesy: Michael Conti Mica, MD

- Use of a burr should be minimized and thoroughly irrigated to diminish risk of HO.
- For use of a CDA without keeled fixation, the bony lip anteriorly of the cephalad vertebra should be maintained if possible. The lip can be resected when using a keeled CDA.
- The bony endplates should be maintained to diminish subsidence. Decortication of the endplates is done with curettes, to avoid exposing cancellous bone.
- Posterior longitudinal ligament (PLL) may be removed at the surgeon's discretion. Removing the PLL is done if there is suspicion of pathology behind the ligament. It is not necessary to retain it for CDA stability.
- Thorough foraminotomy should be undertaken, to minimize recurrent foraminal stenosis. If possible, the foraminotomy should be done with Kerrison rongeurs, as opposed to a high-speed burr, to minimize the risk of HO. If the burr is needed, use copious irrigation and bone wax on bleeding bony surfaces.

CERVICAL DISK ARTHROPLASTY IMPLANTATION

Each implant has specific endplate preparation techniques. The following are general principles of implantation:

- The vertebral endplates should be parallel on both the AP and lateral views to prevent asymmetric placement. Most implants have a distractor to assure the endplates are parallel.
- The implant height should allow an easy fit with the trial. You should not "stuff" the disk space as with an ACDF. If it is difficult to seat the trial, use a smaller implant. Generally most prostheses are 5 mm in height. A larger implant may restrict motion.
- The implant should be large enough in both planes to rest on the cortical rim of the endplates, to avoid subsidence. For safety, the implant should be recessed 1–2 mm on both the anterior and posterior endplates.
- The implant should be placed as posterior as possible to restore normal kinematics and avoid undue stress on the facet joints.
- If keel cuts are required, the surgeon should manually inspect the cuts to assure no bone remains in the cuts, to avoid bony retropulsion, and to assure the implant can be placed as posterior as possible.
- Each step of implantation should be visualized with fluoroscopy.
- After successful implantation, meticulous hemostasis is critical. All exposed cancellous surfaces should be covered in bone wax (especially keel cuts).
- Use copious irrigation and then drain if appropriate.

CLOSURE

Standard for ACDF.

AFTERCARE

- No collar is necessary
- Activities as tolerated
- While HO can occur years after the prosthesis implantation, nonsteroidal anti-inflammatory drugs (NSAIDs) diminish the risk of HO.[3] We recommend 3 weeks of NSAIDs treatment postoperatively if the patient has no contraindications.

REFERENCES

1. Auerbach JD, Jones KJ, Fras CI, Balderston JR, Rushton SA, Chin KR. The prevalence of indications and contraindications to cervical total disc replacement. Spine J. 2008;8(5):711-6.
2. Barbagallo GMV, Assietti R, Corbino L, Olindo G, Foti PV, Russo V. Early results and review of the literature of a novel hybrid surgical technique combining cervical arthrodesis and disc arthroplasty for treating multilevel degenerative disc disease: Opposite or complementary techniques? Eur Spine J. 2009;18 Suppl 1:29-39.
3. Mehren C, Suchomel P, Grochulla F, Barsa P, Sourkova P, Hradil J, et al. Heterotopic ossification in total cervical disc replacement. Spine. 2006;31(24):2802-6.

CHAPTER 9

Pearls of Upper Cervical Spine Trauma Management

Daniel Leas, Barrett S Boody, Rick C Sasso

■ INTRODUCTION

Upper cervical spine injuries, spanning from the occipitocervical junction to the cervical one and two vertebrae, are complex and sometimes intimidating challenges facing the spine surgeon. In this chapter, fundamental considerations of several injury types will be discussed. A review of relevant imaging studies, acute stabilization, and operative or nonoperative treatment modalities will be provided for each injury pattern. These injuries include: Occipitocervical dislocation/dissociation, C1 ring/burst fractures, C1/2 ligamentous instability, and C2 fractures ranging from odontoid fractures to the eponymous Hangman's fracture.

As a matter of general consideration when evaluating patients with upper cervical spine injuries, there is a high rate of concurrent injuries in the neck as well as torso and appendicular skeleton. The most common injuries found in association are fractures of the ribs, sternum, larynx, and/or trachea (19.6%) followed by skull base fractures (7.4%), facial fractures (7.2%), and forearm fractures (5.4%).[1] These patients require a thorough traumatic evaluation by the acute surgical trauma team to ensure appropriate adherence to protocol. Airway, circulatory, and neurologic compromise continue to be common in this patient population.

■ OCCIPITOCERVICAL DISLOCATION/ DISSOCIATION

- *Radiographic evaluation:*
  - Plain radiography:
    - Limited role for acute plain radiographic evaluation:
      - Difficult to perfectly visualize occipitocervical junction on cross-table laterals
    - Basion-dens interval (BDI) **(Fig. 1A)**:
      - Measured as a distance between the tip of the odontoid (dens) and the tip of the basion
      - >10 mm for adults and >12 mm in children should be concerning.
    - Basion-axis interval (BAI) **(Fig. 1B)**:
      - Measured as a distance between the posterior axial line and the basion
      - About 4–12 mm is normal. >12 mm is abnormal.
    - Powers ratio **(Fig. 1C)**:
      - Measured as a ratio between the distance between the tip of the basion to the midpoint of the posterior C1 arch over the distance between the opisthion to the midpoint of the anterior C1 arch.
      - A ratio greater than one is considered abnormal.
      - Only applicable to an anterior dislocation.
  - *Computed tomography (CT)*: Many metrics have been described. Considered the gold standard of diagnostic evaluation
    - Occipital condyle-C1 interval (CCI) **(Fig. 1D)**:
      - Measured at the mid-sagittal point of the OC articulation, space between the occipital condyle and the top of the C1 joint surface
      - >2.5 mm indicative of dislocation/dissociation
    - Condylar sum:
      - Similar to CCI, but a sum of the CCI on the left and the right
      - Abnormal if the sum exceeds 5 mm
  - Magnetic resonance:
    - Not typically indicated for diagnostic confirmation of OC dislocation/dissociation
    - In some cases, stable craniocervical injuries can be identified with either a strain or a unilateral alar ligament avulsion
- *Acute management:*
  - All patients should have provisional immobilization leading up to definitive surgery.
    - Going to the operating room is an emergent goal and should be done in an expedited fashion upon diagnosis. This is life-threatening condition.
  - Early identification of these patients and field collar immobilization has allowed many to survive the pre-hospital phase.

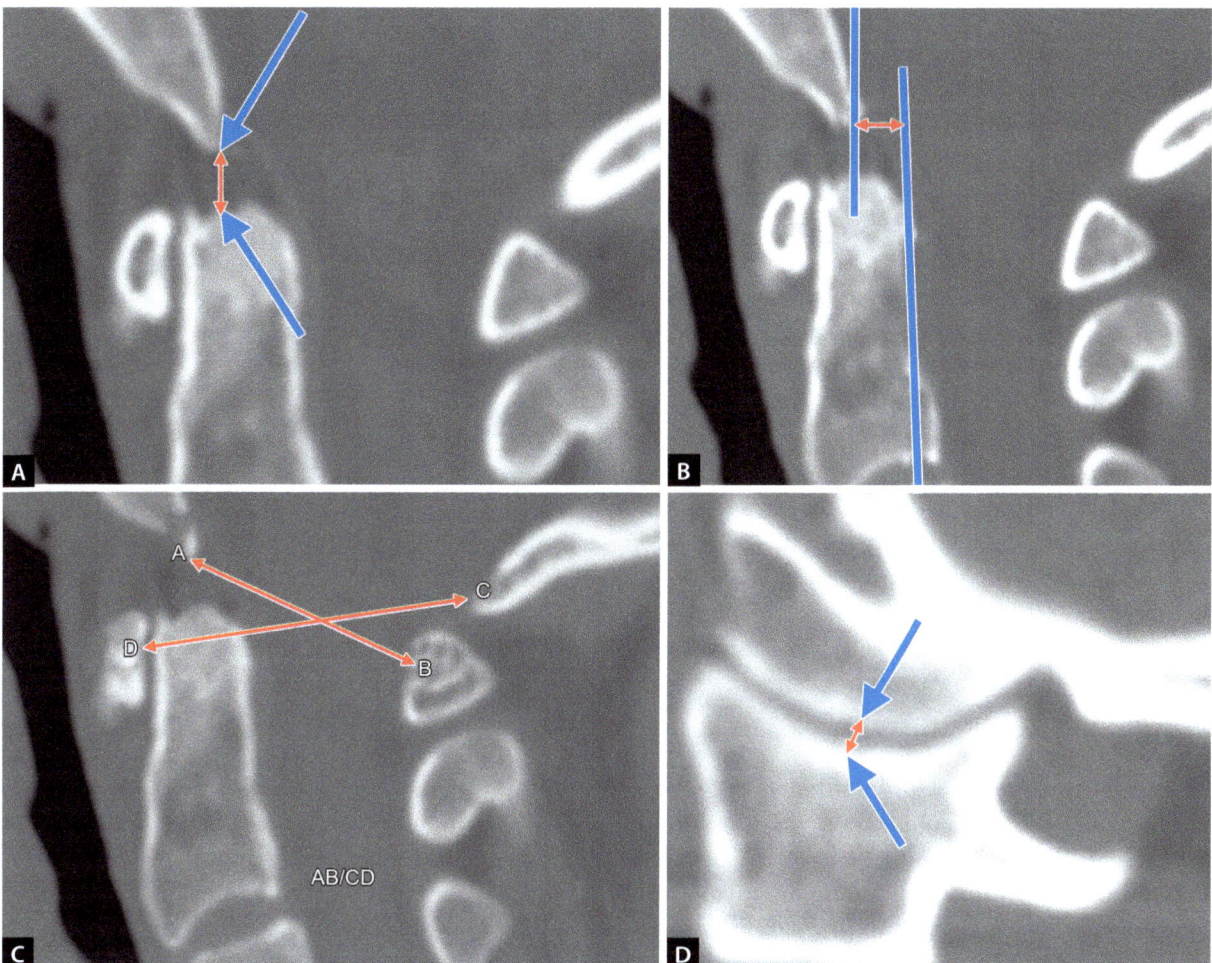

Figs. 1A to D: (A) Basion-dens interval (BDI). The blue arrows point to the tip of both the odontoid process and the basion. The red arrow is the distance measured to determine BDI; (B) Basion-axis interval (BAI). Draw the first blue line in parallel to the posterior cortex of the odontoid process. Draw a parallel line at the most posterior extent of the basion. The distance between these two lines is BAI; (C) Powers ratio. Draw a line from the posterior tip of the basion (A) to the anterior aspect of the C1 posterior arch (B). Draw a second line from the anterior tip of the opisthion (C) to the posterior aspect of the anterior C1 arch (D). Define the ratio of AB/CD. A ratio >1 is considered abnormal; (D) Occipital condyle-C1 interval. Define the largest joint space in the mid-sagittal cut of the right and left occiput/C1 articulation. A perpendicular line is then drawn from the superior endplate of the C1 lateral mass to the inferior cortex of the occipital condyle. A measurement over 2.5 mm or a sum of both the left and right intervals over 5 mm are suspicious for occipitocervical injuries.

- Type of immobilization is somewhat controversial. At a minimum, patients should be maintained in a rigid cervical collar.
  - However, it is important to understand the orthopedic principle of bracing: For the brace to be effective, it must stabilize the region above and below the injury to remove motion at the injured level. Rigid collars do not stabilize the occiput adequately and may benefit from adjunct sandbags next to the head and neck with taping to the backboard. This obviously is not a sustainable immobilization technique and should only be considered for transportation and immediate stabilization in the trauma bay/emergency room (ER) while during the trauma team evaluation and imaging. As a result, operative stabilization or halo placement should be performed urgently.
- For patients too unstable for the operating room, halo vest application is recommended for temporary immobilization. This allows for monitoring of the skull base and avoiding pressure ulcerations. It will also allow access to the neck for airway management (tracheostomy) or increased vascular access (central line). The halo vest is not a good definitive treatment method due to the low healing rate of ligamentous injuries and likelihood of persistent displacement of the atlanto-occipital articulation.
  - *Terminal management:*
    - Definitive management of patients should always consist of rigid occipitocervical fixation.
    - Occipital fixation is typically in the form of low-profile offset screws or an occipital plate. Both should be maintained below the level of the external occipital protuberance.

- The caudal level of fixation is dependent on several factors. The most important factor is maximizing purchase for rigid fixation. In some instances, C2 fixation alone is adequate, and in other cases, the surgeon's prerogative may take the fixation down to C4 or C5 lateral mass.
  - C1 screws can be challenging to integrate into the construct due to the high degree of lordotic rod bend at the OC junction. Typically, the sharp bend is also at the connection point of the C1 screws, further complicating rod placement. Proper utilization of offset connectors can make this transition more fluid.
  - C1 screws can be used for additional fixation points if desired, but make sure to add extra length to the screws so the tulip sits higher, making the rod connection easier. When the C1 tulips are deeper than the C2 screws, rod placement is challenging.
- Wiring constructs are largely a historical treatment method. This has largely been supplanted by screw/rod constructs.
- *Relevant technique pearls:*
  - Neuromonitoring is recommended during positioning due to risks of subluxation and pressure on the brainstem. Signals should be checked supine on the bed prior to prone positioning and again after final positioning before prep and drape. The patient's bed should remain in the room during this phase in the event that they need to be returned to a supine position.
  - Mayfield-type tongs should be utilized for cranial fixation and attached rigidly to the operating room table.
    - If the patient is in a halo frame, the halo can be left in place and used to secure the head to the bed.
  - The goal position of the occipitocervical fusion is for a gaze trajectory approximately 5° below the horizon. Level gaze or gaze above the horizon can be extremely detrimental to patient outcomes due to risks of falling. Short segment fusions allow for some flexibility in the subaxial spine that may accommodate, but every effort should be made at the time of the index surgery.
  - Ensuring the OC junction is reduced at the time of final fixation is paramount in this surgery.
    - Scrutinize the postpositioning X-rays to determine reduction or displacement of injury. Slight changes in head positioning at this time are easier before the patient is prepped and draped.
    - X-rays can be challenging to interpret OC articulation reduction. Consider using intraoperative CT if available to visualize the reduction, looking for seating of the occipital condyles within the C1 superior articular surface on the sagittal images. Subluxation of the OC junction at the time of final fixation increases the risk of construct failure.

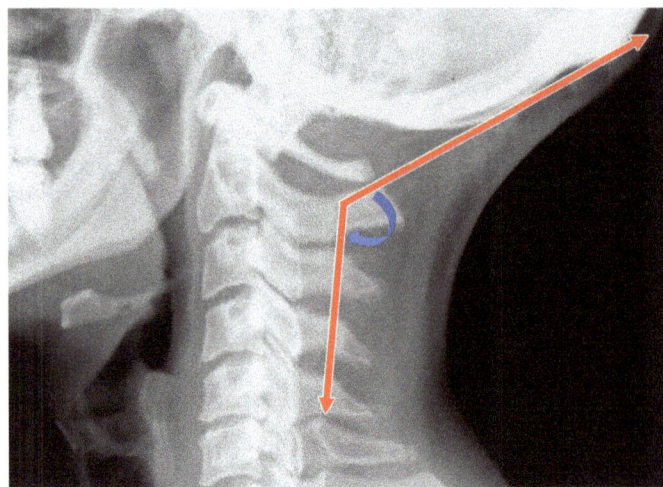

Fig. 2: Occipitocervical angle. A line parallel to the posterior occipital slope is met with a line running parallel to the subaxial spinolaminar junction. The inside angle should be approximately 110°.

  - Additionally, consider using a flat-plate digital radiograph or intraoperative CT as opposed to C-arm radiography to accurately assess the posterior occipitocervical angle (POCA).
    - A line parallel to the posterior occipital slope is met with a line running parallel to the subaxial spinolaminar junction **(Fig. 2)**.
    - A target POCA should be around 108 +/−8° of lordosis.
  - Another helpful relationship to assess the ultimate alignment of your construct is the angle created but a line subtended from the anterior boarder of the cervical spine and the hard palate. Compare this relationship to a preoperative or preinjury film if available. The goal is to restore the patient's natural alignment.
  - Caution should be exercised during the surgical approach to avoid iatrogenic spinal cord injury. Slow exposure of known anatomic landmarks [external occipital protuberance (EOP) and C2 spinous process], meticulous hemostasis, and using blunt, gentle exposure techniques (small cobb or penfield) with bipolar cautery when approaching the spinal canal can avoid potential iatrogenic injury.
  - A C1 and/or C2 laminectomy is likely not required in the absence of preinjury upper cervical stenosis.

ATLAS FRACTURES

- *Radiographic evaluation:*
  - Plain radiography:
    - Limited role for plain radiographic evaluation in the acute setting

- Open-mouth odontoid view can highlight lateral mass displacement relative to the articulation with C2.
- Lateral mass overhang totaling over 8 mm on upright AP odontoid X-ray imaging is associated with concomitant transverse ligament rupture indicating instability.
- Lateral radiographs may show an increase in the atlanto-dens interval (ADI) **(Fig. 3)**, which may be representative of ligamentous injury and resulting instability. When this interval exceeds 3.5 mm, there should be a high suspicion for instability.
- CT:
  - Best for defining fracture morphology
  - Evaluate the status of the anterior arch, posterior arch, and potential ligamentous avulsions of C1 lateral mass. These sections comprise the foundation of Landells atlas fracture classification **(Table 1)**.
  - Sum of lateral mass displacement should not exceed 7 mm on CT scans. This is different from plain radiography due to lack of magnification. Excessive displacement is again indicative of instability **(Fig. 4)**.

- Particular attention should be paid to the retropharyngeal tissues. A typical rule of thumb is "Five at Two and Two at Five" meaning normal soft tissues are approximately 5 mm deep at C2 and 2 cm deep at C5. Excessive swelling may be a surrogate for occult injury prompting additional evaluation with magnetic resonance imaging (MRI) **(Fig. 5)**.
- There is a high (50%+) rate of associated cervical spine injuries, both atlantoaxial and subaxial levels, and all axial, sagittal, and coronal reformats should be evaluated carefully.

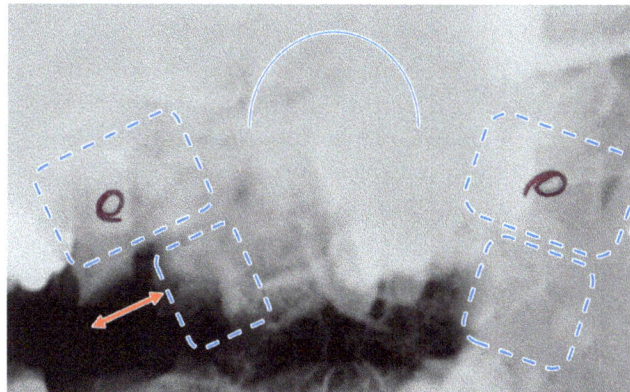

Fig. 4: Lateral mass overhang on anteroposterior (A/P) XR. The C1 lateral masses are highlighted with a drawn "o" in the center. The superior articular process of C2 is highlighted in the dashed box caudally. The red arrow demonstrates unilateral translation of the C1 lateral mass.

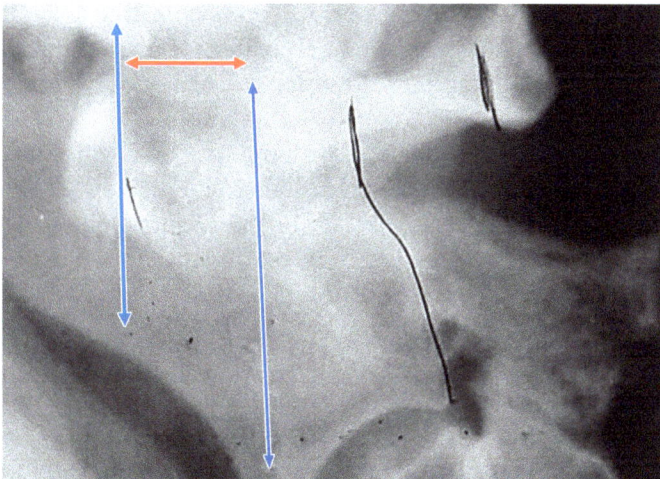

Fig. 3: Increased Atlanto-dens interval. First, draw a line parallel to the anterior cortex of the odontoid. Then mark an additional line parallel to the first, referenced off of the posterior cortex of the anterior C1 arch. The distance between these two is the Atlanto-dens Interval. >3.5 mm is supraphysiologic.

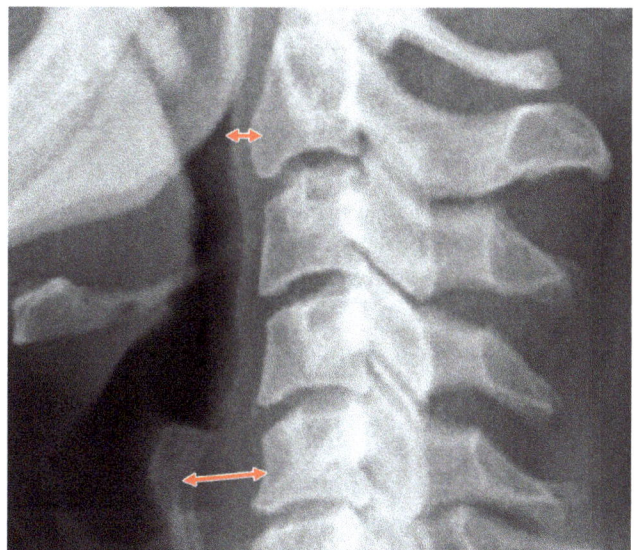

Fig. 5: Soft tissue shadow on lateral C-spine. The red arrows indicate the soft tissue shadow at both C2 and C5. Note the relatively shallow soft tissue shadow at C2 compared to a substantially wider normal shadow at C5.

TABLE 1: Landell's classification of Atlas fractures.

Type I	Isolated anterior or posterior arch fracture. "Plough" type fracture
Type II	Burst-type fracture with bilateral anterior and posterior arch fractures. "Jefferson" fracture. May have associated transverse ligament injury **(Table 2)**
Type III	Unilateral lateral mass fracture. "Floating lateral mass"

TABLE 2: Dickman's classification of transverse ligament injuries.

Type I	Mid-substance or intra-substance tear
Type II	Bony avulsion of ligament with intact ligament mass

- Magnetic resonance:
  - Less common for acute evaluation, but can highlight acute ligamentous injury
  - Sensitivity to order MRI is increased by retropharyngeal soft tissue swelling, or in the setting of a suspicious or equivocal atlanto-dens interval. Typically, 3-5 mm of anterior displacement indicates at least partial ligamentous injury.
  - Carefully evaluate posterior ligamentous complex at all levels with T2 and short tau inversion recovery (STIR) sequencing highlighting water/edema content and T1 sequencing highlighting contiguous or noncontiguous linear collagen fibers
    - Whereas edema (hyperintense T2 or STIR signal) within ligamentous structures is suggestive of soft-tissue injury, disruption or gapping seen on T1 (hypointense signal) is definitive of injury.
  - For patients with confirmed ligamentous injuries, Dickman et al. described a classification highlighting the location of ligamentous insufficiency **(Table 2)**. The presence of a mid-substance tear indicates a lower likelihood of spontaneous recovery.
- *Acute management:*
  - All patients will likely still have a "field" hard collar in place from the trauma evaluation.
  - Once the patient is appropriately stabilized after a thorough primary and secondary survey, they should be transitioned to a well-fitted and well-padded rigid cervical collar. This may be the definitive management based on injury pattern.
    - We find that collars are frequently misunderstood by patients, who treat the collar as a support to simply rest their head on. This leads to jaw pain, skin issues, and increased neck fatigue after collar removal.
    - Instead, we emphasize that patients should continue to work on posture and head control, finding the "center" of the brace when upright, so that their cervical musculature is supporting them, not the collar. We emphasize that the collar to prevent potentially dangerous range of motion during the healing process and is not meant to be a "crutch to rest on."
- *Terminal management:*
  - The decision to operate in the setting of a C1 fracture is almost entirely determined by whether the fracture pattern is stable or unstable.
  - The Landells classification **(Table 1)** was initially designed for therapeutic recommendations. However, recommendations still hinge on whether fractures are associated with disruption of the transverse ligament.
    - The management of >8 mm combined lateral overhang disruption is controversial. Young adults can be reduced in a halo and treated for 3 months in halo immobilization. Elderly adults can be treated in a hard collar with the understanding that displacement may not be improved and significant C1-C2 arthrosis may occur.
  - In the setting of a Dickman type I injury, where the mid-substance of the transverse ligament is disrupted, patients have been shown to have a more successful treatment with C1-C2 fusion.[2]
  - Nonoperative management should consist of a well-fitted rigid cervical collar for a period of 10-12 weeks with routine short-interval radiographs at the initiation of conservative management to ensure no occult instability exists. Nonunion of isolated C1 fractures with nonoperative management has also been described with a rate of 17-27%.[3,4]
    - After 3 months of conservative care of initially "stable" appearing C1 burst fractures, AP instability on flex-ex views is an indication for C1-C2 posterior cervical fusion. It is our experience that this is uncommon.
    - A CT scan can be performed in a delayed fashion for persistent pain to evaluate for nonunion. This can be an indication for surgical management, even in the absence of instability.
  - Surgical management of isolated atlas fractures consists of atlantoaxial fusion.
    - The C2 vertebra is included in the construct as the clinical concern is less about the C1 fracture displacement and more about the potential C1-C2 instability.
  - There have been reported techniques of C1 lateral mass fixation with a transverse connecting rod to reduce the splayed lateral masses and may be considered for bony fragment avulsions of the insertion of the transverse ligament.
    - This, however, is potentially inadequate as the transverse ligament is a primary restraint to anterolisthesis of C1 on C2. Injuries of the midsubstance transverse ligament may not have improved AP stability after C1 osteosynthesis.
    - There have been some limited case series that describe acceptable results with a limited complication profile with both anterior and posterior approach C1 osteosynthesis, but we do not perform this technique.
  - Occipitocervical fusion may be required with severely comminuted lateral masses that do not allow sufficient lateral mass screw fixation.

- Subsidence (commonly asymmetric) of the occipital condyles through the C1 lateral mass toward the C2 superior articulation can additionally be seen, indicating a need for extension to the occiput.
  * This is referred to as a "cock-robin" deformity, with preferential comminution and displacement of one of the lateral masses at C1. Significant coronal deviation may be an indication for C0–C2 fusion. However, patients should understand that correction of the head tilt may come with a significant reduction in cervical range of motion.
- *Relevant technique pearls:*
  - See relevant technique pearls for the C1/2 instability section for C1/2 posterior fixation.
  - Preoperative traction may allow for some residual ligamentotaxis of splayed C1 lateral masses for interval reduction prior to fixation.
  - Occipitocervical fusion may be required in the setting of unfavorable C1 surgical anatomy or inadequate bone stock of lateral masses due to fracture site comminution.

C1/2 INSTABILITY

- *Radiographic evaluation:*
  - Plain radiography:
    * Limited role for plain radiographic evaluation in the acute setting.
    * Lateral view of the upper cervical spine may demonstrate anterior subluxation or dislocation of the C1 ring relative to the odontoid process.
    * Similar to atlas fractures, the atlanto-dens interval can be a clue that there is a degree of instability. The typical threshold is 3.5 mm, though the absence of displacement does not rule out transient dislocation that may have reduced.
    * The posterior atlanto-dens interval (PADI) is representative of the space available for the cord. The distance from the posterior wall of the dens to the anterior aspect of the posterior C1 arch <14 mm is concerning for impending neurologic injury.
    * Rotatory instability is uncommon in an acute traumatic setting and would be difficult to note. There is a small chance that asymmetry would be noted on an open-mouth odontoid view.
    * Open-mouth odontoid views may also highlight an associated atlas ring injury based on lateral displacement of the C1 lateral mass relative to the superior articular surface of C2 (see Atlas Fractures).
    * In asymptomatic patients, flexion/extension views can be considered.
    - We avoid flexion extension views in patients in the ER, patients with neck pain or any neurologic symptoms, or with clear ligamentous injury on MRI scans. This is to avoid catastrophic neurologic injury in patients with unstable injuries in the uncontrolled setting of the ER and trauma bay. Flexion and extension views can be considered in the subacute setting after a comprehensive initial evaluation and imaging with experienced clinicians.
  - CT:
    * Sequential axial cuts through C1 and C2 adjacent to the articulation of the lateral mass of C1 with the superior articular surface of C2 can show relative rotation and/or translation in a fixed dislocation.
    * Comparing parasagittal cuts may allow for demonstration of unilateral relative spondylolisthesis of the C1 lateral mass relative to C2.
    * In the absence of fractures, instability can be a dynamic process and may not be present at the time of the static supine imaging scan.
  - Magnetic resonance:
    * Similar to the discussion regarding atlas fractures, MRI can be a powerful tool to highlight occult ligamentous injuries that may produce clinically significant atlantoaxial instability.
    * The Dickman classification system of transverse ligament injury **(Table 2)** can guide identification of injury morphology, ultimately suggesting terminal treatments.
    * MRI can also identify critical stenosis due to atlantoaxial instability as well as potential mass effect from subacute instability creating a degenerative pannus similar to what is seen in rheumatoid arthritis.
- *Acute management:*
  - As in other acute cervical spine injuries, provisional treatment is always in a hard collar. This will allow adequate stabilization during the acute phase of evaluation and care.
  - Typically, patients arrive with a field collar that should be transitioned to a well-fit, well-padded rigid cervical collar.
  - A firm diagnosis can be obtained with advanced imaging at this point to help determine optimal final treatment.
- *Terminal management:*
  - Definitive management for acute C1–C2 instability is commonly in the form of surgical stabilization.
  - Indications for nonoperative management are only for patients with medical and/or polytrauma comorbidities that preclude safe operative management and require close follow-up with

weekly serial imaging to ensure that progressive displacement has not occurred.
- Halo vest immobilization can be considered for patients with a Dickman Type II transverse ligament bony avulsion.
    * Follow-up flexion and extension X-rays should be performed at 3 months after halo vest removal to ensure stability. Patients should be aware they may still ultimately require surgical management after halo fixation if there is continued instability.
- Intra-substance transverse ligament tears should be treated with rigid fixation of C1–C2. Multiple fixation modalities exist, including a posterior C1–C2 screw-rod construct, transarticular C1–C2 screws, and occipitocervical instrumentation for patients with OC junction injuries or C1 lateral masses that preclude screw placement.
- Operative management should also be strongly considered for patients with fixed displacement. An open reduction from a posterior approach should be supplemented with rigid posterior fixation.
    * Open reduction can be attempted with various techniques such as OR positioning with Mayfield head clamp, exposure and release of the C1–2 joints, and posterior reduction with the C1 screws during rod placement. This can be challenging with longstanding fixed deformity (nonunion of C2 fracture) or patients with inflammatory arthritis (rheumatoid arthritis). In situations with incomplete reduction and continued spinal cord compression at C1–C2 following posterior instrumented fusion, a transoral odontoid resection should be considered.

■ *Relevant technique pearls:*
- See Chapter 2 (C1-2 posterior cervical fusion) for in-depth discussion of C1 and C2 screw placement.
- CT scan may be helpful for defining vertebral artery anatomy relative to instrumentation.
    * Vertebral artery anatomy may prompt the surgical plan to include translaminar or transarticular screws in lieu of a C2 pedicle screw.
        - Most common variant vertebral artery course at C2 is medial and superior, potentially compromising safe placement of C2 pedicle screws.
    * Some studies have shown that intralaminar fixation may be inferior biomechanically to C2 pedicle fixation in the setting of ligamentous disruption. However, as mentioned above, a C2 pedicle trajectory may not be possible depending on patient anatomy. Additionally, laminar and pedicle screws have both been found to provide satisfactory clinical results in our experience.
- An abnormal bony tunnel along the cranial border of the C1 lamina, called the ponticulus posticus or arcuate foramen, can distort intraoperative anatomy. Careful evaluation of preoperative imaging (CT and lateral radiograph) can identify this bony morphology.
    * This highlights the importance of finding and exposing the inferior border of the C1 posterior arch first. We do not find any need to expose the cranial 50% of the C1 posterior arch, as it is unnecessary for screw placement and increases the risk of vascular injury.
- Decompression is rarely required for acute traumatic instability unless patient has pre-existing stenosis.
- Transarticular fixation may require separate caudal stab incisions (commonly around the upper thoracic spine) to allow the surgeon to obtain the proper trajectory intraoperatively from a typical midline approach.
    * Due to the difficulty of exposure, safety issues with vertebral artery anatomy, and difficulty with confirmation of adequate screw purchase in C1 with the transarticular screws, we commonly perform independent C1 and C2 screw placement instead.

ODONTOID FRACTURES

■ *Radiographic evaluation:*
- Plain radiography:
    * An AP, lateral, and open-mouth odontoid view can be helpful in determining alignment for determining operative fixation.
    * Typically, not obtained in isolation, CT recommended in all cases.
    * Open-mouth odontoid view can show subtle extension into the C2 body and C1-C2 articulations, indicating a "Type III" odontoid fracture. This is less sensitive than a CT scan.
- CT:
    * Gold standard for evaluating morphology of odontoid fracture.
        - A true Type I, or odontoid tip, fracture is exceedingly rare. There should be a heightened suspicion for an occipitocervical injury in these patients. An OC injury should be excluded prior to continuing the management and evaluation of these patients (see Occipitocervical Dissociation/Dislocation).
    * Evaluate odontoid tip for a fibrous pseudarthrosis or "os odontoideum" that may mimic a fracture on plain radiographs **(Fig. 6)**.
        - Typically, this is seen as a well-circumscribed bony fragment at the level of the transverse ligament with a mature cortical rim.
        - Fractures in this area are not well-corticated at the junction of the odontoid body and the tip of the odontoid.

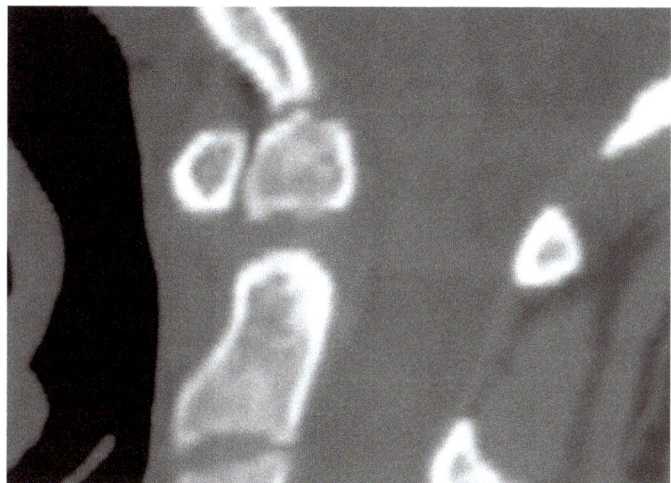
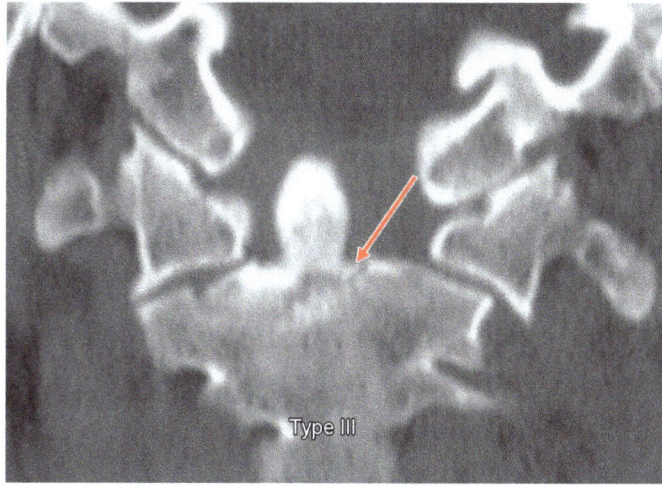

Fig. 6: Os odontoideum. Note the well-corticated junction of the os and the remainder of the odontoid process. This excludes an acute bony injury. However, these patients can still have soft tissue or pseudarthrosis injuries that can be detected by magnetic resonance.

Fig. 7: Type III odontoid fracture. Note the fracture line extending into the vertebral body more anteriorly in the odontoid. Despite a sagittal reformat not showing the fracture in the body, commonly a coronal reformat will show this extension.

- MRI may be useful with T2 and STIR sequencing to determine if there is acute disruption in the setting of an os odontoideum.
* Careful evaluation of the coronal reformats can identify extension into the vertebral body present in a Type III fracture **(Fig. 7)**. This is more difficult to determine on sagittal and axial cuts.
* Fracture obliquity can best be defined on sagittal reformats, which will help determine potential fixation options should the patient require surgical treatment.
* Magnetic resonance:
  - Used primarily to determine whether there is associated soft tissue injury that may correspond to concomitant instability
  - Should be obtained in the setting of neurologic deficit to identify adjacent pathology and spinal cord compression
- *Acute management:*
  * As in other acute cervical spine injuries, provisional treatment is always in a hard collar. This will allow adequate stabilization during the acute phase of evaluation and care.
  * Typically, patients arrive with a field collar that should be transitioned to a well-fit, well-padded rigid cervical collar.
- *Terminal management and relevant technique pearls:*
  * Careful evaluation of the fracture morphology is required when determining the final treatment plan **(Fig. 6)**.
    * Type I fractures, or odontoid tip fractures, can be safely managed with a hard cervical collar for a period of 6–12 weeks depending on the treating physician.
      - We commonly recommend 12 weeks of immobilization.
      - Additionally, we recommend an MRI to rule out occult OC instability with this injury pattern.
    * Type II fractures are the most controversial and will be addressed below.
    * Type III fractures, with extension into the vertebral body, should be treated in a hard collar for a period of 6–12 weeks, similar to the Type I fractures.
      - Similarly, we recommend 12 weeks of immobilization in a cervical collar.
  * Type II fractures are treated across the whole spectrum from hard collars to halo orthoses to some type of internal instrumentation.
    * Selection of collar immobilization can be used for minimally displaced fractures in the elderly patient who is at an increased operative risk. Halo orthoses are strictly contraindicated in these patients.
      - Regular radiographic follow-up should be performed in these patients as displacement is common and may necessitate subacute surgical stabilization.
      - We allow elderly patients without dementia treated in a collar to remove the hard collar for eating to minimize aspiration.
      - Rigid cervical collars are unreliable and potentially dangerous in patients with dementia. Either no immobilization or surgical management should be considered for this population.
    * Multiple studies have debated the improved morbidity and mortality outcomes with surgical management of geriatric odontoid fractures and are controversial.

- However, displaced or distracted fractures, deformity, spinal cord compression, and severe pain are commonly held indications for surgical management.
- Surgical stabilization can also be considered in the subacute setting for continued pain.
- While no data exists to support this, we believe that patients who exhibit subaxial cervical spine stiffness [diffuse idiopathic skeletal hyperostosis (DISH), ankylosing spondylitis (AS), severe degenerative disk disease, etc.] are at higher risk of displacing fractures and having deformity, chronic pain, and increased risk of spinal cord injury. We recommend surgical fixation of geriatric odontoid fractures in these settings, even in minimally displaced injuries. We acknowledge that this is controversial and should be studied further in the literature.
• Younger patients with minimal to nondisplaced fractures can additionally be treated without surgery but should be immobilized with a halo orthosis
    - These patients should be deemed "low risk" for nonunion before deciding on nonsurgical management **(Box 1)**.
    - Regular radiographic follow-up should be performed in these patients as displacement is common and may necessitate subacute surgical stabilization.
• Selection of surgical stabilization depends on the morphology of the fracture:
    - An anterior osteosynthesis screw can be used for fixation of a transverse or reverse obliquity fracture **(Figs. 8A and B)**. This allows for maintained motion of the C1-C2 articulation but does have a higher failure rate when compared to a posterior cervical fusion.
    - C1-C2 transarticular screw fixation or C1-C2 screw/rod constructs are reliable techniques for instrumented stabilization of the C1-C2 joint.
        - C1-C2 transarticular fixation should be avoided in the setting of aberrant vertebral artery anatomy visualized on the initial CT scan.
        - We commonly perform C1-C2 screw/rod constructs for these injuries.
    - Posterior wire-only constructs are largely historical and have been supplanted by modern instrumented fusion techniques.
        - They can be considered in a bail-out setting of suboptimal screw placement but biomechanically are inferior in rotational control.
    - The fracture is commonly somewhat mobile and able to be placed in acceptable position with intraoperative positioning.
        - Anatomic alignment is preferred but not required. Reduction of the C1-C2 joints and ensuring the odontoid fracture fragment is not causing spinal cord compression is the ultimate goal of reduction/positioning for posterior C1-C2 fusion. Overaggressive reduction techniques to achieve anatomic alignment may only increase operative risk without demonstrable clinical benefit.

> **BOX 1:** Risk factors for nonunion with conservative management.
> - Age >50 years
> - Smoker
> - Fracture gap >1 mm
> - Posterior displacement >5 mm
> - Delayed start of treatment >4 days
> - Posterior redisplacement >2 mm
> - Angulation >10°
> - Fracture comminution

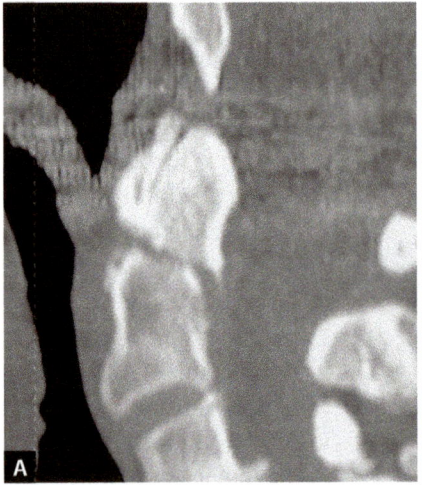 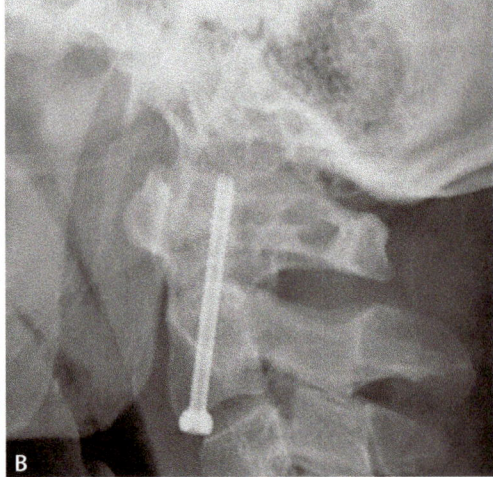

Figs. 8A and B: Transverse odontoid fracture, without (A) and with anterior osteosynthesis screw (B).

- Severe displacement with spinal cord compression may require decompression (C1–C2 laminectomy) along with reduction of the fracture.
  - Positioning with a Mayfield head clamp, reduction with release and mobilization of the C1–C2 joint with a freer or penfield, mobilization within the odontoid fracture with a penfield, and reduction of the C1 screws with rod placement are techniques for fracture reduction. Most commonly, positioning will reduce acute fractures. We recommend reduction with positioning be done before prepping and draping.
  - With an immobile odontoid causing anterior spinal cord compression unable to be reduced or adequately decompressed with the posterior approach, a transoral odontoidectomy may be indicated. Consultation with a surgical otolaryngologist may be helpful for approach.
- *Relevant technique pearls—anterior odontoid osteosynthesis:*
  - The posterior instrumentation techniques at C1–C2 have been discussed in-depth previously.
  - Anterior osteosynthesis of odontoid fractures is an uncommon, but useful technique for odontoid fixation while avoiding fusion of the C1–C2 joint.
    - Optimal patients for this procedure would be a reducible fracture with positioning or light traction, transverse or anterosuperior to posteroinferior fracture line (allows in-line compression with screw placement), and no evidence of osteoporosis or osteopenia. Additionally, kyphotic cervical spines, barrel-chested patients, and/or patients with short necks make the trajectory of the screw challenging and sometimes impossible.
    - The set-up is similar to an anterior cervical discectomy and fusion (ACDF), but a power drill and screw system is required. Options for screw systems include anterior odontoid systems with premade retractors and access instruments or using standard cannulated or solid screw systems (AO small fragment trauma sets or cannulated screw systems).
      - If using one screw technique, a 4.0 mm screw may be used. For two screws, smaller screws may be required.
      - We commonly utilize one screw, as we find more screws increase the surgical complexity of the case without significantly improving outcomes.
  - Positioning is similar to an ACDF, but a flat Jackson frame can be useful to improve visualization with AP fluoroscopy.
    - A radiolucent bite block is placed in the mouth to hold the jaw open, improving AP odontoid visualization.
  - For anterior osteosynthesis, intraoperative navigation or biplanar fluoroscopy is an important tool for safe, accurate placement of the screw.
    - Be aware that navigation may not be accurate if the fracture fragment is mobile. Confirm trajectories and screw placement with frequent C-arm images.
    - If you have access to two C-arms, this can make going between views quicker and more reliable during screw placement.
  - Incisions and approaches should be planned on preoperative sagittal imaging to determine the ideal starting incision location for adequate trajectory of both the drill and the screw.
    - We commonly begin at the C5–C6 level from a right-sided approach, making drilling easier with comfortable position of the dominant hand using the drill.
    - Prolonged retraction has an extremely high (>50%) rate of clinically significant dysphagia, so ensure adequate exposure and dissection before forceful retraction.
    - During dissection, remember to head both down toward the spine and cephalad, to allow for the straight screw trajectory.
    - Starting point is just under the anterior lip of the C2 inferior endplate and this is confirmed with X-ray.
  - To achieve the starting point, a small amount of the superior lip of C3 and C2–C3 disk needs to be removed to ensure the screw begins at the posterior-inferior C2 body.
  - The soft tissue guide is inserted at the start point and confirmed with fluoroscopy, ensuring a midline approach and adequate sagittal trajectory.
    - Take your time finding the start point and trajectory. Once you start drilling, you only have so many chances at drilling the cancellous odontoid before it turns into Swiss cheese and compromises fixation or risks displacing the fracture.
  - *When deciding on screw design, there are two primary options:* Fully threaded and partially threaded.
    - A partially threaded screw allows for compression across the fracture site with a "lag-by-design" function. This works with threads crossing fully to the far fragment and the smooth residual shank permitting unobstructed sliding of the screw in the near fragment. However, this only works if all of the threads are across the fracture site and no residual threads are in the near fragment.
    - A fully threaded screw can still provide compression using a "lag-by-technique" approach with serial drilling. In this case, the far fragment is

drilled to a diameter consistent with the shank of the screw, while the near fragment is overdrilled to the diameter of the screw threads. This acts in a way to allow the threads to piston inside of the near fragment and pull the far fragment in compression with thread bite.
- Cannulated systems:
  - For cannulated systems, utmost care should be taken to control the guidewire. Inadvertent advancement of the guidewire can be catastrophic. For this reason, we do not use guidewire systems.
  - The guidewire is advanced from the starting point to the fracture line. Just as important as where the tip of the screw ends is where the screw passes through the fracture. Passing through the middle of the odontoid at the fracture is important to distributing compressive forces symmetrically throughout the fracture. Erring to a side of the odontoid at the fracture site makes fragment fixation challenging and can displace the fracture with screw placement.
  - The guidewire is advanced into the fracture fragment to the cortical surface.
  - The screw is measured off the guidewire. Make sure the depth gauge is flush with the C2 body, or the screw will be long. We aim to have the threads engaging the far cortex of the odontoid fracture fragment for bicortical fixation. Cancellous-only fixation has a high risk of fracture displacement and hardware failure.
  - The inner sleeve of the drill guide is removed and the outer C2 lip is removed with a reamer through the drill guide to countersink the screw. If tapping is desired, be careful of fracture displacement or guidewire damage/advance. We commonly do not recommend tapping.
  - A short thread partially threaded screw is selected and advanced over the guidewire.
    - Do not push the screw in, let the rotations of the screw pull the screw forward. Forceful screw placement can displace or gap the fracture.
  - Take care to use C-arm liberally throughout this procedure
- Noncannulated systems:
  - The drill guide is advanced to the starting point and trajectory confirmed with fluoroscopy.
  - We utilize a partially threaded 4.0 mm screw, so a 2.5 mm drill is used to drill the path, similar to guidewire placement.
  - A depth gauge is used to determine screw size. Similar to cannulated systems, we aim to use a bicortical screw.
  - The proximal C2 body is countersunk.
  - The screw is carefully placed along the drilled path.
    - This is where minimizing errant passes with the drill is helpful to keep the screw on trajectory.
- A hard collar is used following surgery.
- Gentle active immediate range of motion is encouraged.
- Patients may be discharged from postanesthesia care unit (PACU) to home.

HANGMAN'S FRACTURE

- *Radiographic evaluation:*
  - Plain radiography:
    - Not indicated for first-line evaluation of acute cervical trauma
    - May demonstrate subluxation or instability with flexion-extension studies in sub-acute setting
      - This can be identified by an increase in the apparent space available for the canal between the posterior aspect of the vertebral body and the ventral aspect of the spinolaminar junction.
      - Prevertebral edema can increase sensitivity to occult injury.
  - *Computed tomography:*
    - Fracture morphology most clearly defined with CT **(Figs. 9A to D)**
      - Look for variants with fracture extension into the vertebral body. While commonly C2 traumatic spondylolisthesis is "canal expanding," variants with C2 body fractures exist.

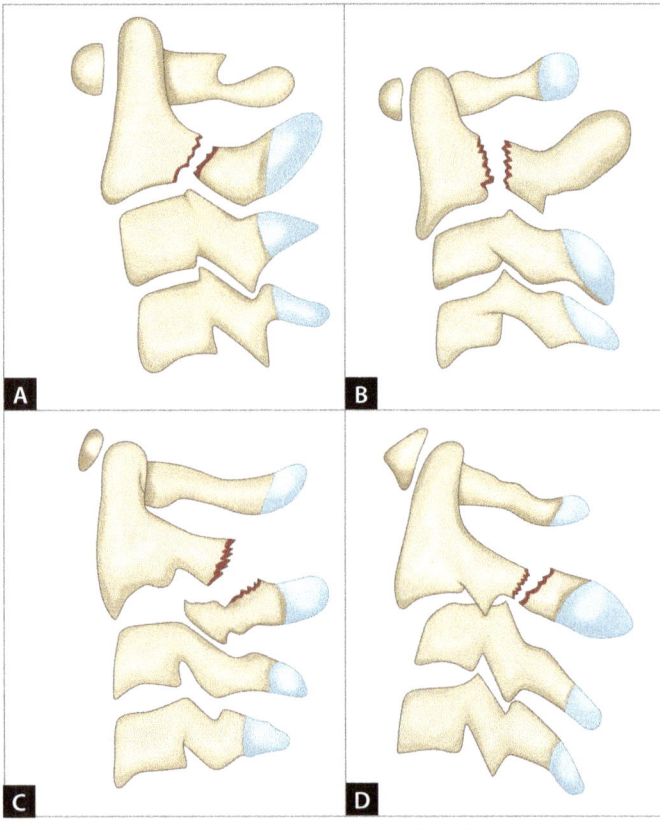

Figs. 9A to D: Fracture morphology as described by Levine and Edwards. Type I (A), Type II (B), Type IIA (C), and Type III (D).

- There is an uncommon fracture variant called the "atypical Hangman's" fracture (Starr-Eismont variant). Typically, fractures exit posterior to the posterior wall of the C2 vertebral body. In some instances, part of the C2 body can be included with the pars fracture. In these rare cases, the fracture is NOT canal expanding and can demonstrate significant compression in the setting of displacement **(Figs. 10A and B)**.
- The relative alignment can be used as a surrogate to understand the energy mechanism that caused the fracture **(Table 3)**.
  - Concomitant injuries can be hypothesized using this classification, however we understand that the cervical spine may have potentially had multiple injurious force vectors at the time of injury and this process may be inaccurate.
- Displacement can be clearly measured to assist with accurate classification.
- Careful evaluation of the transverse foramen may indicate a need for angiography.
- Magnetic resonance:
  - All of the associated soft tissue injuries with the traumatic axial spondylolisthesis can be predicted

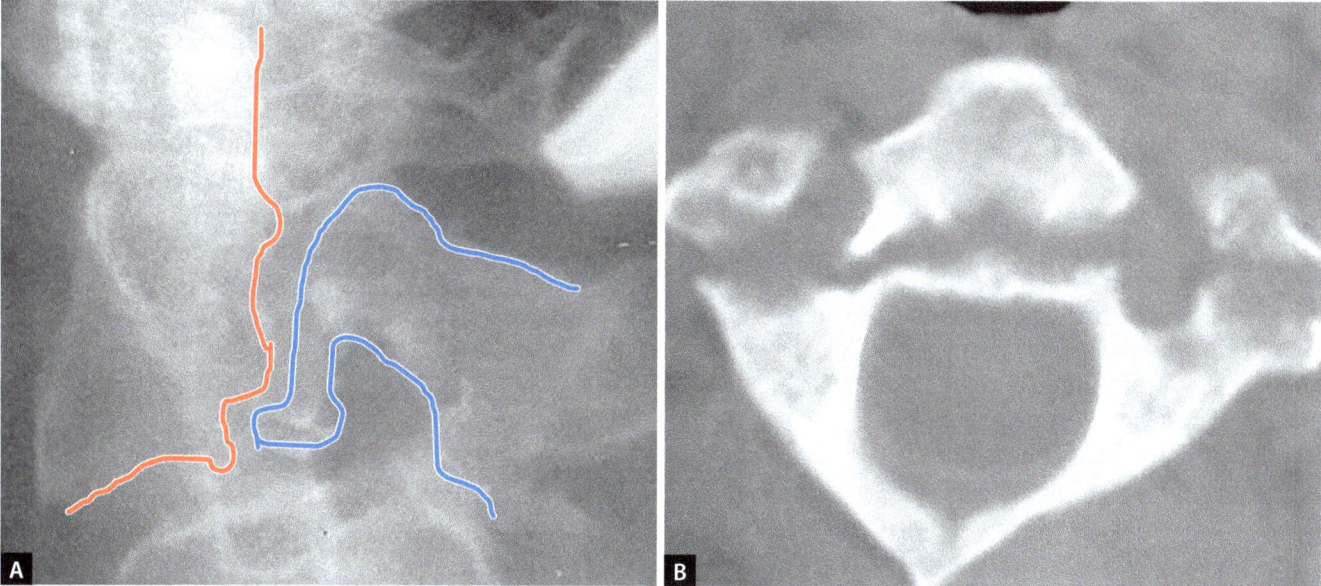

Figs. 10A and B: Atypical Hangman's. (A) The red line outlines the anterior fracture fragment. Note the partial articular involvement of the disk space. The blue line shows the posterior fracture fragment. Most important to note is the section of the posterior wall that is still attached to the posterior elements. This prevents the canal-expanding features classically seen in a traumatic fracture spondylolisthesis of the axis; (B) An axial computed tomography (CT) cut of an "atypical" Hangman's fracture can be seen. This demonstrates a functionally intact spinal canal relative to the fracture line ventral to the posterior wall.

TABLE 3: Levine and Edwards Classification of Hangman's fracture.

Classification	Mechanism of injury	Criteria	Additional considerations
Type I	Hyperextension with axial loading force	Fracture through neural arch with up to 3 mm of displacement and no angulation	• C2/C3 disk remains intact • Stable
Type II	Initial hyperextension followed by axial compression and flexion	Fracture through neural arch with displacement over 3 mm and significant angulation	• C2/C3 disk disrupted • PLL disrupted • ALL may be disrupted • Flavum may be disrupted
Type IIA	Flexion/distraction	Fracture through neural arch without significant displacement, but does have significant angulation	• C2/C3 disk disrupted • PLL disrupted • ALL may be disrupted • Flavum may be disrupted
Type III	Flexion/compression	Fracture through neural arch with bilateral C2/C3 facet dislocations	• C2/C3 disk disrupted • Bilateral facet disruption • PLC disrupted • ALL/PLL disrupted

(ALL: anterior longitudinal ligament; PLC: posterior ligamentous complex; PLL: posterior longitudinal ligament)

based on the degree and angle of displacement of the pedicle-based fracture.
- MRI may be useful for identifying other injuries that can cause neurologic deficits.
  - As this injury is canal-expanding, ongoing compression is uncommon in the absence of C2-C3 facet dislocations or C2 vertebral body fracture variants.

- *Acute management:*
  - As in other acute cervical spine injuries, provisional treatment is always in a hard collar. This will allow adequate stabilization during the acute phase of evaluation and care.
  - Typically, patients arrive with a field collar that should be transitioned to a well-fit, well-padded rigid cervical collar.

- *Terminal management:*
  - Operative or nonoperative management is guided strictly on the stability of the fracture pattern.
  - Using the Levine/Edwards classification, Type I fractures are stable and can be treated with a rigid cervical collar for 6-8 weeks. These are defined by minimal fracture displacement (<3 mm) and no angulation indicating intact ligamentous structures.
    - Patients should have close follow-up to ensure no displacement after initiating nonoperative care.
  - Type II fractures are subdivided into II and IIA categories.
    - Type II is a combination of hyperextension with axial load followed by flexion. This is managed with gentle distraction maintained by a halo orthosis.
    - Type II fractures with >5 mm of displacement should be considered for operative stabilization.
    - Type IIA is unique with its distraction moment and should be treated with axial loading through a halo orthosis. Pure angulation should be seen on imaging studies without displacement of the fracture.
  - Patients with significant disk disruption in higher-grade type II fractures may benefit from a C2-C3 anterior discectomy and fusion. This will allow direct decompression of the cord (if concomitant disk herniation is found) and stabilization of the segment with minimal morbidity.
    - High rate of dysphagia at this level
  - For instrumentation of type II fractures over 5 mm in displacement, an adequate reduction maneuver may allow for direct osteosynthesis screws to be placed in bilateral C2 pedicles.
    - These pedicle screws can be linked with a rod as an additional compressive effect of the posterior ring. By connecting a rod between two bicortical screws and resting the rod along the spinous process, the body can be "pulled back" to the rod.
    - In the absence of successful reduction, a C2-C3 posterior cervical fusion is indicated.
      - Reduction can be difficult to determine with fluoroscopy. Consider intraoperative CT imaging if available.
  - Type III fractures demonstrate maintained bilateral C2-C3 facet dislocations and must undergo open reduction and internal fixation.
    - Repair of the C2 pedicle alone is inadequate for stabilization given the ligamentous disruption.
    - C1 lateral mass coupled with C3 lateral mass screws (and C2 pedicle screws if possible, otherwise, these can be avoided) may be optimal depending on degree of bony comminution of C2 pedicle/body interface to avoid iatrogenically shortened pedicles and resulting canal stenosis.

- *Relevant technique pearls:*
  - Reduction techniques are dependent on the deforming mechanism at the time of injury:
    - *Type II*: Traction alone may be adequate to allow for ligamentotaxis for reduction, but a slight extension moment may be added.
    - *Type IIA*: Gentle extension combined with axial load
    - *Type III*: Facet dislocation should be directly reduced via posterior approach with subsequent instrumented fusion.

REFERENCES

1. Passias PG, Poorman GW, Segreto FA, Jalai CM, Horn SR, Bortz CA, et al. Traumatic fractures of the cervical spine: Analysis of changes in incidence, cause, concurrent injuries, and complications among 488,262 patients from 2005 to 2013. World Neurosurg. 2018;110:e427-37.
2. Dickman CA, Greene KA, Sonntag VK. Injuries involving the transverse atlantal ligament: classification and treatment guidelines based upon experience with 39 injuries. Neurosurgery. 1996;38(1):44-50.
3. Kim MK, Shin JJ. Comparison of radiological and clinical outcomes after surgical reduction with fixation or halo-vest immobilization for treating unstable atlas fractures. Acta Neurochir (Wien). 2019;161(4):685-93.
4. Segal LS, Grimm JO, Stauffer ES. Non-union of fractures of the atlas. J Bone Joint Surg Am. 1987;69(9):1423-34.

CHAPTER 10

Technical Pearls in the Management of Subaxial Cervical Trauma

Edward M DelSole, Michael Yayac, Alexander R Vaccaro

INTRODUCTION

- Surgical management of subaxial cervical trauma focuses on addressing traumatic bony or ligamentous instability as well as spinal canal decompression caused by dislocations, subluxations, disk herniations, and/or fracture fragments causing spinal cord compression and neurologic deficit.
- A distinguishing feature of the surgical management of cervical spine trauma as compared to typical degenerative spine cases is that the surgeon may need to obtain an anatomic reduction of subluxations or dislocations to decompress the spinal cord. Additional challenges that may be present when operating on trauma include extensive bony and soft tissue disruption, which can result in a significant degree of spinal instability, excessive blood loss, and distortion of normal anatomy.
- The AOSpine Subaxial Cervical Spine Classification System provides a common language for these injuries, helping to assess spinal stability after an injury and determine surgical indications. The classification is based upon fracture morphology, facet injury, neurologic status, and case-specific modifiers **(Fig. 1)**.
- AO type A injuries rarely necessitate surgical treatment unless there is disruption of the posterior elements including the posterior capsuloligamentous complex. The exception to this injury type includes A3 or A4 injuries at the cervicothoracic (C-T) junction. Although these injuries may appear innocuous on computed tomography (CT) scan, they may have significant posterior soft tissue disruption and the posterior ligamentous complex should be thoroughly scrutinized on magnetic resonance imaging (MRI).
  - These injuries at the C-T junction, with three column bony and/or soft tissue injury, may benefit from anterior/posterior (360°) fixation due to the increased stresses seen at the cervicothoracic junction.
- AO type B injuries refer to those which have a disrupted posterior and/or anterior tension band while the type C injuries are more devastating as they demonstrate translational instability. These injuries commonly necessitate surgical stabilization due to the instability evidenced by extensive bone and/or soft tissue injury seen on CT and MRI.
- Surgical indications include neurologic injuries, unstable fractures or dislocations, injuries with displacement, facet fractures involving >50% of the articular process. The subaxial injury classification system (SLICS) can be used as an adjunct to the AOSpine classification to score the severity of injuries and help guide surgical indications.
- In our practice, the Halo vest is not the preferred management for any subaxial injury pattern because it does not adequately stabilize the subaxial spine.
- Spinal cord injury secondary to cervical spine injury may necessitate urgent surgical decompression.
  - Our preference is to perform decompression and stabilization for all spinal cord injuries, including incomplete and complete injuries, as soon as the patient can safely undergo surgery, preferably within 24 hours of injury.

ANTERIOR SURGERY VERSUS POSTERIOR SURGERY

- The decision to perform surgical decompression and stabilization from an anterior or posterior approach is controversial. In general, decision-making is influenced by a comprehensive evaluation of patient and surgical factors, including surgeon experience, location of bony and/or soft tissue injury, location within the spine (upper subaxial versus CT junction), presence of associated vascular or visceral neck injuries, and presence of ventral compressive disk herniations or fracture fragments.

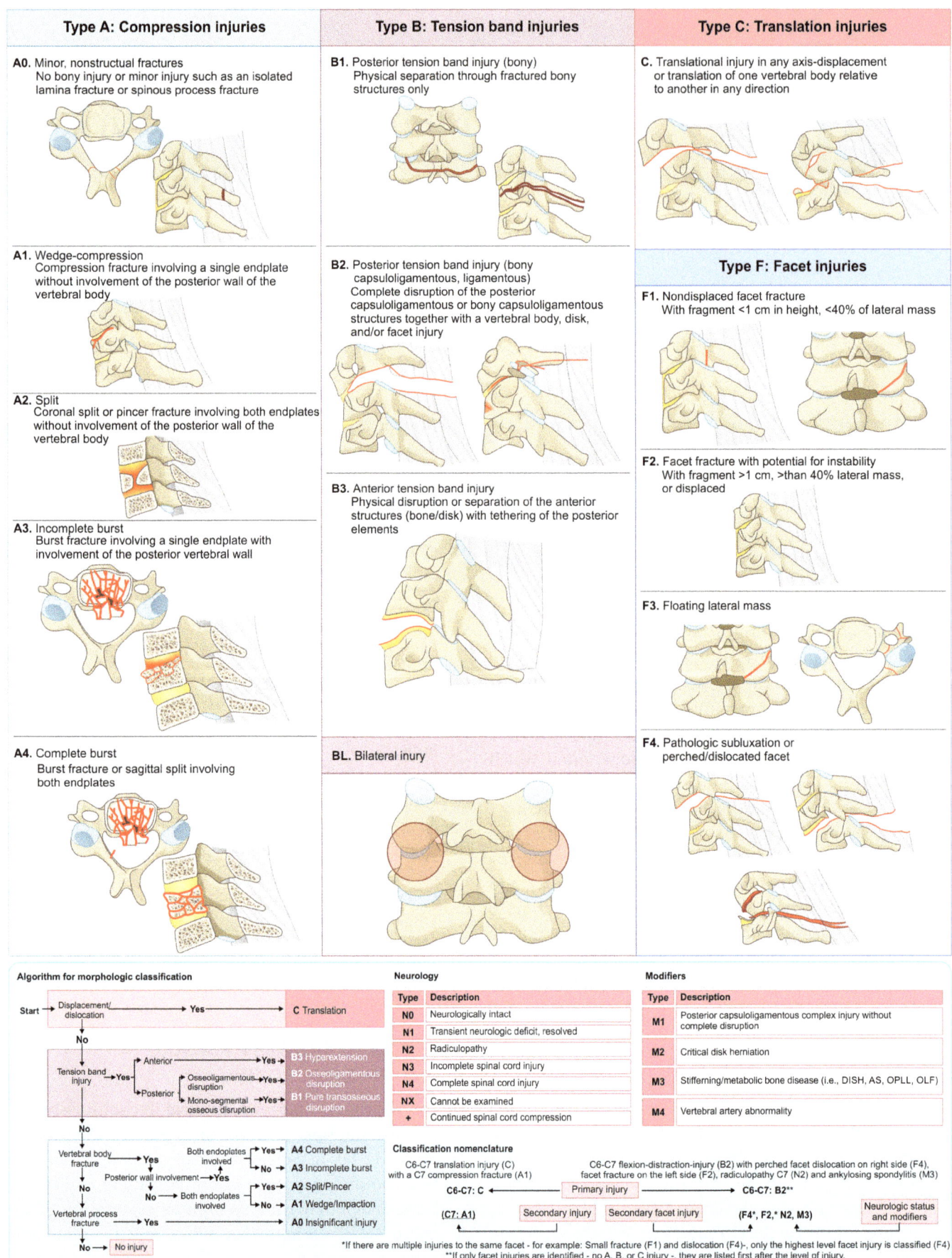

Fig. 1: The AOSpine Subaxial Cervical Spine Classification System.
Source: Vaccaro AR, Koerner JD, Radcliff KE, Oner FC, Reinhold M, Schnake KJ, et al. AOSpine subaxial cervical spine injury classification system. Eur Spine J. 2016;25(7):2173-84.

- B1 and B2 injuries occur through a flexion-distraction type mechanism with a violation of the posterior tension band and may be suitable for posterior surgery alone. These injuries may however demonstrate a dislocation injury that spontaneously reduced. Therefore, if B1 and B2 injuries are combined with a compressive injury to the vertebral body or compressive disk herniation, anterior or circumferential stabilization may be required.
- B3 injuries, which occur through extension-distraction mechanisms, may be suitable for anterior surgery alone.
  - However, the surgeon should take extreme care to evaluate for ankylosing spine conditions, such as diffuse idiopathic skeletal hyperostosis (DISH) or ankylosing spondylitis (AS), which would indicate an unstable injury and require a long posterior construct and anterior grafting of the residual injury gap.
- Displaced type C type injuries, in which the anterior and posterior stabilizing structures are disrupted, may warrant 360° stabilization **(Figs. 2A to D)**. The presence of large compressive anterior disk herniations and degree of translation (facet perch/subluxation, unilateral dislocation, bilateral dislocation) commonly dictates approach.
  - A simplified approach to these injuries is to first identify any compressive disk herniation. If present, the anterior approach would be performed first and a subsequent posterior approach can be performed for reduction of residual translation or for enhanced stability for bilateral dislocations. Therefore, a posterior-only approach would be appropriate in the setting of minimal or absent anterior disk herniations.
- Due to the unique and increased mechanical stress at the C-T junction, it is generally recommended that injuries at this location undergo 360° stabilization.

PATIENT POSITIONING AND PRESURGICAL PLANNING

- Intraoperative neurophysiologic monitoring (IONM) should be used for any unstable cervical injury.
- Motor-evoked potentials are checked prior to and after endotracheal intubation. Alternatively, awake fiberoptic intubation can be performed followed by a motor examination before anesthetic induction to ensure intact postintubation neurologic function.
- Motor-evoked potentials are also performed prior to and after the patient is positioned in order to obtain clear prepositioning and presurgical baselines and establish a safe patient position for surgery.
- *Anesthesia*: As compared to awake fiberoptic intubation, a rapid-sequence intubation will eliminate ability for motor-testing by IONM until paralytic agent is metabolized or medically reversed.
- *Anterior surgery*:
  - Supine on a standard orthopedic table. A flat Jackson table can also be used to facilitate intraoperative fluoroscopy.
  - Interscapular bump or inflatable blood pressure bag to facilitate neck extension
  - Gardner-Wells tongs and a Mayfield Horseshoe may be useful as a reduction tool in type C injuries (unilateral or bilateral jumped facets). Gardner-Wells tongs allow traction to be applied, while the Horseshoe controls the spatial location/position of the head, which influences cervical spine alignment as well as affects the vector of traction.
    - Make sure to evaluate the occipital cervical junction both prior to and following application of traction to ensure there is no occult occipital-cervical injury.

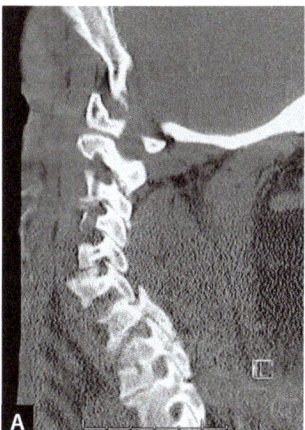 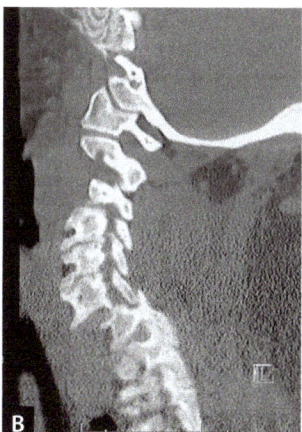 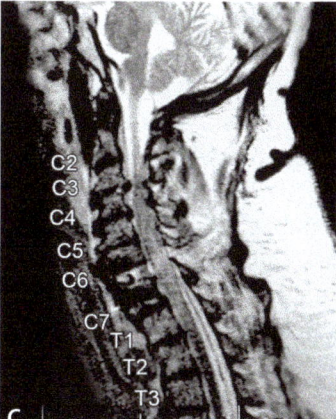 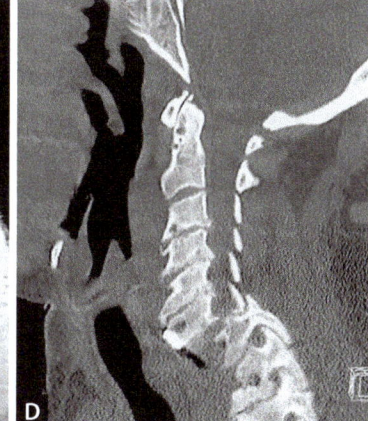

Figs. 2A to D: The imaging is of a 48-year-old female ASIA A at the C6 level secondary to a displaced AO type C injury (A and B) treated at an outside hospital with closed reduction and anterior cervical discectomy and fusion (ACDF); (C) The patient was transferred from an outside hospital on postoperative day 4 with new deltoid weakness. Computed tomography scan revealed fixation failure and subsequent displacement; (D) The patient was subsequently treated with revision ACDF with supplemental posterior cervical instrumented fusion to obtain maximal stability in this highly unstable injury pattern.

- Shoulders can be depressed with tape to facilitate imaging.
- X-ray or fluoroscopy images should be obtained after final positioning to ensure the fracture and alignment characteristics have not changed substantially.
  - Obese patients and low subaxial cervical spine injuries may not be well-visualized with lateral intraoperative X-rays and the surgeon should anticipate this preoperatively. If you are relying on fluoroscopic confirmation of a reduction intraoperatively, you may require the use of O-arm or plan for a second, posterior approach for direct visualization and final reduction/stabilization of the injury.

■ *Posterior surgery:*
- Prone on a standard orthopedic table with chest rolls and a Mayfield attachment
- Mayfield vice head holder
- If instrumentation is to be carried to the occiput, C1, or C2, then the table can be rotated around its base 180° with the head opposite to the anesthesia machine in order to facilitate fluoroscopic guidance.
- Shoulders depressed to facilitate radiography
- An alternative position would be prone on an open Jackson frame with the head in a Mayfield vice controlled by a "C-flex" apparatus (Allen Medical Systems, Acton, MA). Positioning in this fashion is advantageous for patients of high body mass index. A potential disadvantage of this is the possibility of "hanging" the patient by the Mayfield vice once the table is put into reverse Trendelenburg position. This may be dangerous for patients with severe myelopathy or traumatic cervical spine injuries.

TECHNICAL PEARLS FOR SPINE EXPOSURE AFTER SUBAXIAL TRAUMA

- The spine is exposed using the standard techniques for either anterior or posterior surgery.
- The midline can be difficult to identify due to deformity and displacement of fractured bone. The surgeon should use all available noninjured anatomic landmarks to ensure a safe dissection to the spine. Especially for the posterior approach, we recommend early identification of the traumatic pathology (loose spinous processes, soft tissue disruption, etc.) and exposure of normal levels to be included in the instrumentation above and below the injury to orient your approach. Beginning with exposure of the injured levels can be dangerous due to distorted anatomy.
- Care should be taken when using a bovie during a posterior approach in the setting of fractured and displaced laminae as the spinal cord may be exposed in unexpected locations. Preoperative imaging will help determine at-risk areas of the exposure and strict subperiosteal dissection is required to reduce the risk of iatrogenic spinal cord injury.
- Traumatic injuries to the spine are associated with significant bleeding from disrupted soft tissue and osseous structures. Blood should be immediately available in the operating room. The surgeon should also consider the use of tranexamic acid as well as Cell Saver (Haemonetics Corp., Braintree, MA) or a similar erythrocyte salvage technology.
- Hemostatic technologies should be readily available including bovie electrocautery, bipolar electrocautery, Aquamantys (Medtronic, Minneapolis, MN), Floseal (Baxter International, Deerfield, IL), or Fibrillar (Ethicon Inc., Somerville, NJ) to name a few.
- In general, unstable spine fractures can result in traumatic durotomy. In these cases, cerebrospinal fluid (CSF) may be encountered. Extravasation from the dural injury can be controlled using cottonoids with plan for an attempted primary dural repair with 6-0 goretex or potentially a dural patch for large, irreparable defects. Dural repair can be augmented with a resorbable collagen matrix such as DuraGen (Integra Life Sciences, Plainsboro, NJ) or liquid dural sealants such as DuraSeal (Integra Life Sciences, Plainsboro, NJ).
- If CSF is encountered, the fascia is closed using #1 Vicryl suture in figure-of-8 fashion, followed by running nonabsorbable suture to prevent premature wound breakdown should the tensile strength of Vicryl deteriorate in the CSF environment.
- Postoperative management of traumatic durotomy involves retention of subfascial drains for 72 hours. If we are confident with the dural repair, we do not impose head-of-bed (HOB) restrictions. If necessary, we will keep the HOB <30° for 24 hours followed by a trial of physical therapy. If symptoms persist, a lumbar drain can be inserted.

TECHNICAL PEARLS FOR POSTERIOR SUBAXIAL INSTRUMENTATION

- In brief for posterior surgery, our order of operations is typically the exposure of the relevant levels, fracture reduction, drill/tap for instrumentation, perform any necessary decompression, place instrumentation, confirm alignment fluoroscopically, place rods, and lastly decorticate and bone graft in the gutters lateral to the hardware.
- Posterior osseous fixation can be achieved in all levels except for those in which the lateral mass is "floating" (ipsilateral lamina and pedicle fractures, AO subtype F3). In this scenario, fixation must span the injured level if a posterior approach is chosen. For example, for a C5–C6 dislocation with a floating right-sided C5 lateral mass,

instrumentation can be placed in C4 and C6 as well as on the left side of C5.
- Our preference is for lateral mass screw fixation in the C3–C6 levels and for pedicle screw fixation in the C7 and T1 level. Make sure the pedicles are of sufficient size for screw fixation on preoperative CT prior to attempting screw placement. For experienced surgeons, a freehand technique can be used.
  - A safe technique for placement of C7 pedicle screws utilizes a burr to create a laminoforaminotomy at the C6–C7 level to allow for palpation of the C7 pedicle with a nerve hook to safely determine screw start point and trajectory. The pedicle is then cannulated using a 1.7 mm high-speed burr, stopping intermittently to palpate the bony corridor with the burr. Burr to a depth of 18–20 mm is safe. The pedicle trajectory is then tapped with a 3.5 mm tap, palpated with a ball-tipped probe, and a 4.0 mm screw may be inserted. The typical length of this screw is 18–20 mm. The same procedure can be performed for the T1 pedicle, with a laminoforaminotomy performed at C7–T1 as a guide.

SURGICAL MANAGEMENT OF SUBAXIAL BURST FRACTURES (AO TYPE A3 OR A4 INJURIES)

- The goals of surgery on A3 or A4 injuries include direct spinal cord decompression, reconstruction of the anterior column, and osseous fusion.
- Scrutinize the preoperative MRI and CT at the levels of the corpectomy, looking for vertebral artery aberrancy or injury as well as location of fracture fragments. Also look for fracture fragments that involve the walls and potentially the vertebral artery. If these are inadvertently removed carelessly, you may create a vertebral artery injury.
- Additionally, plan your graft height preoperatively, using intact levels caudad and cephalad to predict the intended graft size. This can help prevent undersizing, resulting in potential kyphotic deformity, or "overstuffing" the corpectomy, as the posterior structures may be disrupted and may overdistract during Caspar distraction and/or Gardner-Wells tong traction.
- Corpectomy is performed with the patient supine as previously described with Gardner-Wells tongs and 5–10 lb of weight. This allows the application of a light but consistent distractive/stabilizing force to the spine. Caspar pins can be placed in cephalad and caudad vertebra for additional distraction.
- Ventral spinal cord decompression commonly involves corpectomy of the affected level with discectomy above and below (e.g., C5 corpectomy includes C4–C5 and C5–C6 discectomy). Interbody grafts must then span from C4 to C6.
- We recommend beginning with discectomy above and below the corpectomy segment prior to the corpectomy. This allows identification of the uncovertebral joint to determine the midline for safe trough creation of the corpectomy. Additionally, the posterior longitudinal ligament (PLL) is exposed at the disk levels to provide orientation of depth of the corpectomy. Identifying these landmarks prior to corpectomy allows for safe performance of the corpectomy trough.
- Our corpectomy trough is typically 16 mm in width, and never extends laterally past the uncovertebral joint. Cut a 16 mm length of plastic ruler and use it intraoperatively to guide your corpectomy. Common mistakes are "coning in," meaning the width is appropriate superficially, but narrows as the trough is deepened, as well as erring the direction of the trough away from the surgical approach side. Make sure the trough maintains width as you deepen the trough and that it stays midline as determined by the exposed uncovertebral joints. The corpectomy is deepened using a combination of rongeur, high-speed burr, and Kerrison punch. Be careful using rongeurs initially in the traumatic setting, as unlike degenerative corpectomies, you may inadvertently compress the spinal cord with the downward force of the rongeur.
- In the cephalad and caudad endplate of the anticipated corpectomy site, the burr can be used to sculpt an elevated lip in the posterior cortex of each vertebral body to help serve as a barrier to posterior migration of the graft.
- The surgeon should expect high blood loss during corpectomy, especially in the setting of fracture. You should be actively communication with your anesthesia team during this part of the case and the operating room should be equipped with (or have readily available) cell saver and topical hemostatic agents. Hemostasis is critical at the conclusion of the corpectomy trough creation, as you will not have access to the epidural space or walls of the corpectomy after the graft is placed.
- Allograft (both iliac crest and fibula, depending on size requirements) is an acceptable option for interbody graft choice. We recommend the graft be slightly taller anteriorly instead of a purely rectangular shape to prevent posterior migration with early graft settling. We use a reciprocating saw for the initial cut and a burr for final modifications.
- Interbody grafting should be carefully planned such that a graft of appropriate height and depth is used. In unstable injuries, a graft of excessive height can cause inadvertent distraction of unstable facet joints or cause a malreduction. Use preoperative imaging to template roughly what the desired graft height will be. Additionally, we recommend using intraoperative X-ray

to ensure that the graft is placed appropriately. Make sure to understand the depth of the graft prior to insertion, as excessively posterior placement of the graft can risk injury to the spinal cord.
- The graft should be sized that it only requires gentle impaction at most into the defect. Avoid aggressive impaction of the graft in traumatic injuries, as the graft is likely too large and needs further modification. Be patient with graft sizing, as several modifications of graft sizing are commonly required.
- Our preference is to use a plate to stabilize the graft in the setting of these unstable injuries.
- For these unstable injuries, we nearly always perform posterior stabilization and fusion in conjunction with the corpectomy.

SURGICAL MANAGEMENT OF SUBAXIAL FLEXION-COMPRESSION INJURIES (AO TYPE B1 AND B2 FRACTURES)

- AO type B1 and B2 injuries are disruptions of the posterior tension band. B1 injuries are defined as a tension band injury only through a bony structure. B2 injuries are defined as complete disruption of the posterior capsuloligamentous complex along with the vertebral body, disk, and/or facet. B2 injuries are destabilizing to a motion segment and may require surgical reduction and fixation.
- These injuries are best treated with reduction of any residual displacement or angulation, posterior instrumentation, and posterior fusion. This approach reconstructs the disrupted posterior tension band.
- Due to the injury mechanism, type B injuries are commonly associated with compression or burst fractures of the vertebral body (AO type A). Severe burst fractures are a contraindication to an isolated posterior approach due to the need to reconstruct anterior column and ventrally decompress the spinal cord through a corpectomy of the fractured body.
- B1 and B2 fractures at the C-T junction often require anterior column support due to the high flexion moment across this transitional zone.
- We recommend avoidance of the standard chin-tuck for exposure due to the highly unstable nature of the injuries and instead place the patient prone in a neutral position. To assist with holding the head and neck stable during the flip, the cervical collar can remain on the patient after the flip until the Mayfield clamp is secured to the bed. As a result, the length of exposure and skin incision may need to be increased as compared to a degenerative posterior cervical spine approach.
- The fracture reduction is typically performed by positioning the patient prone and applying a gentle extension moment only if necessary to the cervical spine through a Mayfield vice. The B-type injuries may not have translation like C-type, but may demonstrate a similar amount of instability despite the initial appearance on MRI and CT. Care should be taken not to hyperextend the spine, which could cause further destabilization or neurologic injury. The reduction should be confirmed with fluoroscopy prior to instrumentation and fusion.
- To facilitate closure of the wound, we recommend the skull be positioned in a chin tuck position. This can be facilitated through the Mayfield head positioner.

SURGICAL MANAGEMENT OF SUBAXIAL SUBLUXATIONS AND DISLOCATIONS (AO TYPE C FRACTURES) (FIGS. 2A TO D)

- These unstable injuries present with varying degrees of displacement. The injury involves disruption of the posterior capsuloligamentous complex, the intervertebral disk, and often the anterior longitudinal ligament (ALL).
- AO type C fractures (including F subtypes 2-4, or facet fracture/dislocations) have historically undergone closed reduction with traction in the emergency room (ER). These are the traditional "jumped facet" type injuries with anterior translation. This procedure was historically advocated for an awake, neurologically intact patient, provided that a reliable physical examination could be conducted during the procedure, and that the procedure could be halted should neurologic deterioration be observed.
- Our current practice has evolved to now foregoing closed reduction of these injuries in the ER. Instead, we proceed directly to MRI with subsequent surgical intervention. The rationale is that these patients will ultimately need to go to the operating room for stabilization, and we prefer to perform the reduction in the controlled environment of the operating room. If closed reduction is attempted but fails, then open reduction can be performed right away.
- For patients physiologically suitable for surgery, closed or open reduction in the operating room under anesthesia with neurophysiologic monitoring is a convenient alternative for both the patient and the surgeon.
- Open reduction techniques may vary from direct anatomic reduction of bone, such as facet fractures, versus indirect reduction of fractures such as type A3 or A4, which can occur with specific positioning, distraction, and fixation strategies.
- For facet dislocations without an associated disk herniation, our preference is to approach the injury from posterior. The patient is positioned prone on a standard orthopedic table with the head positioned in a Mayfield vice.
- Frequently the cranial facet is locked ventral to the caudal facet, effectively preventing a reduction. Depending on the degree of soft tissue injury, a variety of reduction techniques can be utilized. For bilateral

facet dislocations, commonly there is significant soft tissue injury and occasionally the facets can be relocated with towel clips placed on the cephalad and caudad level of injury spinous processes, with a gentle flexion and distraction force initially to disengage the facets followed by a gentle posterior translation of the cephalad segment to reduce the facets. If trauma has occurred to the pedicle, lamina, or spinous process of one of the levels in question, reduction forces should not be directly applied at that level. Frequently, the spine reduces quickly after the facets are unlocked. If this does not work, the facets can be unlocked using a high-speed burr to incrementally remove the cranial aspect of the caudal facet superior articular process until the inferior articular process is visualized and released. The reduction can then be fine-tuned with the towel clip technique as needed described above. The surgeon should be mindful of how much superior articular facet is removed since this may affect the residual lateral mass available for lateral mass screw fixation at that level. Unilateral facet dislocations do not commonly have the significant soft tissue injury seen with bilateral dislocations and simple reduction with towel clips is commonly unsuccessful.

- Additionally, a two-person technique is useful for difficult reductions. One person applies a dorsally directed force to the towel clip attempting to reduce the spine, while applying counterforce directed ventrally at the levels caudal. A second person unscrubs, unlocks the Mayfield vice, and applies an extension moment to the cervical spine. This can be done several times, each attempt achieving a higher degree of reduction.
- Once anatomic reduction is achieved, posterior fixation is performed, typically with lateral mass screws. The surgeon should be aware that you can lose reduction between the reduction maneuver and final instrumentation. Use intraoperative X-ray to confirm the reduction after final posterior instrumentation is secured.
- In the presence of an associated large disk herniation, the injury is approached anteriorly first in order to remove the disk and prevent neurologic injury during a posteriorly based reduction.
- In the setting of traumatic disk herniation, the PLL should be resected in its entirety in order to confirm the ventral dura is adequately decompressed.
- Following discectomy, reduction may be achieved from the anterior approach if there is significant soft tissue injury posteriorly. Reduction from the anterior approach is similar to the closed reduction technique. Incremental amounts of traction using a slight flexion vector can be applied with the Gardner-Wells tongs with motors run after increases in weight along with continuous lateral X-ray images to evaluate for degree of facet distraction. Additionally, Caspar distraction and intervertebral spreaders can be used to apply distraction as well. If the facets are able to be perched, an extension moment can be created by inflating a pressure bag beneath the shoulders, gentle posterior pressure on the cephalad vertebra, and/or changing the traction vector on the Gardner-Wells tongs. Unilateral facet dislocations may require a rotational maneuver of the Gardner-Wells tongs, similar to closed techniques, to create initially a gentle anterior force (head rotation opposite of the facet dislocation) to unlock the perched facet, followed by a posterior force (head rotation toward the facet dislocation) to reduce the inferior articular facet after it has cleared the superior articular facet.
- If reduction is able to be achieved, interbody grafting and anterior plating with screws in cephalad and caudad vertebral bodies can be performed. A supplemental posterior approach can then be performed per surgeon preference.
- In the event that the reduction cannot be adequately achieved from the anterior surgery, the surgeon has two options. The wound may be closed following discectomy, the posterior procedure is performed, and a final anterior surgery is performed for placement of graft and instrumentation. Alternatively, the surgeon can place an undersized graft with a plate secured to the cephalad segment only with screws. Then the posterior approach is performed with final reduction and instrumentation. This approach obviates the third anterior approach, but may limit the success of the posterior reduction maneuvers. Our approach is to perform the discectomy without graft placement and perform a third anterior approach following posterior reduction for final anterior graft placement.

SPECIAL CONSIDERATIONS

- Diseases that stiffen the spinal motion segments, namely AS and DISH, merit special consideration. Fractures in the setting of a stiffened spine increases the mechanical force at the fractured segment due to the presence of an atypically long, rigid lever arm above and below the fracture level. These patients typically suffer distraction-extension type injury mechanisms that may involve all both anterior and posterior spinal columns (AO type B). Within the AOSpine classification system, these diseases are appended the modifier M **(Figs. 3A to D)**. For these injuries, we commonly perform an extensive posterior instrumented fusion of three or more levels above and below the level of injury with an anterior approach used subsequently for graft placement in any residual gap left at the site of injury.
- As previously mentioned, the cervicothoracic junction requires special consideration. Injuries in this region

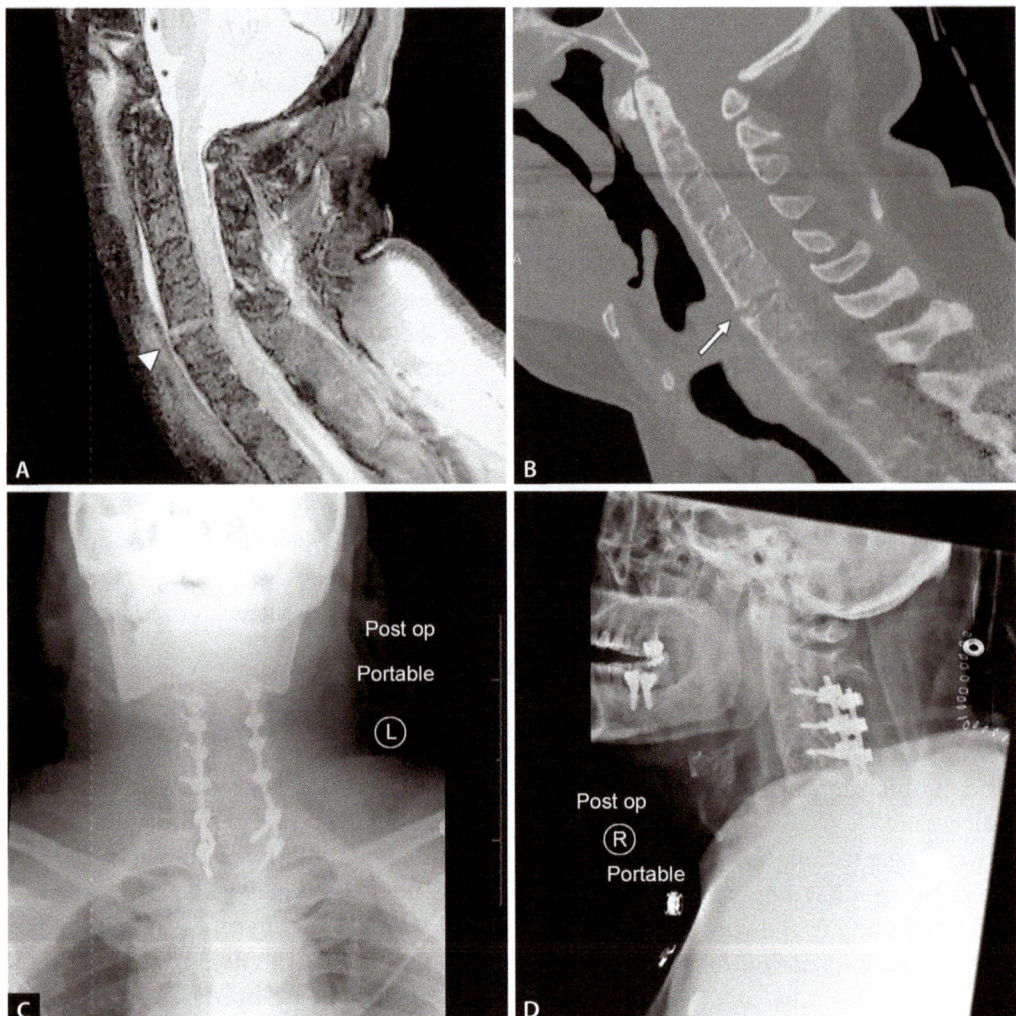

Figs. 3A to D: A 49-year-old male with ankylosing spondylitis sustained an extension-distraction type injury (AO type B3-M) as a result of a motor vehicle accident. (A) The T2-weighted sagittal magnetic resonance imaging (MRI) with prevertebral swelling and edema through the C5–6 disk space (arrowhead); (B) The sagittal computed tomography (CT) scan demonstrating disruption of the ossified anterior longitudinal ligament suggestive of an extension injury (arrow). Due to the highly unstable nature of this injury, the patient underwent posterior stabilization; (C and D).

often require surgical stabilization, and often with a combined anterior/posterior approach.

POSTOPERATIVE CARE

- Fractures requiring surgical stabilization are treated in a hard cervical collar for 6 weeks, even with internal fixation.
- Patients are seen in the office at 2 weeks postoperatively for a wound check and radiographs. They are seen subsequently at the 6-week, 12-week, 3-month, 6-month, and 12-month follow-ups in the office with X-rays.
- Serial radiographs will not necessarily confirm fusion, but can identify hardware complications or alignment changes that may be secondary to nonunion.

ACKNOWLEDGMENTS

The authors would like to acknowledge the AO Foundation for the permission to reprint the subaxial classification system artwork. AOSpine is a clinical division of the AO Foundation—an independent medically guided nonprofit organization. The AOSpine Knowledge Forums are pathology focused working groups acting on behalf of AOSpine in their domain of scientific expertise. Each forum consists of a steering committee of up to 10 international spine experts who meet on a regular basis to discuss research, assess the best evidence for current practices, and formulate clinical trials to advance spine care worldwide. Study support is provided directly through AOSpine's Research department and AO's Clinical Investigation and Documentation unit.

SECTION 2

Thoracolumbar

- **Thoracic Transpedicular Decompression and Costotransversectomy**
  Preetpaul S Bagi, Glenn S Russo, Shirvinda A Wijesekera

- **Anterior Thoracic Discectomy/Corpectomy/Anterior Instrumentation**
  Yoji Ogura, John R Dimar, Leah Y Carreon

- **Technical Pearls in the Management of Spinal Oncology**
  Mostafa El Dafrawy, Jacob Buchowski

- **Percutaneous Thoracolumbar Pedicle Screw Fixation**
  Barrett S Boody, Glenn S Russo, Greg Anderson

- **Thoracolumbar Osteotomies: Posterior Column, Pedicle Subtraction, and Vertebral Column Resection**
  Daniel R Rubio, Sean M Rider, Munish C Gupta

- **Thoracolumbar Instrumentation**
  Ron Lehman

- **Sacral and Pelvic Instrumentation**
  Barrett S Boody, Glenn S Russo, Joseph D Smucker

- **Transforaminal Lumbar Interbody Fusion**
  Barrett S Boody, Glenn S Russo, Jeffrey Rihn

- **Technical Pearls in the Management of Adult Scoliosis**
  Lawrence Lenke, James D Lin

- **Anterior Lumbar Interbody Fusion Technique**
  Barrett S Boody, Glenn S Russo, Mark Kurd

- **Technical Pearls in the Surgical Management of Thoracic and Lumbar Trauma**
  Ashley R Strickland, Rohan Gopinath, Samuel Q Li, Jael E Camacho, M Farooq Usmani, Steven C Ludwig

- **Open Microdiscectomy and Laminectomy**
  Tyler Kreitz, Howard An

CHAPTER 11

Thoracic Transpedicular Decompression and Costotransversectomy

Preetpaul S Bagi, Glenn S Russo, Shirvinda A Wijesekera

■ INTRODUCTION

- The thoracic transpedicular approach and costotransversectomy both provide access to the lateral spinal canal, neural foramina, intervertebral disks, and posterolateral vertebral body. Costotransversectomy allows for additional access to the costovertebral joint and extended access to the anterior aspect of the thoracic vertebral body. These approaches also allow for single-stage surgery with the ability to decompress and stabilize the anterior and posterior spine simultaneously.
- Indications include lateral or paracentral thoracic disk herniations, canal decompression for fractures, bony or epidural tumor resection, discitis or osteomyelitis, and deformity. Access to the midline anterior dura is limited, and spondylectomy or en bloc resection for tumor is possible, but challenging, via these approaches.

■ SURGICAL PLANNING AND IMAGE REVIEW

A posterior approach to the ventral aspect of the thoracic spine requires thorough review of the patient's neurologic symptoms, comorbidities, and imaging. A magnetic resonance imaging (MRI) and a computed tomography (CT) allow for identification of the pathology of interest and its relationship to important surrounding structures. Radiographs allow determination of sagittal and coronal alignment. Short tau inversion recovery (STIR) and contrast-enhanced T1-weighted MRI images can help determine bony infiltration by tumors, and CT imaging can define bony characteristics, and differentiate osteophytes from soft disks and delineate lytic from sclerotic lesions.

Suggested Equipment

- Jackson table or radiolucent table with gel rolls
- Intraoperative fluoroscopy
- Intraoperative multimodal neuromonitoring

■ NEUROMONITORING

Baseline and intraoperative motor evoked potential (MEP) and somatosensory evoked potential (SSEP) monitoring are recommended for all cases.

■ POSITIONING

- The patient is positioned prone on a rotating Jackson table with chest, thigh, and hip pads, and a ProneView head positioner. Care is taken to offload pressure from the eyes during head positioning. The rotation of the bed allows increased visualization for resections performed across midline. In high thoracic pathology (T1-T4), the arms can be tucked along the patient's body to prevent the surgeon from leaning over the arm board. For lower thoracic pathology (T5-T12), the arms can be extended on arm boards (superman position) with care taken to appropriately abduct the shoulders ~30°, flex the elbows ≤90°, and position the forearms in neutral rotation.
- If a rotating Jackson table is used, care must be taken to secure the patient to the table with at least two safety straps.
- Position the chest and hip pads to allow adequate decompression of the abdomen, which will reduce the abdominal pressure and epidural bleeding.
- Positioning of the pads will also help facilitate closure of an osteotomy if that is part of the intended procedure.
- Taping of the shoulders is quite helpful for the purposes of positioning stability, radiographic visualization, and reduction of skin folds in upper thoracic cases.
  - On each side two segments of tape are utilized. One strip travels along the horizontal skin surface overlying the trapezius toward the lateral aspect of the deltoid and then down the lateral contour of the arm to the end of the bed. A second strip of tape beginning ventrally on the upper chest traveling dorsally over

the top of the shoulders to the foot of the bed should also be applied.
- A three-pronged head clamp (Mayfield) is useful for upper thoracic levels and can facilitate correction.

Localization

- Accurate localization in the thoracic spine can be challenging and requires careful attention to fluoroscopic technique and anatomic landmarks. Upright radiographs and CT should be reviewed preoperatively to determine total number of ribs, number of lumbar vertebra, and any abnormalities should be carefully noted. Only after this review is performed should intraoperative fluoroscopy be used to count cephalad from S1.
- Diagnosis of fracture or tumor is often easily identified by direct visualization of the pathology in addition to radiographic counting of fixed structures. For example, facet fractures or disruption are often easily seen. These observable findings do not replace the need to obtain radiographic confirmation as well, but will serve to aid in rapid localization of the appropriate level. In the absence of easy visual identification, it will be useful to count ribs and transverse processes (TPs) from the cervicothoracic junction or thoracolumbar junction.

APPROACH

- Mark the planned incision running vertically over the posterior midline spine centered at the level of pathology.
- Take care to achieve meticulous hemostasis during the superficial dissection. Self-retaining Weitlaner retractors can be used to place the underlying tissue under tension to more easily identify the midline plane.
- Continue dissection through the thoracolumbar fascia and then subperiosteally with Cobb elevators and/or electrocautery. Dissection should be continued laterally to expose the spinous process, lamina, facet joints, and TPs. Subperiosteal dissection minimizes blood loss and muscle damage.
- At this stage, superficial retractors can be exchanged for deep Gelpi retractors.

PEDICLE SCREW PLACEMENT

- Depending on the extent of planned anterior and middle column resection, pedicle screws are placed one or two levels above and below the index level. The afflicted level, such as in the setting of tumor or fracture, may not lend itself to instrumentation.
- To place free-hand screws, a Leksell rongeur is used to remove the cortex at the junction of the TP and lamina 3 mm medial to the lateral margin of the pars interarticularis. If it is difficult to adequately open a starting point with a rongeur, a straight curette is useful to gradually widen the cortical opening. Starting points in the thoracic spine will vary depending upon location in the thoracic spine. Resecting a portion of the inferior articulating process of the cephalad level will help to expose the start point and facilitate decortication for purposes of fusion. A blush of cancellous bleeding can often be seen originating from the cancellous bone of the underlying pedicle.
- Place the tip of a straight thoracic probe at this location and angle perpendicular to the lamina in the sagittal plane and medialize approximately 15° in the coronal plane. Place gentle downward pressure while gently rotating the probe to cannulate and expand the pedicle. Use a ball-tipped probe to palpate the ventral floor and all four walls of the pedicle for breaches. Use of the ball tip probe should be careful and gentle, rather than a vigorous motion. Neurologic injury can result from a medial breach that is vigorously probed. A tap undersized by 1 mm is then used prior to screw placement. The tapped screw path should be evaluated again with the ball-tipped probe.
- Fluoroscopy can be an important tool in patients with small pedicles to find an accurate starting point and trajectory. The desired start point can be prepared and located with a short starting awl placed in the left and right pedicles. Then, under an anteroposterior (AP) image, the start point can be evaluated for cephalad, caudal, medial, and lateral position. This will increase confidence prior pedicle cannulation.

TRANSPEDICULAR DECOMPRESSION

- *Posterior decompression:*
  - The superior and inferior interspinous ligaments are removed with a Leksell rongeur at the level of the pediculectomy and any additional levels needed for the treatment of stenosis.
  - The ligamentum flavum will become visible as the rongeur is used to resect the interspinous ligament. A raphe is usually visible in the midline between the left and right aspects of the flavum. Often a bit of epidural fat can be seen in this raphe.
  - One of two techniques for laminectomy can be considered depending on the magnitude of compression.
  - With one method, a laminectomy is performed by creating bilateral troughs through the lamina using a high-speed side cutting drill such as a 3-mm AM-8. Care must be taken not to place downward pressure on the underlying spinal cord. The trough can be completed through the far cortex with the use of a diamond burr, to mitigate the risk of dural tear. Intermittent irrigation should be used to control the heat from the burr.

- At the caudal aspect of the laminectomy, the ligamentum flavum at the inferior aspect of the index lamina is removed medial to lateral using a Kerrison rongeur. Light upward traction should be applied with a towel clip or Kocher clamp and the bone and soft tissue can be dissected off the dorsal aspect of the lamina with a Woodson elevator or small Kerrison rongeur. Lysis of adhesions and attachments to the dura can be conducted by direct visual inspection. The upward traction minimizes the introduction of instruments into the spinal canal.
- Alternatively, the lamina can be thinned with a high-speed burr or Leksell rongeur. Subsequently, a Kerrison 2 or 3 can be used to gently remove the residual lamina from a caudal to cephalad position in a piecemeal fashion.
- Finally, residual ligamentum flavum should be removed with a Kerrison.
- The laminectomy should be extended in the cephalad and caudal direction to allow access to the area of interest whether it be the disk space or the retrovertebral area. To properly access the disk space, we have found that generous bony resection cephalad to the pediculectomy is often needed.
- Facetectomy can be conducted with a Kerrison rongeur.
- Decompression should appear wide enough to visualize the lateral margin of the dura, and the existing roots should be visible.
- A unilateral screw rod construct is useful at this juncture for provisional stability. We favor a construct capturing two levels above and two levels below the lesion.

- *Pedicle cannulation:*
  - The pedicle and neural foramen can be identified caudal to the level of the superior facet with a nerve hook or Woodson elevator.
  - The inferior facet at the index level is removed using a high-speed drill. This can also be performed using a Leksell rongeur or an osteotome.
  - Next, the pedicle is skeletonized using a small Kerrison rongeur to remove the superior articular facet and identify the cephalad and caudad neuroforamina. The lateral margin of the dura is easily appreciated along with the exiting root. The mouth of the pedicle can be opened with a rongeur or high-speed burr.
  - The cancellous cavity of the pedicle is cannulated either with the use of a large tap or a burr. If needed, intraoperative fluoroscopy can be used to aid in depth of resection and safely guide the surgeon down the pedicle. A wide posterior decompression will provide clear visual landmarks of the pedicle. However, given the extent of posterior element resection, the depth to which the pedicle is cannulated should be carefully observed to prevent anterior breach through the vertebral body.
  - The use of a large tap will create a cavity through which decancellation can be performed. Once the cancellous portion of the pedicle has been removed, the remaining cortical wall can be thinned with a burr and eventually removed with a pituitary rongeur. A small cottonoid can be used to protect the spinal cord and exiting nerve root from the rongeur.
  - In the classic approach, only the medial and superior aspect of the pedicle are removed, but the entire pedicle can be resected if needed. We favor removal of the entire pedicle to the level of the posterior aspect of the vertebral body. Of note, tumor invasion of the pedicle can soften the bone to the point where pituitary forceps can be used to complete the transpedicular approach without the need for a burr.
  - A Woodson elevator can be used to develop and define the epidural space anterior to the spinal cord. Development of this plane is important and will help mitigate the risk of traction injury during the course of further anterior decompression.

- *Anterior decompression:*
  - Bleeding during this portion of the case can increase significantly. Thus, the anesthesia team should be made aware so that preparations from a surgical and anesthetic standpoint can be made.
  - We find the inside sleeve of a pool suction to be useful at providing suction while minimizing the issue of clogging during this portion of the case.
  - Decompression within the disk space or vertebral body is performed with a curette working in a circular manner from the lateral to medial direction. Once a cavity within the vertebral body is created, further undermining with a curved curette can widen the cavity within the vertebral body. As bone or lesion material is mobilized, straight and forward biting pituitary rongeurs are useful to retrieve the loose material. In the setting of tumor, be mindful of bony defects in the posterior aspect of the vertebra. If not recognized, the curettes and forward biting pituitary can protrude through these defects and place the dura at risk.
  - Once a cavity has been created within the space of the vertebral body, the posterior aspect of the vertebra can be resected. This will remove ventral material that compresses the cord. Make sure to sweep ventral to the dura to ensure it is free and there are no residual tethers.
  - Next, a 45° or 90° down pushing Epstein curette is useful for resection of the posterior cortex. A

Woodson can also work well, depending on the quality of the bone. Often, gentle hand pressure, rather than a mallet, is all that is required for resection of the posterior wall. Care must be taken to ensure that the dura is free from the instruments. If we are at all unsure of the retraction of the dura, we consider placing a cottonoid ventral to the dura, and thus between the curette and dura.
- Bleeding can be controlled with hemostatic agents of choice. Packing the defect with cottonoids is also helpful. Balancing bleeding with expedient decompression is important. If needed, consider pausing to allow the anesthesia team to catch up with resuscitation. We generally favor achieving maximal decompression and pause once we are sure the neurologic structures are safe. It is important for the surgeon to recognize their abilities when pursuing a speedy decompression.
- If additional access is required to sufficiently decompress the canal, exposure can be increased by performing a costotransversectomy.

COSTOTRANSVERSECTOMY

- *Approach:*
  - Several different incisions can be used to perform a costotransversectomy and the decision ultimately depends on the underlying indication for the procedure. A curvilinear incision 8 cm lateral to the spinous process of the index level that is 10-12 cm in length has classically been described.
  - However, given the familiarity with the approach and given that most procedures require concurrent laminectomy and/or stabilization, a midline posterior approach as described above is most common. The midline incision also allows for complete subperiosteal dissection, identification of neural structures, and avoids transection of the erector spinae musculature. This is the authors' preferred technique.
  - Continuing from the dissection described above in the approach section, further subperiosteal dissection is carried posteriorly and laterally along the TP until the corresponding rib is encountered. Taking care to remain on the bony surface of the rib, dissection is carried out further laterally. Depending on the extent of exposure desired, the cephalad and caudal level can also be exposed. The rib will angle ventrally toward the spine, and this inflection point is usually located 4-6 cm lateral to the lateral edge of the TP.
- *Rib disarticulation:*
  - The authors utilize a small straight curette to dissect the periosteum off the rib edge both superiorly and inferiorly at the angle of the rib. Next, with either the small curved curette or a Woodson, a plane can be developed between the rib and the neurovascular bundle at the inferior costal groove. The pleura is preserved with this dissection by carefully developing the plane along the ventral aspect of the rib. The cephalad and caudal ribs are similarly exposed and will provide the desired window in the retropleural space. A longer cottonoid can be helpful for blunt dissection. If the pleura is inadvertently entered, a Raytec or cottonoid is helpful at limiting further extension of the defect.
  - Once the rib has been dissected circumferentially, a 4 mm Kerrison rongeur or a rib cutter can be used to cut through the rib at the posterior inflection. Bone wax is used to seal the medial cut end of the rib.
  - Use a Woodson or curette to detach the soft tissue around the TP. Next, use a Leksell rongeur to remove the superior and lateral aspect of that TP. This will transect the costotransverse ligament which connects the transverse costal facet of the TP to the tubercle of the rib.
  - Next, to remove the rib from the costovertebral junction, gently manipulate the rib to tension the soft tissues, utilize a series of Cobb elevators or curettes to gradually release the soft tissue attachments in a controlled fashion. Note that the radiate ligament which surrounds the costovertebral joint is particularly robust and heavier instruments, such as a Cobb, may be needed to leverage the forces required to disarticulate in a controlled manner. After disarticulation, the rib segment will be free and can be gently lifted away from the underlying pleura. The resected portion of the rib should be used as bone graft material. It can be morselized or split into strips.
    - Of note, the pleura lies in close proximity to the superior margin of the rib and a pleural defect can occur during dissection. If the pleura is inadvertently violated, continue with removal of the rib as above and then perform a repair. The authors prefer to perform a primary repair with a running, locking 2-0 Vicryl suture. If a large tear is present, the repair can be performed over a red rubber catheter. After only a small defect in the pleura remains, the red rubber catheter can be sealed with a purse string suture. Perform a Valsalva maneuver to force air from the pleural space, remove the red rubber catheter, and synch and tie the purse string. It is important to note the patient will have a small pneumothorax postoperatively that should resolve spontaneously. Monitor postoperatively with upright chest radiographs.

Corpectomy

- Prior to proceeding with a destabilizing corpectomy, a temporary rod should be in place on the side contralateral to the approach. We typically recommend engaging two or three levels of fixation above and below the intended corpectomy site.
- *Nerve root sacrifice:*
    - For ventral tumor excision or interbody implant/graft placement, nerve root sacrifice may be necessary. Two nerve roots may be needed to place a large static corpectomy cage at one level. The authors' preferred technique is to resect a single root and consider the use of an expandable device and shortening of the spinal segment.
    - Prior to nerve root sacrifice, the mean arterial pressure (MAP) should be maintained >80 mm Hg and baseline MEP and SSEP readings should be obtained.
    - A bulldog clip should be applied to the spinal artery traveling in conjunction with the index nerve root. Neuromonitoring should be observed for about 10 minutes while checking MEPs to ensure blood supply from the artery is not critical for spinal cord perfusion. If no changes in spinal cord monitoring are noted, final silk ties can be placed followed by transection of the nerve root. If both the left and right roots are to be resected, both roots should be temporarily clamped, and MEPs should be conducted.
        + The ties are typically placed lateral to the dorsal root ganglion (DRG).
        + Placing the ties too close to the axilla runs the risk of a cerebrospinal fluid (CSF) leak.
        + Placing the ties too far leaves a remnant nerve root that is long and will fall into the working corridor. However, by leaving the tie long, the remnant nerve root can be gently retracted out of the field of view.
- *Exposure:*
    - Use a Penfield 4 or Woodson elevator to continue subperiosteal dissection along the lateral aspect of the vertebral body ventrally until the anterior margin of the vertebral body is reached. The authors prefer to use these instruments as opposed to larger Cobb's because we feel that their size allows for better visualization during exposure, more control, and are therefore safer. It is important to avoid injury to the segmental vessel or sympathetic trunk. A malleable retractor can be placed to protect and allow safe displacement of the pleura and aorta ventrally. There are a number of commercially available retractors that facilitate exposure as well. However, the authors favor the malleable retractors as they are readily adjustable.
    - Dissection should be carried cephalad and caudal along the lateral margin of the vertebral body. The cephalad and caudal disk will be exposed and aid in orienting the surgeon to the three-dimensional anatomy.
- *Decompression:*
    - If the pathology allows, removal of the disk first can help to isolate the bone and reduce blood loss as the disk is avascular. Incise the disk with an 11 blade scalpel to open the annulus and expose the underlying nucleus.
    - Debulk the disk space with a series of straight and forward angled pituitaries. The endplates of the remaining vertebral bodies should be cleared with straight and curved curettes.
    - After the disk is debulked, the annulus can be resected with Kerrison rongeurs. Elevating the dura along the posterior aspect of the annulus will allow for removal of the annulus across the spinal canal. A pituitary rongeur is useful for resection of the lateral margin of the annulus. Down pushing curettes are useful at reaching the far side endplates.
    - As the discectomy proceeds, a larger surface area of the endplates will become visible, allowing for further preparation of the endplates. Using the retropleural exposure will allow for more direct visualization across the disk space to the contralateral anatomy.
    - Depending on the nature of the pathology, the resection of the ventral most aspect of the annulus may not be necessary. This may help to mitigate the risk to the great vessels.
    - Once the discectomy is complete, the corpectomy can be conducted. A quarter inch or half inch osteotome can be used to resect the vertebral body. Aim at an angle toward the empty disk space and take an adequate section that will allow for removal with a pituitary. Once larger portions of bone have been removed, the use of a curette is advised to resect within the exposed cancellous surface. Once the ventral cortex is exposed, a pituitary or Kerrison should be used to resect the bony structure. The pathology being pursued will dictate to what extend the ventral aspect of the cortical shell needs to be resected. Often, the anterior cortical rim of the vertebral body can be left in place. As it will be thin, the ventral cortex will collapse during correction with compression if needed for deformity correction.
    - An angled down pushing Epstein curette is used to push bony material away from the thecal sac to complete the corpectomy.
    - Mean arterial pressure should be held over 90 mm Hg and frequent MEP checks are advised during this portion of the case, and these should be continued through the remainder of the case, including closure, as delayed motor changes can occur.

- Initial correction can be applied through the rods. Once the final alignment is approximated, the cage can be placed.
  - When significant correction is planned and the patient has poor bone quality, two rods can be placed, one engaging three screws above the osteotomy site, the other engaging the three screws below the osteotomy site. A side-to-side connector can be used to place an additional rod lateral to each of the cranial and caudal rods. These secondary rods can be overlapped and connected to one another via a side-to-side connector. With this construct, deformity correction can be obtained by loosening the side-to-side connector on the secondary rods. This further has the benefit of manipulating the osteotomy by using a block of pedicle screws; thus, increasing control and reducing the risk of screw pull-out or loosening.
- *Cage placement:*
  - Cage reconstruction will contribute to mechanical stability by load sharing through the anterior column.
  - A variety of implant choices exist, including cortical struts, static, and expandable cage options. The authors favor a static cage in the upper thoracic spine, and an expandable cage in the mid to lower thoracic spine. In the event that an expandable cage is not available, a traditional titanium mesh cage is quite useful. These cages are easily customized to a given defect and are readily handled with the use of a tonsil clamp.
  - Cages should be packed with local autograft when possible; however, bone substitutes may be used in tumor or infection cases when using local bone is not an option.
  - Measuring the defect can be done with a caliper or ruler. The authors' preferred method is to cut a portion of the disposable ruler that accompanies the marking pen. Then this shortened flexible segment can be placed into the defect and a measurement of the defect is easily accomplished. An undersized implant is most helpful to allow safe and easier placement of the cage in the anterior space. Subsequently the defect can be closed compressed on the cage facilitating contact and loading across the anterior column.
  - In the upper thoracic spine, a cervical corpectomy cage is often the correct size implant. As it will be placed from the posterior side, the lordosis of the cervical cage can be helpful, as it will be in kyphosis. In the upper thoracic spine, the expandable cage options may have too large of a footprint to be safe or useful.
  - In the mid thoracic and lower thoracic spine, the authors favor an expandable cage option. The smallest footprint is usually best suited to ventral placement from a posterior approach. Depending on the device selected, the expandable cage will span a range of vertical sizes. Select a cage that is smaller than the measured defect to allow for expansion to fill the defect.
  - When placing the cage, exploit the space created in the retropleural location to allow delivery of the cage into the anterior column. Be mindful of the tail of the sacrificed root, as impingement upon this may drag the thecal sac with it and place neural structures at risk.
  - With the cage in the desired position, compress through the instrumentation to secure the cage. After positioning, and prior to release of the insertion handle, a fluoroscopy image should be used to verify satisfactory placement. The cage should be placed midline on AP radiograph and the posterior edge of the cage should remain anterior to the posterior cortex of the superior and inferior vertebral bodies on lateral radiograph. The insertion handle can be removed prior to imaging but recognize that the cage may need adjustment. Without the handle, cage adjustment may be more challenging. If the handle has been moved and the cage requires repositioning, a tonsil clamp can be used to hold the cage while distraction is applied on the instrumentation. Then with the cage mobile, the tonsil clamp can aid in minor adjustments.
  - The authors favor more ventral cage placement to allow more space between the thecal sac and the posterior aspect of the cage. This also allows for additional bone graft to be applied around the cage for fusion purposes.

Final Posterior Instrumentation and Bone Graft Placement

- Rods and set screws should be placed on each side and final tightened. A cross-link is not necessary with unilateral rib removal.
- Copiously irrigate the wound with normal saline and perform a Valsalva maneuver under irrigation to evaluate for occult pneumothorax.
- Following suction of irrigation, a final Valsalva maneuver should be performed to assess the ventral dura and nerve root stump for sources of CSF leak.
- The available posterior bony elements should be decorticated to provide a wide fusion bed and bone graft (local autograft versus cancellous allograft chips and bone substitute) should be placed. The authors favor placement of a sheet of gelfoam over the decompressed thecal sac to limit bone graft fragments from falling into the decompression window.

Closure and Postoperation

- Apply topical vancomycin powder and then remove retractors and obtain careful hemostasis.
- If desired vancomycin powder can be mixed in a one to one mixture with saline, such that 1 g of vancomycin is mixed with 1 cc of saline. It can be mixed with a Penfield 4 until the consistency of bone wax is achieved. Initially it will appear that there is not enough saline but continued stirring will achieve the desired consistency. The doughy consistency can allow the vancomycin to be placed away from the decompression window.
- A multilayered closure is desired. First, a subfascial medium Hemovac drain is placed. The local muscle is then elevated and reapproximated in two layers. First with #0 Vicryl suture in an interrupted fashion and followed with an additional running #1 Vicryl more superficial in the muscle layer. Fascial closure is performed with a running #1 Vicryl suture reinforced with interrupted figure-of-8 #1 Vicryl suture. A subcutaneous flap is raised superficially along the fascia to minimize tension on the suture repair. A superficial medium Hemovac drain is then placed.
- This is followed by buried, deep dermal, interrupted 2-0 Vicryl stitches. Evenly spaced superficial skin staples are then placed.
- An occlusive sterile dressing is placed.
- An upright chest radiograph should be performed in the recovery room to evaluate for pneumothorax.

CHAPTER 12

Anterior Thoracic Discectomy/Corpectomy/Anterior Instrumentation

Yoji Ogura, John R Dimar, Leah Y Carreon

■ INTRODUCTION

The ability to perform an anterior approach to thoracic spine is a critical skill to develop when there is anterior pathology of the thoracic spine, which includes vertebral body tumors, anterior central herniations, burst fractures, osteomyelitis, excessive kyphosis, certain other deformities, and any lesion that causes anterior cord compression that cannot be addressed using a standard posterior approach. The anterior approach via a thoracotomy provides superior access and visualization of the entire anterior vertebral body to easily facilitate a central thoracic discectomy or complete corpectomy from T3 to T12. The traditional anterior transpleural approach was first reported in 1969.[1] This approach provides excellent exposure to the anterior column. However, it has several disadvantages including postoperative pain, pulmonary complications, and the need for chest tube placement.[2,3] The retropleural approach was developed to address these issues,[4] with a smaller incision, and less violation of the pleura and diaphragm. A thoracoscopic approach has also been developed,[5] but it has a steep learning curve and requires specialized equipment and has fallen out of favor. In general, a retropleural approach offers advantages over other anterior thoracic transpleural approach when the pathology can be addressed with a limited exposure to the lateral aspect of the vertebral body. However, when the pathology requires extensive visualization of the pathology or it involves multiple vertebral segments, the transpleural approach remains the gold standard and is recommended. The chapter is limited to adult conditions that require an open approach acknowledging that minimally invasive techniques are also available for adolescents for anterior release, fusion, and tethering and for adults for specific pathologies.

Indications

- *Anterior compressive lesions:*
  - Tumor
  - Thoracic disk herniation
  - Ossification of posterior longitudinal ligament (OPLL)
  - Burst fractures and bony fragments resulting from trauma
  - Primary thoracic stenosis (PTS)
- Pyogenic osteomyelitis
- Tuberculosis, fungal, and granulomatous disease
- Deformities including Scheuermann's kyphosis and severe scoliosis.

■ CONTRAINDICATIONS

- Posterior compressive lesions
- Significant pulmonary compromise
- Circumferential instability (consider addition of posterior instrumentation)
- Pleural scarring
- Prior surgery
- Pulmonary embolus.

■ PREOPERATIVE EVALUATION

- Medical comorbidities that preclude single-lung ventilation such as severe pulmonary disease or prior pulmonary resection.
- Disk location (central, paracentral, or lateral)
- Nature of disk (calcified or not)
- A calcified disk often causes intradural invasion due to dural erosion. Although without absolute certainty, a magnetic resonance imaging (MRI) or thoracic myelogram/computed tomography (CT) may help delineate this problem.
- Extent of herniation (intra- or extradural). Loss of continuity of the posterior longitudinal ligament (PLL) in sagittal acquisitions and the "hawk-beak" sign in axial T2 acquisitions were reported to be associated with intra-dural disk herniation. However, at times, a preoperative diagnosis of intradural disk herniation is difficult.

- Determine the range of adjacent corpectomies for safe excision of calcified or migrated disk.
- Number of ribs, lumbar, and thoracic segments involved.

Preoperative Diagnostic Modalities

- Plain thoracic radiographs—all patients
- *MRI scanning*: Counting views with continuous sagittal reconstructions from C2 or sacrum to the operative level are critical for intraoperative level identification in the thoracic spine. We commonly obtain preoperative counting views with MRI and/or CT scans and correlate to intraoperative X-ray or CT scans.
- CT scanning with three-dimensional (3D) reconstruction
- Bone scan (specific indications, e.g., skeletal screening for cancer)
- *CT-guided biopsy:* All anatomic and radiographic modalities are used to identify the correct level of pathology or areas of surgical planning.
- Pulmonary function testing (PFT) when indicated by preoperative evaluation. Risk stratification is helpful for identifying patients who may not tolerate single-lung ventilation.

INSTRUMENTS SUGGESTED

- Double-lumen endotracheal tube
- A pivoting radiolucent Jackson table with axillary roll, kidney rests, and arm rests
- *Intraoperative CT scanning*: Guidance for levels, screw placement, and resection margins
- Intraoperative fluoroscopy per surgeon preference and unavailability of other modalities
- Intraoperative neuromonitoring [motor evoked potentials (MEPs), somatosensory-evoked potentials (SSEPs), and pre- and postflip baseline signals]
- Specialized long chest instruments, thoracotomy instruments, and retractors (curettes and rongeurs)
- Scalpels (long handles), curettes, Kerrison, pituitary rongeurs, rib cutters, and high-speed drills
- Interbody constructs such as autograft, allograft, or synthetic fixed or expandable cages [polyetheretherketone (PEEK), titanium, and composite]
- Screw-rod or screw-plate specialized anterior instrumentation systems
- Drains and chest tubes. We place 15 French Hemovac drains in the retropleural space and No. 32 chest tubes in the pleural space.

POSITIONING

Great attention must be paid to positioning. A true lateral decubitus X-ray allows accurate orientation and subsequent screw placement in an appropriate position. We recommend creating a perfect lateral image by adjusting patient position and/or bed while keeping the fluoroscope in the standard upright anteroposterior (AP) position. The surgeon typically stands behind the patient. C-arm, O-arm, and displays are set up on the opposite side. Mayo and back table are set up above the patient's knee. The positioning of the fluoroscopy into the room is done before the incision. The variable of a specific operating room (OR) will ultimately determine how it is employed during surgery and differs from facility to facility.

- A double-lumen endotracheal tube is inserted to allow for selective deflation of one lung if needed.
- Neuromonitoring is set up and baseline signal is obtained after intubation before transfer to OR bed.
- Positioned on a radiolucent table in the lateral decubitus position (left side up) with an axillary roll placed under the dependent axilla to protect the brachial plexus.
- Secured with kidney rests placed at the xiphoid process, pubic symphysis, and lumbosacral junction (we do not use a collapsible bean bag support because it interferes with radiographic imaging and locks the patient too rigidly on the table preventing raising the kidney rest and jack-knifing the bed to aid in exposure).
- Padding of all bony prominences is required to prevent compressive neuropathy and pressure necrosis. Care should be taken especially in the dependent axilla, the ulnar nerve at the elbow, and the peroneal nerve at the fibular neck.
- Hips and knees are slightly flexed to secure the position using padded straps or wide tape (4″). Patients must be perpendicular to the floor **(Fig. 1)**.
- Approach side is determined based on the level and location of the lesion. If neither side is predominantly involved by the lesion, approach from left-sided is preferential for mid to lower thoracic lesions (T6–12) to avoid the inferior vena cava (IVC) and the liver **(Figs. 2 and 3)**, whereas approach from the right side is preferable for upper thoracic lesions to avoid the aorta and aortic arch (above T5), but care must be to not damage the azygous vein and to triple tie the vein if needs to be sacrificed **(Fig. 4)**. Deformity cases are typically approached from convex side because the curvature of the spine presents the apex close to the incision aiding in easier access, typically thoracic curves are right-sided, hence this is the most frequent approach.

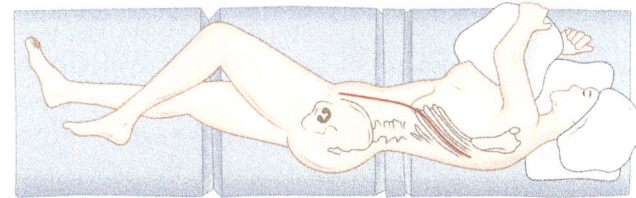

Fig. 1: *Positioning.* Left thoracic approach. Hips and knees are slightly flexed to secure the position. Patients must be perpendicular to the floor.

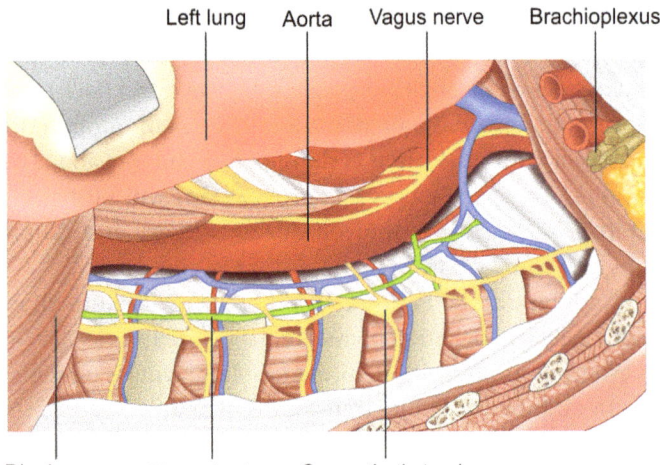

Fig. 2: *Left thoracic approach.* Lateral view of left thoracic spine with sympathetic chain and segmental vessels located deep to the parietal pleura. Be aware of the existence of thoracic duct as chyle leak of lymph into thorax is a rare but potentially devastating consequence of thoracic duct injury.

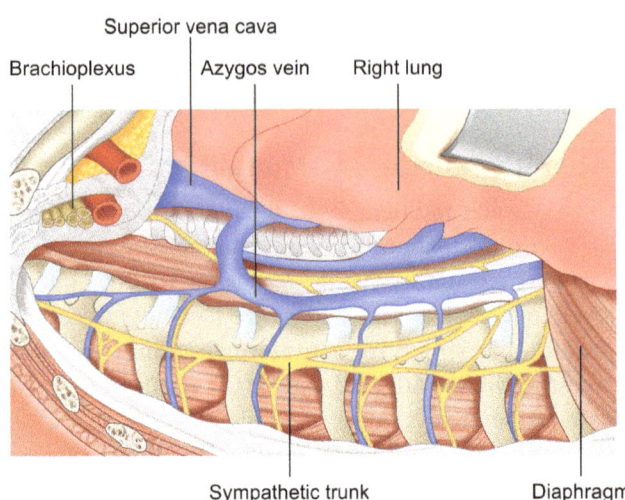

Fig. 4: *Right thoracic approach.* Lateral view of right thoracic spine with sympathetic chain and segmental vessels located deep to the parietal pleura. Dissection should be done with maximum care as vena cava is more fragile than aorta and hard to repair. Triple tie azygos vein to prevent loss of control.

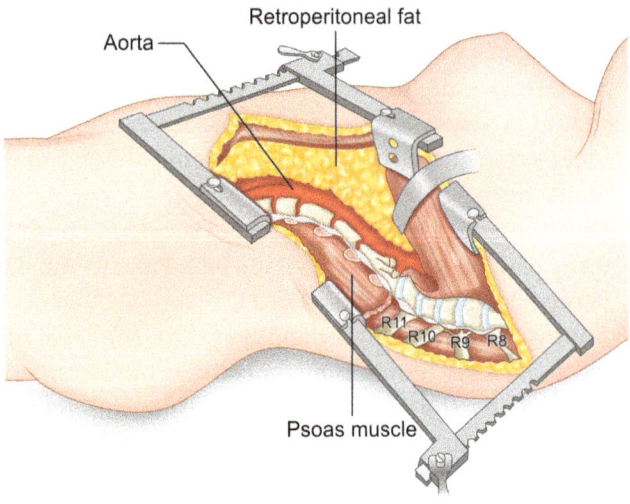

Fig. 3: *Left thoracolumbar approach.* After resecting the 10th rib and reflecting the diaphragm from the lower ribs and the crus from the side of the spine, thoracic and abdominal cavities converge and wide exposure is obtained.

- Regular AP and lateral radiographs or a lateral view of fluoroscopy are used for level localization. The rib overlying the level of pathology in the midaxillary level (usually one to two ribs above) is resected. For example, remove seventh or eighth rib for T9 corpectomy. For single-level discectomy cases, the rib resection is not necessarily required, but rib resection, typically one rib resection is enough per one level of vertebrectomy, improves exposure. Additional ribs may be cut to improve exposure. A rib head originating from the affected disk space needs to be resected during a discectomy to expose the foramen and posterior annulus; e.g., remove seventh rib head for T6–T7 discectomy.

- We always prefer a posteroanterior (PA) view to save on breast and thyroid X-ray exposure but it may be necessary to use an AP view due to the area of surgery or body habitus. A true lateral decubitus position is best obtained without trunk rotation or tilt. Check coronal alignment as well.

- Wrong level procedure is not an uncommon problem[6] in thoracic spine surgery. Always count the number of ribs and nonrib lumbar vertebrae, and determine the size of the end rib. Correlate the number of ribs from preoperative X-rays and CT scan with the number of ribs palpated on the patient. The 12th rib may not be felt, and the most inferior rib palpated can be the 11th rib. We always evaluate preoperative X-rays, MRI, and CT scanning prior to surgery. Intraoperatively we use plain radiographs, fluoroscopy, or if necessary, an intraoperative CT scan which is potentially more accurate in identifying thoracic levels. However, all studies should be used synergistically. We use all modalities (X-rays, CT, and MRI) for counting. We typically use fluoroscopy and AP + lateral X-rays to correspond preoperative images including the patient's X-rays, CT, and MRI to identify levels.

Approach

- Author prefers transpleural approach in case a broad exposure (corpectomy or multilevel discectomy) is necessary, or pleural adhesions are suspected. The lung can be deflated to improve visualization combined with decreasing the depth of respirations (tidal volume) concurrent with increasing the number of breaths during this in a standard transpleural approach.

- *Drape widely*: Entire hemithorax, including the neck cranially and the iliac crest caudally.

CHAPTER 12: Anterior Thoracic Discectomy/Corpectomy/Anterior Instrumentation

- A 12-15 cm skin incision is made, extending from a lateral border of paraspinal musculature to the dorsal axillary line over the selected rib. Extension of the incision toward costochondral junction is required in some cases to expand ventral access.
- After skin incision with a scalpel, electrocautery is used to dissect subcutaneous tissues and superficial periosteum. The latissimus dorsi is transected carefully, while the anterior serratus muscle should be preserved and retracted, only being transected under special circumstances when an extensive exposure is required. Its edges should be marked and meticulously repaired when closing. The periosteum is elevated circumferentially around the rib with a Cobb or Alexander elevator. Then, achieve circumferential subperiosteal dissection with careful attention to neurovascular bundle using Doyen rib dissector. Carefully preserve the neurovascular bundles running inferior to each rib. If unintentional injury occurs, we have to tie off the artery to avoid excessive blood loss. We always separate and preserve the intercostal nerve. The tip for subperiosteal dissection is to proceed posterior to anterior on the superior edge of the rib and anterior to posterior on the inferior edge of the rib in the direction of the intercostal muscle fibers for ease of dissection.
- The amount of liberated rib variable depending on the extent of the desired exposure and as a general rule, the more extensive the number of vertebral bodies and disks addressed, the longer the resection, sometimes extending posteriorly and resulting in resection of the rib head. The longer resection also provides more potential autogenous bone graft when required. The resected rib also can be shaped or bundled together to provide structural bone graft. The rib is cut with a rib cutter as far ventrally and dorsally as possible to obtain a good exposure. Bleeding from the rib can be controlled with bone wax. Remove all sharp rib tip fragments. The rib resection may not be required if a single thoracic disk is to be addressed. In that case, divide the intercostal muscles between two ribs.
- Incise the rib bed in line with the resected rib without violation of the parietal pleura and the neurovascular bundle (If choosing transpleural approach, incise both the rib bed and parietal pleura here, which allows entry into the thoracic cavity). The underlying parietal pleura is bluntly freed from the rib bed using fingers and Kittner dissection. The rib bed incision is continued proximally and blunt dissection of the pleura off the proximal rib head extends dorsally to expose the lateral aspect of the vertebral bodies and disks.
- Parietal pleura is relatively thick posteriorly, but becomes thinner laterally. Carefully dissect lateral aspect. Keep in mind that pleura is fragile in elderly patients. A small violation (<2-3 mm) of pleura can be left alone or suture with absorbable suture.
- Insert a self-retaining rib retractor. Cover the lung with moist lap sponges and gently retract medially and ventrally with a wide malleable or wisp retractor taking care not to puncture the lung parenchyma.
- Once the pleura overlying the disks and vertebral bodies is identified, it is split caudal and cephalad to expose the areas of interest after it is isolated with a right angle using a scissors or bovie. The segmental arteries should be conserved, but often due to encasement in tumor or infection may require ligation with 2-0 long silk ties backed up by hemoclips.
- Localization is done by inserting an easily visualize marker or needle into disk space and identify the correct level using fluoroscopy or plain radiographs. The spine looks like hills and valleys from the lateral exposure, where hills are disks. The disk is more prominent and whiter than the adjacent vertebral bodies but may become collapsed and spondylosed with aging making the identification difficult. In the face of pathology such as infection, fracture or tumor the landmarks can be severely obscured requiring careful dissection until an intact disk level or body can be identified well enough to properly identify the level. With these processes, the marker, often a Penfield No. 2, can be used to palpate the area of interest and will often fall into a cavity of phlegmon or tumor where the body or disk has been destroyed.
- If it is necessary to ligate a segmental identify the vessels around the midpoint of the vertebral body and preserve them whenever possible to prevent a watershed injury to the cord, ligate them firmly in the middle of vertebra and not foraminally when required. Adamkiewicz artery is one of the concerns when operating the lower thoracic area and its location is variable. Potential spinal cord ischemia has been traditionally argued with its ligation, though some suggest no evidence of spinal cord ischemia and neurologic deficit with up to three levels of bilateral embolization or ligation. Nevertheless, all segmental vessels should be preserved to avoid a rare but catastrophic neurological deficit.

Considerations Specific to the Upper Thoracic (above T5) Spine Approach

When the thoracotomy is performed proximal to T5, the scapula will need to be mobilized in a cranial and medial direction. Draping the ipsilateral upper extremity into the surgical field is necessary to help manipulate the scapula and assist in retraction. A curved incision that follows the medial and inferior scapular border is used **(Fig. 1)**. After skin and subcutaneous tissue are incised, division of the serratus anterior and trapezius at the inferior border of the scapula may be necessary for adequate scapular retraction.

The serratus anterior must be divided as distally as possible to avoid iatrogenic injury of the long thoracic nerve. Then, it becomes possible to rotate and retract the scapula cranially and medially with the scapular retractor. Once the scapula has been mobilized and the appropriate rib is identified, exposure can proceed as previously described. The third rib is typically excised, which allows exposure of the lateral aspect of the spine from T1 to T5. However, the visualization can be poor for T1–T3. The authors recommend a sternal notch resection or "trap door" sternotomy combined with a standard ventral cervical approach to visualize T1 through T3.[7] Transverse incision along the lower cervical skin crease and vertical incision along the midline are made. After the strap muscles are divided, the precervical fascia and pretracheal fascia are incised at the level of the sternal notch. The notch is resected or the sternum is split and retracted laterally. After the exposure of the pericardium and thymus, the thymus is retracted to the right. The working space is between the left common carotid artery and the innominate artery, thyroid, esophagus, and trachea. Retraction of these structures exposes the ventral aspect of the vertebrae. Excellent visualization of T1 to potentially T4 can be obtained by this technique that is commonly used by thoracic surgeons for access to this area.

Considerations Specific to the Thoracolumbar Junction (T10–T12) Approach

- The retropleural approach is modified for the approach to these levels because of diaphragm attachment.
- After the rib removal, the diaphragm remains in the rib bed at the lowest three rib levels. Detach the diaphragm approximately 2 cm from its peripheral attachment to the chest wall using electrocautery after carefully separating the retroperitoneal fat from the bottom of the diaphragm. If further exposure is necessary, detachment of the diaphragm by dividing the medial and lateral arcuate ligaments and the crus of the diaphragm can be performed after splitting the costochondral cartilage tip to visualize **(Figs. 3 and 5)**. Mark the diaphragm with suture to allow for accurate reapproximation.
- After the vertebral and disk procedures, the diaphragm is reattached with suture using a running number one absorbable suture reapproximating the edges lining up the previously placed 3-0 silk marking sutures followed by a standard rib approximation and latissimus dorsi repair with number one interrupted or running absorbable suture.

■ DISCECTOMY

- Rib heads articulate with vertebral bodies and transverse processes and can obscure the posterior disk space. Partial or entire rib head resection may be necessary

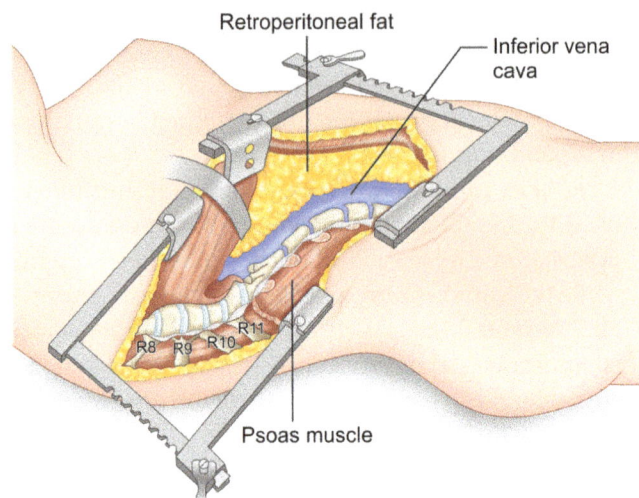

Fig. 5: *Right thoracolumbar approach.* After resecting the 10th rib and reflecting the diaphragm from the lower ribs and the crus from the side of the spine, thoracic and abdominal cavities converge and wide exposure is obtained.

  to expose disk spaces. We typically use a rongeur or osteotome for rib head resection.
- The precise midline of the lateral disk annulus fibrosus when feasible is sharply incised using No. 15 blade knife on long handle. Make sure to identify the midpoint of the disk space before this to avoid cord or vascular injury. Get an X-ray if you are unsure where you are in the AP plane. The disk is removed with curettes and pituitary rongeurs. The adjacent endplate and disk margins are removed using a long-nosed high-speed drill, creating a space into which the herniation can be pushed posteriorly away from the spinal cord using down-turn curettes.
- In case of large, calcified disk herniation, direct decompression is deferred until adjacent partial corpectomy is performed. Occasionally the top of the pedicle is burred down to increase central canal and foraminal exposure. Excision of calcified disk, osteophytes, and complete spinal cord decompression is performed last under magnified direct vision to avoid a spinal cord contusion or dural tear. Calcified disks can adhere or erode through the dura so care must be taken to tease it off and repair or sealing may be required.
- Cranial and caudal partial corpectomies are performed to adequately gain visual exposure, particularly when there is concurrent spondylosis present, to safely directly decompress the spinal cord. Otherwise, durotomy and neurologic injury can occur due to poor visualization to the pathology and due to a limited working surgical portal and field. Normally there is only a minimal caudal/cephalad corpectomy required but if there is a question of stability, the discectomy should be full and the defect should have an anterior interbody fusion (AIBF), a structural cage placed and potentially a follow-up posterior stabilization and fusion done. The tips here are

to start decompression with the shallow side but keep the decompression incomplete. Next, we decompress the contralateral side (deep side) and come back to the shallow side to complete decompression. If the shallow side is completely decompressed first, the visualization becomes poor because of the dura mater distention.
- All maneuvers such as curetting and Cobb work that require force are directed away from the spinal cord to avoid pressure on the ventral thecal sac. But be aware the aorta and IVC is on the other side. The anterior longitudinal ligament (ALL) should be preserved to protect these structures and only removed at the end when required.

CORPECTOMY

- Removal of one or more vertebral bodies may be necessary in some cases such as trauma, infections, or tumors. Identification of the segmental vessels may be difficult in these cases, and exposure of the spine should start at the intervertebral disk, which is less vascular.
- Always start with a complete discectomy to define the cephalad and caudal extent of the body at the level above and below where the selected vertebrae is to be performed before complete removal of vertebral body. This serves to define the margins of the resection and prepare the endplates above and below the resection for later interbody support placements. Remove the cartilaginous endplate using a Cobb elevator and curettes meticulously to provide solid support during reconstruction.
- Care must be taken to protect the anterior and anterolateral structures, such as aorta, vena cava, azygos vein, sympathetic chain, and thoracic duct, to prevent inadvertent injury. Always first identify ALL and perform each procedure dorsally to ALL.
- First identify posterior wall of the vertebral body whose border is marked by the foramen by continuing the reflection of the pleura, removal of the rib head, and palpating the foramen using a Penfield #2. The posterior margin of the corpectomy is identified by the pedicle, foramen, and posterior edge of the disk while the anterior border is identified by the anterior curvature of the disk and the ALL. The corpectomy is accomplished using osteotomes, curettes, various rongeurs, from pedicle to pedicle completely until reaching the opposite cortical wall. An important point here is to make sure to establish the borders of the corpectomy before going deeper (go wide before going deep). This avoids "coning down" and helps to make sure your graft will fit well in the depth of the corpectomy. Also, it improves visualization when working at the deeper aspects. You can also confirm depth with a lateral X-ray to make sure you are all the way down. The amount of resection depends on the type of pathology and exposure.
- Bleeding can be controlled with electrocautery, gelfoam, Floseal™, Surgicel™, and packing. Intraoperative bleeding can be brisk when doing corpectomies so thoughtful, preoperative consideration should be done to assess how much bleeding the surgeon should expected for a specific problem, i.e., infection or tumor, etc. Assessment by the surgeon can therefore be made as to what preventative methods to take preoperatively (e.g., embolization) and intraoperatively.
- When a suspicious lesion is noted, it should *always* be biopsied and sent for cultures.

INTERBODY SPACER AND SPINAL INSTRUMENTATION

The rationale for using anterior instrumentation is to allow for the reconstruction and immediate stabilization when the anterior and middle column integrity is lost. An essential element of anterior reconstruction is to anatomically place the interbody spacer into the corpectomy defect. It must fit into the defect and restore the ideal spinal column alignment. Then, surgeons must determine the type of spinal instrumentation (anterior or posterior instrumentation) based on all the clinical information and pathology. Certain materials, cage shapes, profile, and what is the pathological process will determine material selection. Fortunately there are a variety of interbody space options to meet this goal including structural bone graft (humeral and femoral shaft, patellar wedges, etc.), synthetic static, and expandable cages some with variable endplate caps (PEEK and titanium mesh) from a wide variety of commercial carriers. We commonly utilize autologous iliac crest bone graft (ICBG) but will consider titanium mesh cages for filling defects. For correction of kyphotic alignment, we utilize expandable cages.

Interbody Spacer

- *Bone graft*: Structural tricortical ICBG **(Fig. 6)**, local autograft, allograft (humeral and fibular shafts), and

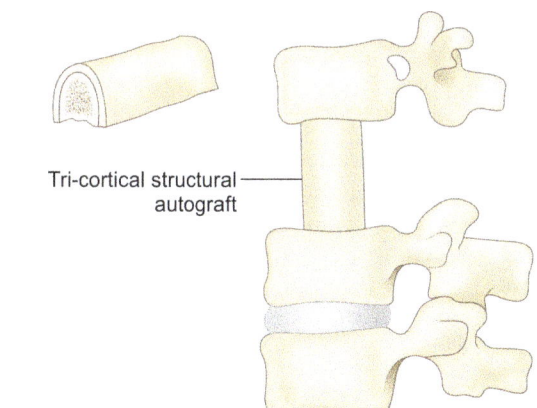

Fig. 6: *Tri-cortical structural autograft.* Iliac crest is trimmed and placed into the corpectomy defect.

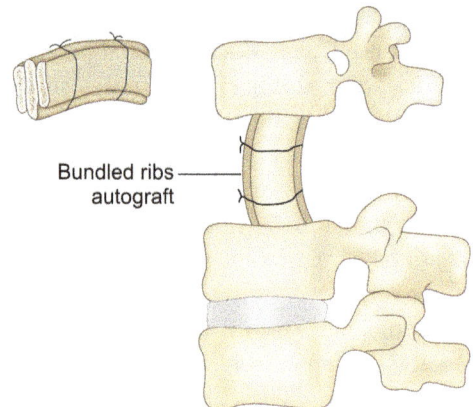

Fig. 7: *Bundled resected ribs autograft.* Bundled resected ribs can be placed into the corpectomy defect.

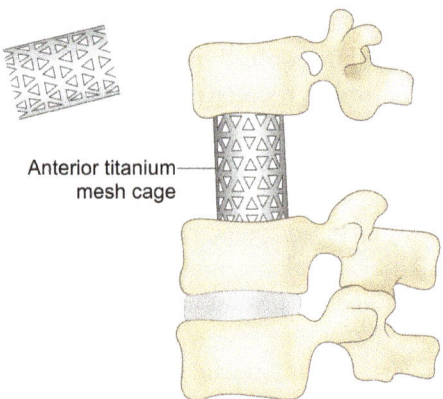

Fig. 8: *Titanium mesh cage.* An appropriate length of titanium mesh cage is placed into the defect. We typically use a titanium mesh cage when we need to fill a defect.

biologic adjuvants. Bundled resected ribs **(Fig. 7)** may also be used. The use of auto graft is limited by the size of the corpectomy and tricortical iliac crest is generally limited to just one level. Allograft materials come in a wide variety of shapes and sizes and are not limited by size or volume obtainable as autograft.

- *Cage sizing*: The cage diameter is determined based on preoperative imaging. Interbody cage or structural bone graft height is determined by measuring with caliper. Maximizing the size of the cage will improve its endplate contact area support and strength.
- *Cage types*: PEEK and titanium mesh cages **(Fig. 8)** or modular cages are available in a wide variety of shapes, diameters, and lengths making them useful for both discectomy and corpectomy. Stout, thicker wall titanium cages are preferred since earlier mesh cages have experienced compression failures in the face of nonunions.
- The authors would not recommend the use of PEEK cages ever in osteomyelitis since the material is prone to the formation of glycocalyx, and instead would recommend autograft, allograft, or titanium which has bacteriostatic properties.
- Modular cages provide variability in diameter and angulation to match the endplate geometry along with expansile functions to fill the corpectomy defect. Expandable cages have many advantages since they allow for a precise fit and easier insertion. It is still important to preserve sturdy endplates to prevent subsidence. Caution should also be exercised to not over expand the cage through the adjacent endplates causing cage subsidence. Cage size is usually 17–23 mm in diameter, but determined using an intraoperative trial. Endcaps may decrease the rate of subsidence and have the added benefit of building in kyphosis which is occasionally useful for multilevel corpectomies, rarely for single level ones.
- Local ICBG, autograft, allograft preparations, and bone morphogenic proteins can be inserted into cage for grafting, although bone morphogenic proteins are an off-label usage and this should be fully explained to the patient and consent granted for its use. It is beneficial for the cage to have a portal to allow for the insertion of more bone graft when necessary, particularly expandable cages.
- *Cage insertion*: Cage is placed at the appropriate place with inserter. Expand the cage height in case of an expandable cage, and then remove inserter. Plain radiographs, fluoroscopy, or on occasion with large individuals or upper thoracic cages an intraoperative CT is done to confirm cage placement to confirm the proper placement of the cage in an appropriate position.
- Anterior column cages and grafts are best placed in compression to prevent migration, subsidence, and increase fusion rates. Various commercially available distraction devices are available, generally as part of an anterior instrumentation set, to expand the corpectomy site if needed to place an anterior graft or cage; however, this is rarely required due to postural reduction. Compression is obtained by flattening out the bed and dropping kidney rest on Jackson table. Also, by applying distraction force before inserting a cage, compression can be obtained when distraction forces are removed. We can add compression force when using anterior instrumentation system and/or a posterior follow-up stabilization. Preserving a residual anterior cortical rim of bone can aid this goal and prevent anterior displacement.

Anterior Instrumentation

Anterior instrumentation can provide immediate stability to the spine following reconstruction of the anterior column along with avoiding the potential need for second posterior fusion with spinal instrumentation. Although not as strong as a combined anterior and posterior stabilization construct, anterior instrumentation is useful in patients with normal bone but should be avoided in patients with osteoporosis due to an elevated chance of failure at the bone-instrumentation interface. It is pretty rare to apply anterior plate/rod system since pedicle screw systems have been developed and somewhat dangerous because of their high profile and proximity to the great vessels. This is particularly true of left thoracotomies where in the past they have eroded through the aorta causing death. Generally, anterior instrumentation should be reserved for patients that have severe 360° injury or bone destruction where the anterior instrumentation is employed to provide temporary fixation until pedicular instrumentation is applied posteriorly or to hold the interbody implants is due to a poor bone implant interface. The followings circumstances may be suitable for anterior instrumentation:

- Unstable fractures, tumors, infections that and cannot wait for posterior instrumentation.
- Burst fracture, especially at L1, L2, or L3 where the plate is lateral in the psoas muscle and the aorta has migrated anteriorly to the spine.
- Adolescent idiopathic scoliosis (AIS) with a type 5C curve.

There are multiple options available for anterior instrumentation. Single or dual screws as well as compression or locking plates are available. The basic principle of this technique is connecting the vertebral body screws above and below the corpectomy site by a rod or plate. The options include a single-rod construct, a dual-rod construct, or a plate. Dual-rod constructs or a plate provide more rigid stability than single-rod constructs. Dual-rod systems or plates should be the first choice, although single-rod systems are indicated in case of smaller vertebrae sized at the time of surgery, which varies based on the sex and the size of the patient body habitus.

It is important to have measured all of the potential and planned vertebra coronal (width) diameters to determine the screw lengths and place it on a picture archiving and communication systems (PACS) monitor for reference during surgery. Make sure to notice any concurrent body level pathology (fractures) since it may affect your fixation. Both poly-axial and fixed head screws (the author prefers fixed) may be placed into the vertebral bodies through a staple, plate, or washers which improves their resistance to toggling of the screw in the relatively soft cancellous bone **(Fig. 9)**. Bicortical fixation is best as this technique allows more rigid stability of the screw-vertebral body bone interface. Identification of foramen with a Penfield #4 and posterior adjacent vertebral margin allows for accurate screw placement in a proper position in the center of the vertebral body. Maintaining your screw direction perfectly vertical, parallel to the posterior and anterior vertebral body margins, will help avoid the breach of a posterior screw into the spinal canal. Fluoroscopy can aid significantly in placement.

For single-rod constructs, the entry hole of the vertebral body screw is created at the junction of the pedicular origin and the vertebral body with a high-speed drill or a sharp awl. A straight probe is then directed toward the surgeon's

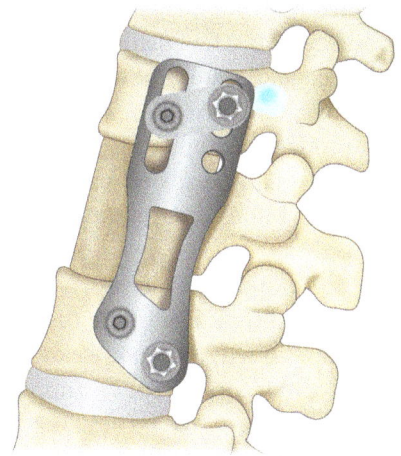

Fig. 9: *Anterior thoracic plate.* Screws are placed into the vertebral bodies through a staple or plate which improves their resistance to toggling of the screw.

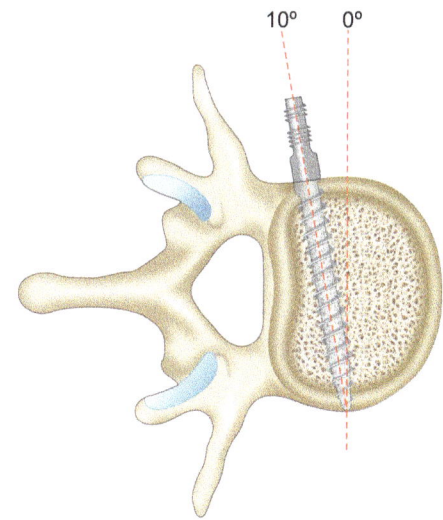

Fig. 10: *Bicortical screw purchase:* It should be obtained whenever feasible. Care must be taken that posterior screw does not intrude spinal canal.

finger on the contralateral side of the body. The trajectory crosses the center of the vertebral body and parallel to the endplates. Bicortical screw purchase should be obtained when feasible **(Fig. 10)**. Preoperative measurement using CT helps to determine the screw length. The tip here is bluntly dissecting vascular tissues from vertebra and put surgeon's finger on the contralateral side to avoid vascular injury with screw insertion maneuver.

For dual-rod constructs, which are less commonly employed, a two-holed vertebral staple is implanted as posterior as possible. Then insert two screws per a vertebra. Posterior screw is placed directly parallel to cord side to side in vertebral bodies. Make sure that posterior screw does not intrude spinal canal. Anterior screws are typically angled slightly posterior to converge and triangulate with posterior screws. The placement of vertebral body screws in triangular alignment decreases the risk of screw pullout. Several current systems vertebral body staple will fix this angle.

Bicortical purchase is ideal especially in osteoporotic cases. The surgeon can use distraction instruments when inserting the bone graft or cage. Removal of distraction allows mild compression of cage. Rods are then placed in position, and slight compression can be applied to the anterior column support, which eventually leads to a solid construct with optimal alignment. Finally, connect the dual rod with transverse connectors.

There are some important caveats worth mentioning concerning dual rod system use in the thoracic spine in a standalone fashion and why to be very careful in choosing this option. First, the available space and vertebral body footprint becomes progressively smaller in the upper thoracic spine, making the placement of dual rod constructs challenging due to space limitations. The rib heads will need to be resected almost universally to fit the plate also causing potential problems later in life. Additionally, the bodies are more triangular shaped and narrower limiting fixation and the likelihood of placing an errant screw in the canal. Finally, the presence of any metabolic bone disease, which is quite common in patients requiring anterior surgery (tumors, osteoporosis, and fractures), will severely limit the bone screw interface fixation and these anterior systems have been shown to have a very high standalone failure rate, even with the use of autograft, of over 20%. Therefore, except for specific instances, they should be an adjunct to posterior pedicular fixation.

CLOSURE

- After thorough irrigation and meticulous hemostasis, the pleura is inspected, and inadvertent pleural tears should be sutured with running suture using 3-0 Vicryl or staple. The ribs are approximated with 5-6 #2 Vicryl™ sutures and a rib approximator. Chest tube is necessary in transpleural approach, whereas it is not usually required in retropleural approach. When air leak is recognized in a retropleural approach or in case of transpleural approach, a No. 32 chest tube is placed and brought out through a separate stab incision. The chest tube is maintained until no leak is identified on cough, and the drainage is less than 30 mL over a 24-hour period.
- Closed suction drain is placed in the retropleural space and brought out 1–2 interspace caudal to incision.
- Closure is then performed in layers in order: Ribs using #2 Vicryl™, rib bed, innermost intercostal muscle, internal intercostal muscle, external intercostal muscle using #1 Vicryl™, subdermal tissue using 2-0 Vicryl, and subcuticular tissue using 3-0 Vicryl™.
- The anterior serratus and latissimus dorsi muscles are closed with interrupted and running #1 Vicryl™ sutures.
- The chest tube is secured with a #2-0 silk suture and the subcutaneous tissue is approximated with inverted and interrupted #3-0 Vicryl™ in layers if required. We prefer a #3-0 subcutaneous closure but this is an individual surgeon choice.

REFERENCES

1. Perot PL Jr., Munro DD. Transthoracic removal of midline thoracic disc protrusions causing spinal cord compression. J Neurosurg. 1969;31(4):452-8.
2. McCormick PC. Retropleural approach to the thoracic and thoracolumbar spine. Neurosurgery. 1995;37(5):908-14.
3. Fessler RG, Sturgill M. Review: complications of surgery for thoracic disc disease. Surg Neurol. 1998;49(6):609-18.
4. Otani K, Yoshida M, Fujii E, Nakai S, Shibasaki K. Thoracic disc herniation. Surgical treatment in 23 patients. Spine. 1988;13(11):1262-7.
5. Rosenthal D, Dickman CA. Thoracoscopic microsurgical excision of herniated thoracic discs. J Neurosurg. 1998;89(2):224-35.
6. Vanichkachorn JS, Vaccaro AR. Thoracic disk disease: diagnosis and treatment. J Am Acad Orthop Surg. 2000;8(3):159-69.
7. Sundaresan N, Shah J, Feghali JG. A transsternal approach to the upper thoracic vertebrae. Am J Surg. 1984;148(4):473-7.

CHAPTER 13

Technical Pearls in the Management of Spinal Oncology

Mostafa El Dafrawy, Jacob Buchowski

■ STAGING, BIOPSY, AND PROGNOSTICATION

Spinal metastases are a common first presentation for cancer patients. Appropriate work up and thorough evaluation is the first step in the treatment plan. To determine prognosis in those patients, one must identify the extent of the disease burden, performance status, spinal stability, and neurologic function. Treatment options are varied and should be considered in the context of the patients' prognosis.

■ STAGING AND WORK UP

The goal of the work up is to confirm origin and extent of metastatic disease, rule out a primary spinal tumor, and to determine staging and prognosticating. Since primary spinal tumors are exceedingly rare, they are sometimes overlooked during the initial evaluation. Maintaining vigilance and adhering to a standard work up can help avoid this pitfall **(Flowchart 1)**.

- *History:* Is there a known history of metastasis? Is there a history of malignancy and how was it managed (i.e., chemotherapy, radiation, and/or surgery)?
- Complete physical and neurologic examination
- *Imaging:*
  - Magnetic resonance imaging (MRI) of the whole spine with and without contrast
  - Computed tomography (CT) of the chest, abdomen, and pelvis. However, only a CT of the chest is needed in a young patient (<30 years) with a spinal lesion more suspicious of a primary tumor
  - Skeletal survey when multiple myeloma is suspected or bone scan for other skeletal lesions
  - Plain films of the whole spine, standing to assess alignment with physiologic loading, or individual regions C/T/L spine when patient is unable to stand.

Laboratories: Complete blood count (CBC), metabolic panel, serum protein electrophoresis (SPEP), urine protein electrophoresis (UPEP), prostate-specific antigen (PSA),

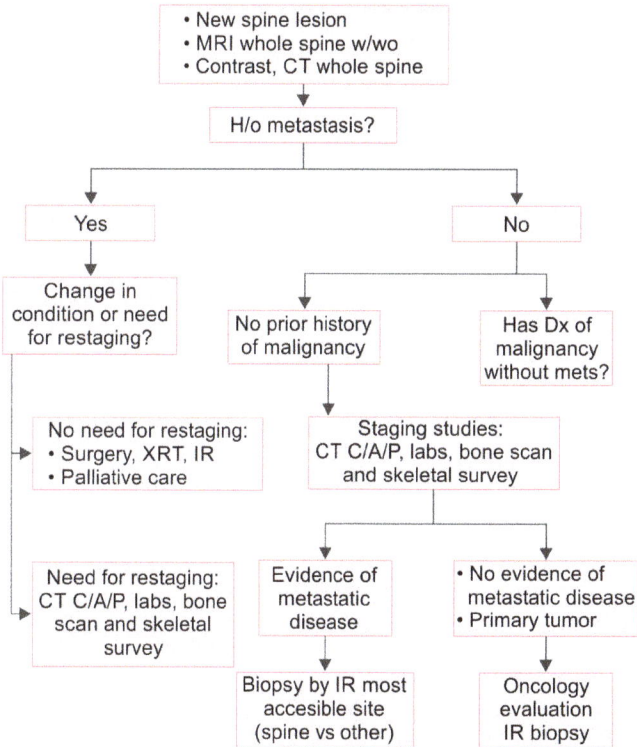

Flowchart 1: Algorithm for work up of new spinal lesions.

(CT: computed tomography; IR: interventional radiology; MRI: magnetic resonance imaging; XRT: external beam radiation therapy)

liver function test (LFT), thyroid panel, metabolic panel, erythrocyte sedimentation rate (ESR), C-reactive protein (CRP), prothrombin time (PT), partial thromboplastin time (PTT), and lactate dehydrogenase (LDH) and other indicated laboratories per medical oncology team to determine source of primary.

■ BIOPSY

Biopsy is an integral part of the diagnosis and treatment of neoplastic disease. Tissue diagnosis is required for a new spinal lesions with no known primary to rule out a primary spinal tumor. Biopsy is also required in patient with a known primary but no biopsy-confirmed metastasis, in such cases, either visceral or spinal lesions can be sampled, whichever is more accessible. In a patient with history of biopsy-proven metastatic disease, a repeat biopsy is usually not required unless there is suspicion of a new tumor based on imaging findings.

To optimize the outcome, the biopsy should be planned with the definitive surgery in mind and should be carried out by or in concert with the team that will ultimately treat the patient.

Biopsy should always be performed in conjunction with the staging studies recommended above (in other words, obtaining a biopsy should never preclude appropriate staging).

Patients may initially present with an isolated spinal lesion with no known primary who presents with neurodeficit either from collpase of a spinal segment and focal kyphosis or rapidly progressive myelopathy or cauda equina syndrome from compression by tumor. In those cases, we resort to the following algorithm for management of unknown isolated spine lesion with neurodeficit **(Flowchart 2)**.

The Musculoskeletal Tumor Society staging system (MSTS) recommends that the biopsy is performed by the treating center to reduce errors in diagnosis, complications, and changes in the course of treatment, noting a 2 to 12-fold increase in errors if the biopsy was performed at the referring institution.[1] A percutaneous transpedicular biopsy by interventional radiology (IR) is usually done through a paramedian approach. The biopsy entry site and pathway are considered contaminated and should be aligned with the plane of incision for the surgery.

Biopsy Pearls

- *The choice of biopsy technique depends on several factors:* Location of the lesion, surrounding structures and bony elements, proximity of the spinal cord and nerve roots, as well as consistency of the lesion. Usually IR guided biopsy is the first choice, open biopsy is needed if the pathologist requires more tissue for a definitive diagnosis.
- It is best to discuss location and choice of biopsy with medical oncologist first.
- Antibiotics should be held prior to biopsy and all patients should have a sample sent for cultures.
- Highest yield biopsy site is the advancing edge of lesion or extraosseous portions.
- Avoid biopsy of the center of the tumor, often necrotic with minimal diagnostic yield.
- Biopsy multiple sites of the lesion if possible
- Avoid disrupting planes as biopsy tract should be excised at the time of surgery.
- Meticulous hemostasis
- Discuss with pathologist to ensure adequate representative tissue has been obtained intraoperatively.

There are three biopsy techniques, choice of technique depends on location and accessibility of lesions and availability and expertise of interventional radiology at the institution.

1. *Fine needle aspiration biopsy (FNA):* Overall accuracy is highest in giant cell tumors 83% and drops to 72% if the suspected lesion is malignant and 23% in benign tumors.[2,3]
2. *Core needle biopsy:* The overall diagnostic accuracy of a core needle biopsy is 89%, with a false-negative rate of 11%.[2,3] The diagnostic yield is higher in patients

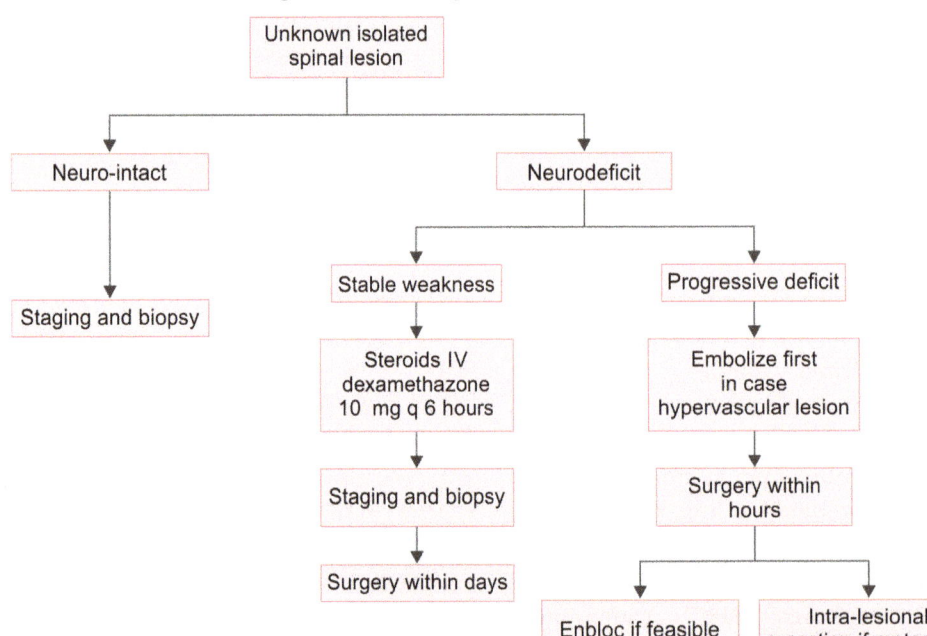

Flowchart 2: Algorithm for management of unknown isolated spine lesion.

with metastatic disease (100%) as compared to those with primary bone lesions (46–76%). The diagnostic yield is lowest in patients with bone lesions caused by hematological malignancies (58%). The diagnostic yield is higher in lytic lesions (88–93%) versus sclerotic bone lesions (46–76%). In addition to lower diagnostic yield, almost a quarter of the sclerotic lesions biopsied (24%) yield a false-negative finding.
3. *Open biopsy:* Image-guided biopsy has replaced open surgical biopsy. Overall accuracy of CT-guided biopsy is ~89% with better accuracy in lytic (93%) than sclerotic lesions (76%).

PROGNOSTICATION

Given the short life expectancy, the benefit of any potential treatment should be weighed against the risks of the intervention and disease burden of patients with spinal lesions. Longevity is highly dependent on the primary tumor histology, overall disease burden, neurologic, and performance status.

The long-term benefits of an invasive, timely, or costly procedure might not become apparent in patients with a short life expectancy (<3 months). An overly aggressive treatment approach might cause more harm than benefit. Patients who are candidates for surgery should have anticipated life expectancy of ≥3 months, and patients undergoing external beam radiation therapy (XRT) should have anticipated survival ≥1 month.

Several frameworks have been developed to determine prognosis and provide key principals and general guidance to treatment. Those frameworks take in consideration important concepts and decision points in the management of spinal lesions including neurological, oncological, mechanical, and systemic patient factors.

Prognostication frameworks determine three main categories:
1. *Performance status:* Karnofsky performance status (KPS) **(Table 1)**[4] and Eastern Cooperative Oncology Group (ECOG) **(Table 2)**[5]
2. *Survival and overall burden of disease:* Revised Tokuhashi, Tomita, and neurologic, oncologic, mechanical, and systemic (NOMS) criteria
3. *Spinal stability:* Spinal instability neoplastic score (SINS) system and neural elements compromise and compression [epidural and spinal cord compression (ESCC) scale].

Tokuhashi score **(Table 3; Flowchart 3)** is a scoring algorithm to guide surgical therapy in patients with spinal metastases. It incorporates tumor histology, neurologic deficit, number of extraspinal bone metastases, extent of visceral disease, performance status, and the extent of vertebral metastases.[6]

Tomita score: The Tomita grading scales **(Table 4)** is commonly used to aid in selecting operative candidates

TABLE 1: Karnofsky performance status (KPS).

Karnofsky	100%	Normal, with no complaints or signs of disease
	90%	Capable of normal activity with few signs or symptoms of disease
	80%	Normal activity with some difficulty, some signs or symptoms of disease
	70%	Self care; incapable of normal activity and work
	60%	Requires some help but can fulfill most personal requirements
	50%	Requires frequent help and medical care
	40%	Disabled; specialized care needed
	30%	Severely disabled; hospital admission indicated; death is not imminent
	20%	Very ill; urgent hospital admission and treatment required
	10%	Moribund with rapidly progressive fatal disease processes

TABLE 2: Eastern cooperative oncology group (ECOG) scale.

Measurement of performance status		
Scale	Grade	Description
ECOG	0	*Fully active:* Able to carry on all predisease activities without restriction
	1	Restricted in strenuous activity; ambulatory; able to perform light work
	2	Ambulatory; able to perform self care; unable to work; bedridden ≤50% of the time
	3	Limited self care; bedridden ≥50% of the time
	4	Completely disabled; incapable of self care; bedridden

to facilitate matching the therapeutic strategy to the life expectancy and predict the patient's survival time.

The Tomita score includes tumor histology, considered the single strongest predictor of postoperative survival, and the extent of visceral and bone metastases.[7]

NOMS framework: NOMS is a decision framework for spinal metastasis that stands for neurologic, oncologic, mechanical instability, systemic disease. NOMS paradigm integrates modern radiation and surgical options and provides evidence-based criteria for treatment of metastatic spinal tumors. Based on the main decision points, NOMS evaluates the patient's systemic disease, sensitivity to oncologic treatments, neurologic symptoms, and mechanical stability to select optimal treatment.[8]

Risk factors: A recent retrospective study identified risk factors associated with survival that should be considered in prognostication of patients with metastatic spine disease.[9]

Poor prognostic factors were as follows:
- Age of >65 years
- ECOG performance status (score 3–4)

TABLE 3: Tokuhashi score.	
Characteristic	**Score**
General condition (performance status):	
• Poor (PS 10–40%)	0
• Moderate (PS 50–70%)	1
• Good (PS 80–100%)	2
No. of extraspinal bone metastases foci:	
≥3	0
1–2	1
0	2
No. of metastases in the vertebral body:	
≥3	0
2	1
1	2
Metastases to the major internal organs:	
• Unremovable	0
• Removable	1
• No metastases	2
Primary site of the cancer:	
• Lung, osteosarcoma, stomach, bladder, esophagus, pancreas	0
• Liver, gallbladder, unidentified	1
• Others	2
• Kidney, uterus	3
• Rectum	4
• Thyroid, breast, prostate, carcinoid tumor	5
Palsy:	
• Complete (Frankel A, B)	0
• Incomplete (Frankel C, D)	1
• None (Frankel E)	2
Criteria of predicted prognosis: Total score (TS) 0–8 = >6 mo; TS 9–11 = ≤6 mo; TS 12–15 = ≤1 yr.	

TABLE 4: Tomita score.	
Prognostic factors	**Points**
Primary tumor:	
• Slow growth (breast, thyroid, etc.)	1
• Moderate growth (kidney, uterus, etc.)	2
• Rapid growth (lung, stomach, etc.)	4
Visceral metastases:	
• Treatable	2
• Untreatable	4
Bone metastases:	
• Solitary or isolated	1
• Multiple	2

Spinal stability: Stability is a significant driver in the decision-making process and requires surgical intervention and is rarely improved by radiotherapy (RT) alone. The following criteria are considered indications for impending spinal instability and collapse:[10]

- ≥3 columns destroyed or >1 column in adjacent vertebrae
- ≥20° kyphosis or ≥50% collapse
- About 50–60% vertebral body involvement in the T-spine, or costovertebral joint destruction + 25–30% vertebral involvement
- About 35–40% vertebral body involvement in the thoracolumbar or lumbar spine or posterior element/pedicle destruction + 25% vertebral involvement.

Spinal Instability Neoplastic Score

Spinal instability neoplastic score is a scoring system specific to patients with cancer, based on six radiographic or clinical categories that are weighted by their contributions to spinal instability. Spinal instability neoplastic score is the most widely used scoring system to determine spinal stability in patients with spinal lesions (**Fig. 1 and Table 5**).

The six component scores are combined with total scores ranging from 0 to 18 to categorize spinal stability as either stable (0–6), potentially unstable (7–12), or unstable (13–18). A score of 0–6 is classified as a stable spine, and no action is needed. A score of 7–12 means stability is indeterminate, warranting surgical consideration. A score of 13–18 indicates spinal instability which requires surgical stabilization.

Spinal stability: SINS and ESCC scale (**Fig. 1 and Table 6**).[11]

Preoperative Embolization

Preoperative embolization of hypervascular tumors such as renal, thyroid, melanoma, hemangiomas, and aneurysmal bone cysts (ABCs) has been shown to reduce intraoperative blood loss and allow for a more complete resection.[12] Traditionally gelatin products have been used, however many other embolic materials are available today, including detachable coils and injectable embolic agents [e.g., Onyx, an ethylene vinyl alcohol copolymer; polyvinyl alcohol

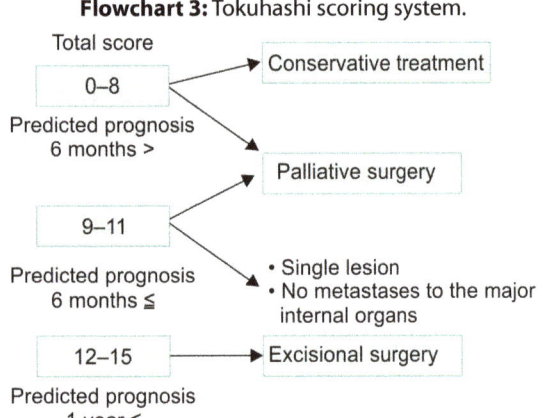

Flowchart 3: Tokuhashi scoring system.

- Primary cancer other than lymphoma, breast cancer, multiple myeloma, kidney cancer, prostate cancer, or thyroid cancer
- >1 spine metastasis
- Metastases to lung or liver or brain
- Previous systemic therapy
- White blood cell count of 11,000/mL
- Hemoglobin level of <10 g/dL.

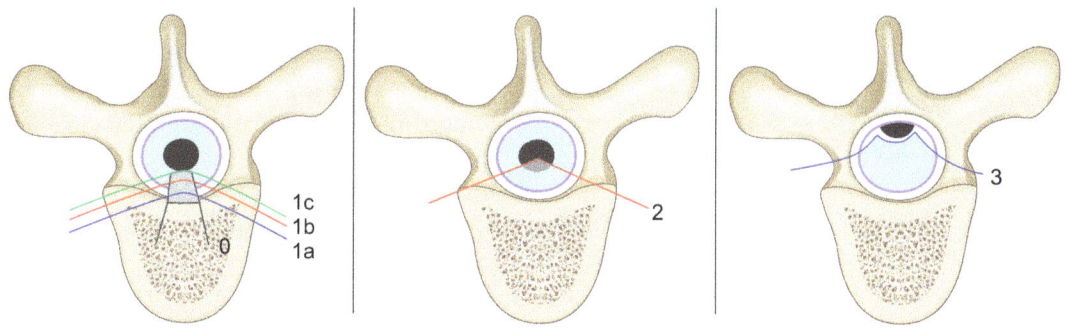

Schematic representation of the 6-point ESCC grading scale

Grade 0 Bone-only disease
Grade 1a Epidural impingement, without deformation of thecal sac
Grade 1b Deformation of thecal sac, without spinal cord abutment
Grade 1c Deformation of thecal sac, with spinal cord abutment, without cord compression
Grade 2 Spinal cord compression, with cerebral spinal fluid (CSF) visible around the cord
Grade 3 Spinal cord compression, no CSF visible around the cord

Fig. 1: Epidural spinal cord compression (ESCC) scale.

TABLE 5: Spinal instability neoplastic score (SINS).

	SINS
Location within the spine:	
• Junctional (occiput-C2, C7–T2, T11–L1, L5–S1)	3
• Mobile spine (C3–C6, L2–L4)	2
• Semi-rigid (T3–T10)	1
• Rigid (S2–S5)	0
Pain relief with recumbence and pain with movement or loading of the spine:	
• Yes	3
• No (occasional pain but not mechanical)	1
• Pain-free lesion	0
Bone lesion quality:	
• Lytic	2
• Mixed lytic or blastic	1
• Blastic	0
Radiographic spinal alignment:	
• Subluxation or translation present	4
• De-novo deformity (kyphosis or scoliosis)	2
• Normal alignment	0
Vertebral body collapse:	
• >50% collapse	3
• <50% collapse	2
• No collapse with >50% body involved	1
• None of the above	0
Posterolateral involvement of spinal elements (facet, pedicle, or costovertebral joint fracture or replacement with tumor):	
• Bilateral	3
• Unilateral	1
• None of the above	0

TABLE 6: Treatment applications of the epidural spinal cord compression (ESCC) scale.

	Radio sensitive tumors	Radio-resistant tumors
Low grade ESCC Grade 0 or 1	Conventional external beam radiation therapy	Stereotactic body radio therapy
High grade ESCC Grade 2 and 3	Conventional external beam radiation therapy	Surgery and stereotactic body radio therapy

(PVA), n-butyl cyanoacrylate (nBCA)]. A 2016 systematic review and meta-analysis[13] of preoperative embolization of 37 studies with a total of 1,305 patients with spinal tumors showed 68.3% rate of complete devascularization for all tumor types. Renal cell carcinoma (RCC) was the most commonly embolized tumor comprising 47.4% of all tumor embolizations. The overall complication rate of embolization was 3.1%. Neurologic injury, either transient or permanent, was the most common related to inadvertent embolization of the spinal cord circulation causing vascular injury or postprocedural tumor swelling and worsening of compression. At our institution, a CT angiogram and IR consultation are performed as part of a tumor meeting. All hypervascular tumors are considered for preoperative embolization.

Another meta-analysis of six pooled studies showed that preoperative embolization can be effective in reducing intraoperative blood loss in spinal metastases surgery in both RCC and mixed primary tumor groups, with a mean decrease in blood loss of 1,226 mL and a significant difference in the pooled outcomes.[14]

The efficacy of preoperative embolization to reduce intraoperative blood loss and improve visibility and resectability of the lesion depends on several factors, including tumor type, surgical approach, and tumor location. Preoperative embolization is also helpful in defining the vascular anatomy.

Embolization can also be used as a palliative measure in patients with unresectable spinal tumors after the failure of

TABLE 7: Hypervascular spinal tumors.		
	Malignant	
Benign	**Primary**	**Metastatic**
Hemangioma	Chordoma	Renal cell carcinoma
Aneurysmal bone cyst	Osteosarcoma	Thyroid carcinoma
Giant cell tumor	Chondrosarcoma	Hepatocellular carcinoma
Osteoid osteoma	Ewing sarcoma	Breast cancer
Osteoblastoma	Plasmacytoma/ multiple myeloma	Sarcoma
Paraganglioma	Giant cell tumor	Melanoma
Osteochondroma	Hemangiopericytoma	Neuroendocrine tumor
Chondroma	Lymphoma	

chemotherapy or RT, palliative embolization is performed to relieve pain and improve neurologic symptoms **(Table 7)**. Embolization reduces the mass effect and relieves spinal cord compression by causing tumor necrosis and shrinkage. Moreover, tumors previously considered unresectable may be respectable after embolization.

ROLE OF CEMENT AUGMENTATION

Vertebroplasty and kyphoplasty are effective palliative procedures for painful vertebral compression fractures in patients with malignant spinal lesions. Percutaneous cement augmentation is common for the treatment of spinal metastases, particularly lytic lesions such as breast cancer. The main objective is pain relief, not indicated as primary treatment for neurologic dysfunction due metastatic epidural spinal cord compression (MESCC) or for gross spinal instability. Pain is relieved by the structural support of the vertebral body by polymethyl methacrylate (PMMA) preventing microscopic movement and macroscopic collapse, as well as exothermic ablation of nerve endings.[15]

Contra-indications:[16,17]
- ≥75% of vertebral body height loss
- ≥20% spinal canal compromise due to epidural disease
- Posterior vertebral body cortex violation
- >3 levels to be treated
- Radiculopathy
- Uncorrected coagulopathy.

Outcomes: In a recent systematic review, patient of cancer-related compression fractures[18] were collected from 2 randomized controlled trials (RCTs), 16 prospective studies, 44 retrospective studies, and 25 case series. A pool of 33,426 patients who underwent vertebroplasty or kyphoplasty were reviewed for improvement in visual analog scale (VAS) for pain, Oswestry disability index (ODI), KPS, and associated complications. At the earliest follow-up, there were clinically relevant improvements in pain, ODI, and KPS scores. Cement leakage was seen in 37.9% and 13.6% of patients treated with PVP and kyphoplasty, respectively, while other symptomatic complications were rare.

ROLE OF RADIOFREQUENCY/ CRYOABLATION

Image-guided spinal tumor ablation is another palliative treatment option for painful spinal metastases. Multiple types of locally ablative techniques can be performed by IR, including radiofrequency ablation, microwave ablation, cryoablation, laser interstitial thermal therapy, and thermal ablation. Local ablative techniques can be done as primary treatment, but are most commonly used as a salvage treatment option in cases where previous RT has been delivered and reirradiation is unlikely to be safe or effective. One study showed that salvage radiofrequency ablation after previous RT decreased pain scores from 7.7 to 3.3 in 1 month, with approximately 50% of patients having a reduction in opioid usage.[19]

Percutaneous cryoablation and radiofrequency ablation are a relatively new minimally invasive techniques for the management of spinal metastases. The role of radiofrequency ablation (RFA) and cryoablation for metastatic disease is currently evolving. Both techniques are useful for treatment of smaller lesions, which if left untreated could ultimately result in fracture and/or neural compression. RFA and cryoablation are frequently combined with vertebroplasty/ kyphoplasty.[20]

Cryoablation: This is performed through formation of a hypoattenuating ice ball, which is readily identified by CT, causing thermal injury to the tumor cells. A liquid gas, commonly argon, is usually used to cool the tip of the cryoprobe. Multiple probes can be used in various orientations to achieve additive overlapping ablation zones. Cryoablation is effective in the treatment of osteoblastic metastases when high impedance often renders RFA or microwave ablation ineffective.

Radiofrequency ablation involves placing a percutaneous needle within the tumor and high-frequency alternating current is passed through the needle, which causes frictional heating and necrosis of the surrounding tissue.[21] RFA or microwave ablation techniques are effective in reducing pain due to spinal metastasis,[22] the main limitation is that the ablation margin cannot be visualized with CT, potentially causing more pain in the post-treatment period.

SURGICAL OPTIONS

Surgery for the treatment of primary and metastatic tumors requires planning and a multidisciplinary approach by surgeons experienced in treating patients with neoplastic spine disease **(Flowchart 2)**.

Selection of the operative technique depends on surgeon familiarity with the various surgical approaches to the spine and treatment goals, location of the lesion, and need for complex spinal reconstruction. Although metastatic spine disease is more prevalent than primary spinal tumors, it is important to recognize the operative approaches and goals of treatment for both. These treatment options are usually palliative and need to strongly consider the patient and their families' wishes. The recovery from any procedure should not be longer than the patient's remaining life span.

DORSAL APPROACHES VERSUS VENTRAL APPROACHES

The goal of surgical decompression is to achieve adequate decompression that allows expansion of the dura and affected nerve roots. Different approaches have been used on the basis of the spinal level of the lesion, bone involvement, and surgeon preference.

The choice of anterior versus posterior or combined approach is a complicated decision that is beyond the scope of this chapter. An anterior tumor location does not require a formal anterior approach. Costotransversectomy and lateral extracavitary approach are options for thoracic anterior decompression and grafting from a posterior-based access. Similarly, transpedicular approaches allow access to the vertebral body for corpectomy with root preservation in the lumbar spine.

Lateral approach allows easier access to the vertebral body and provides anterior column support; however, canal decompression is challenging through lateral exposure. Additionally, anterior thoracic or retroperitoneal lumbar resections may still require posterior fixation.

Pearls

- Instrument long, at least two levels above the tumor level for durable structural support as fusion often does not occur in those patients
- Skip the tumor level
- Arthrodesis often does not occur as most patients are treated postoperatively with RT and/or systemic therapy which will likely prevent fusion.
- Consider large diameter rods and/or multirod constructs.
- Cement augmentation of screws in osteoporotic bone is a potential option.
- Choice of material is important as it will affect the MRI quality later if needed (titanium alloy has better MRI characteristics than cobalt chrome).
- Consider consultation with plastic surgery for closure when postoperative XRT planned or need for flap for a tension free closure.

ANTERIOR APPROACHES

- *Craniocervical junction:* Transnasal, transoral, and transmandibular
- Transcervical craniocervical approach and anterior subaxial cervical approach
- *Cervicothoracic approach:* Manubriotomy and sternotomy
- Posterolateral thoracotomy
- Minimally invasive thoracoscopic approach
- Thoracoabdominal for tumors of the thoracolumbar spine
- Retroperitoneal and transperitoneal anterior lumbar and lumbosacral approach.

POSTERIOR APPROACHES

- Occipital-cervical and posterior subaxial cervical approach
- Transpedicular, costotransversectomy, lateral extracavitary approaches for intralesional resection and en bloc resection. Costotransversectomy approach is one of the most commonly employed approaches in surgical management of spinal oncology including metastatic and primary pathologies. It is considered the work-horse approach for the thoracic spine and the extracavitary approach for the lumbar spine. The technique and pearls are described in detail in a separate chapter. The transpedicular approach is by far the most versatile of these techniques, and can be safely used for a 360° decompression, minimizing the number of procedures patients need.
- Minimally invasive approaches, minimal access, and tubular access from posterior approach
- Posterolateral approach to thoracolumbar metastases—separation surgery
- *Minimally invasive techniques:* (Thoracic and lumbar): Cement augmentation, percutaneous stabilization.
- *Posterior lumbar and sacral approach and stabilization:* Intralesional lumbar resection.

RADIATION THERAPY (EXTERNAL BEAM RADIATION THERAPY, STEREOTACTIC BODY RADIOTHERAPY, STEREOTACTIC RADIOSURGERY) AND SEPARATION SURGERY

Radiation therapy is considered in the management of nearly all patients with spinal metastases, except for the small number with highly chemosensitive tumors or those undergoing enbloc excision **(Flowchart 4)**.

Based on the treatment response to conventional external beam radiation therapy (cEBRT), tumors are classified as either radioresistant or radiosensitive.[23]

- Highly radiosensitive tumors include most hematologic malignancies (i.e., lymphoma, multiple myeloma, and plasmacytoma), as well as selected solid tumors such as seminoma.
- Intermediate sensitivity breast cancer prostate cancer

Flowchart 4: Radiation therapy options.

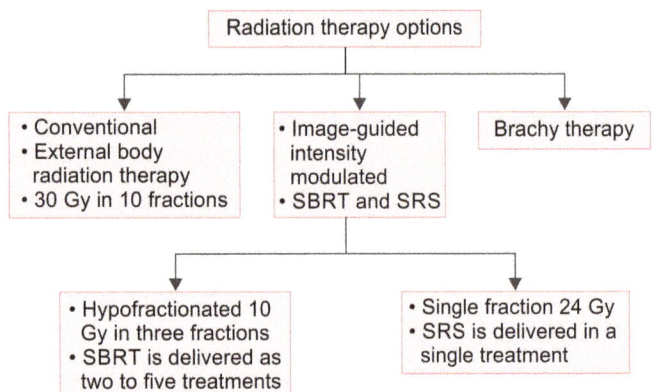

(SBRT: stereotactic body radiotherapy; SRS: stereotactic radiosurgery)

- *Radioresistant:* Most other solid organ malignancies, RCC, colon, nonsmall-cell lung carcinoma (NSCLC), thyroid and hepatocellular carcinoma; melanoma; and sarcoma.

Spinal cord tolerance varies with dosing regimens from 45 to 50 Gy in 180 cGy fractions or 30–33 Gy in 300 cGy fractions. Ideal radiation treatment protocol is not clearly defined, although 30 Gy in 10 fractions is a common treatment algorithm.

Historically, treatment responses for osseous tumors to systemic therapies were limited, and, thus, cEBRT, often defined as 30 Gy in 10 fractions, was the mainstay of treatment for spinal tumors.[24-26]

Technical advancements in patient immobilization, image-guided radiation therapy (IGRT) delivery systems, and sophisticated planning software facilitated the integration of stereotactic body radiotherapy (SBRT) into treatment algorithms and have been a true paradigm changer for the treatment of spinal metastases.

Stereotactic body radiotherapy provides reliable tumor control regardless of tumor histology, volume, and prior radiation. High-dose SBRT for radioresistant tumors overcomes the radioresistance seen in cEBRT. Evidence shows excellent outcomes with SBRT for traditionally radioresistant tumors such as RCC,[27] sarcoma,[28] and melanoma.[29]

Separation surgery provides an alternative to standard open corpectomy and tumor excision. This technique is best employed for patients with significant epidural extension with compression of the thecal sac or cord and radioresistant tumors not amenable for resection. Separation surgery is a single-stage approach, usually posterolateral transpedicle, for epidural decompression, and fusion for treatment of spinal metastases.[30] The goal is to resect enough epidural tumor, creating a 2 mm or more boundary or "safe zone" between cord and the residual tumor. This separation between the tumor and the spinal cord allows high radiation doses (15 Gy[31]) administered with SBRT to the entire tumor margin without risking spinal cord injury. In a series of 186 patients undergoing separation surgery, Laufer et al. reported <5% local progression rate at 1 year with low rates of instrumentation failure.[32] Separation surgery followed by stereotactic radiosurgery provides durable tumor control without the need for extensive tumor excision durable symptomatic responses.

ANTERIOR COLUMN RECONSTRUCTION TECHNIQUES

The debate how to reconstruct the anterior column after corpectomies is still ongoing. The choice of bone graft used in the reconstruction as well as the construct design is controversial. There is very little evidence in the literature to provide guidance on the use of bone graft in metastatic tumor reconstruction. Bony union usually does not occur given the shorter life expectancy of those patients, associated comorbidities, and radiation treatment inhibiting bone fusion.

Factors affecting choice of anterior column reconstruction include patient age, tumor histology, likelihood of achieving clear margins, life expectancy, anatomic location, history of preoperative chemotherapy, history of radiation therapy, bone quality, adequacy of soft tissue coverage, need for local tumor surveillance, graft cost, and graft availability.

The choice of material for reconstruction depends on the nature of the tumor and the patient's life expectancy. Options for anterior column reconstruction include structural iliac crest, structural allograft, commercially available cages, PMMA bone cement, and vascularized fibula or rib. In a survey of spine surgeons treating tumors, structural allograft was most popular for anterior reconstruction, followed by cage reconstruction, and PMMA bone cement.[33] In relatively long-life expectancy (2 years or more), reconstruction was performed using allograft. If the ilium is not involved with tumor, autograft could be considered. In patients with metastatic disease and a short life expectancy, reconstruction using PMMA can be considered. Expandable cages are becoming popular option for reconstruction as they provide immediate stability and allow correction of deformity by dialing in angulation as needed (lordosis or kyphosis).

Technique of PMMA Anterior Column Support

A small trough is hollowed out in the vertebral bodies adjacent to the resection. A piece of silastic tubing or K-wire is used to bridge the area of resection, and the ends of the tubing or wire are inserted in the trough made in the adjacent vertebrae. The tubing or resection site is filled with methyl methacrylate, which is allowed to harden. Additional methyl methacrylate is then used to surround this tubing and fill the area of vertebral body resection.

ROLE FOR EN BLOC RESECTION

There is no defined role for oncologic resection for metastases, however, carefully selected patients with oligometastatic resectable disease may be candidates for wide margin surgery. En bloc resection is considered for solitary metastatic lesions, long disease-free interval with acceptable morbidity, and for radiation-resistant tumors. Other patient factors favoring this technique include excellent patient performance status, favorable tumor histology, and feasibility/low morbidity of resection.

A recent systematic review[34] of 229 cases of primary tumors and 77 cases of solitary metastatic tumors showed median time to recurrence was 113 months for the primary group and 24 months for the metastatic group. Disease-free survival rates at 1, 5, and 10 years were 92.6, 63.2, and 43.9%, respectively, for the primary group. Disease-free survival rates at 1, 5, and 10 years were 92.6%, 63.2%, and 43.9% for the primary group and 61.8%, 37.5%, and 0% for the metastatic group, respectively.

REFERENCES

1. Mankin HJ, Mankin CJ, Simon MA. The hazards of the biopsy, revised: For the members of the Musculoskeletal Tumor Society. J Bone Jt Surg Am. 1996;78(5):656-63.
2. Wu JS, Goldsmith JD, Horwich PJ, Shetty SK, Hochman MG. Bone and soft-tissue lesions: What factors affect diagnostic yield of image-guided core-needle biopsy? Radiology. 2008;248(3):962-70.
3. Nourbakhsh A, Grady JJ, Garges KJ. Percutaneous spine biopsy: A meta-analysis. J Bone Jt Surg Am. 2008;90(8):1722-5.
4. Switlyk MD, Kongsgaard U, Skjeldal S, Hald JK, Hole KH, Knutstad K, et al. Prognostic factors in patients with symptomatic spinal metastases and normal neurological function. Clin Oncol (R Coll Radiol). 2015;27(4):213-21.
5. Bollen L, van der Linden YM, Pondaag W, Fiocco M, Pattynama BP, Marijnen CA, et al. Prognostic factors associated with survival in patients with symptomatic spinal bone metastases: a retrospective cohort study of 1,043 patients. Neuro Oncol. 2014;16:991-8.
6. Tokuhashi Y, Matsuzaki H, Oda H, Oshima M, Ryu J. A revised scoring system for preoperative evaluation of metastatic spine tumor prognosis. Spine. 2005;30(19):2186-91.
7. Tomita K, Kawahara N, Kobayashi T, Yoshida A, Murakami H, Akamaru T. Surgical strategy for spinal metastases. Spine (Phila Pa 1976). 2001;26(3):298-306.
8. Barzilai O, Laufer I, Yamada Y, Higginson DS, Schmitt AM, Lis E, et al. Integrating evidence-based medicine for treatment of spinal metastases into a decision framework: Neurologic, oncologic, mechanical stability, and systemic disease. J Clin Oncol. 2017;35(21):2419-27.
9. Paulino Pereira NR, Janssen SJ, van Dijk E, Harris MB, Hornicek FJ, Ferrone ML, et al. Development of a prognostic survival algorithm for patients with metastatic spine disease. J Bone Joint Surg Am. 2016;98(21):1767-76.
10. Tanechi H, Kaneda K, Takeda N, Abumi K, Satoh S. Risk factors and probability of vertebral body collapse in metastases of the thoracic and lumbar spine. Spine. 1997;22(3):239-45.
11. Bilsky MH, Laufer I, Fourney DR, Groff M, Schmidt MH, Varga PP, et al. Reliability analysis of the epidural spinal cord compression scale. J Neurosurg Spine. 2010;13(3):324-8.
12. Nair S, Gobin YP, Leng LZ, Marcus JD, Bilsky M, Laufer I, et al. Preoperative embolization of hypervascular thoracic, lumbar, and sacral spinal column tumors: technique and outcomes from a single center. Interv Neuroradiol. 2013;19(3):377-85.
13. Griessenauer CJ, Salem M, Hendrix P, Foreman PM, Ogilvy CS, Thomas AJ. Preoperative embolization of spinal tumors: A systematic review and meta-analysis. Thomas1 World Neurosurg. 2016;87:362-71.
14. Luksanapruksa P, Buchowski JM, Tongsai S, Singhatanadgige W, Jennings JW. Systematic review and meta-analysis of effectiveness of preoperative embolization in surgery for metastatic spine disease. J Neuro Intervent Surg. 2018;10:601-6.
15. Fourney DR, Schomer DF, Nader R, Chlan-Fourney J, Suki D, Ahrar K, et al. Percutaneous vertebroplasty and kyphoplasty for painful vertebral body fractures in cancer patients. J Neurosurg. 2003;98(1 Suppl):21-30.
16. Cotten A, Boutry N, Cortet B, Assaker R, Demondion X, Leblond D, et al. Percutaneous vertebroplasty: state of the art. Radiographics. 1998;18(2):311-20; discussion 320-3.
17. Deramond H, Depriester C, Galibert P, Le Gars D. Percutaneous vertebroplasty with polymethylmethacrylate. Technique, indications, and results. Radiol Clin North Am. 1998;36(3):533-46.
18. Sørensen ST, Kirkegaard AO, Carreon L, Rousing R, Andersen MØ. Vertebroplasty or kyphoplasty as palliative treatment for cancer-related vertebral compression fractures: a systematic review. Spine J. 2019;19(6):1067-75.
19. Greenwood TJ, Wallace A, Friedman MV, Hillen TJ, Robinson CG, Jennings JW. Combined ablation and radiation therapy of spinal metastases: a novel multimodality treatment approach. Pain Physician. 2015;18(6):573-81.
20. Wallace AN, Greenwood TJ, Jennings JW. Radiofrequency ablation and vertebral augmentation for palliation of painful spinal metastases. J Neurooncol. 2015;124(1):111-8.
21. Rybak LD. Fire and ice: thermal ablation of musculoskeletal tumors. Radiol Clin North Am. 2009;47(3):455-69.
22. Dupuy DE, Liu D, Hartfeil D, Hanna L, Blume JD, Ahrar K, et al. Percutaneous radiofrequency ablation of painful osseous metastases: a multicenter American College of Radiology Imaging Network trial. Cancer. 2010;116(4):989-97.
23. Rades D, Fehlauer F, Schulte R, Veninga T, Stalpers LJ, Basic H, et al. Prognostic factors for local control and survival after radiotherapy of metastatic spinal cord compression. J Clin Oncol. 2006;24(21):3388-93.
24. Gerszten PC, Mendel E, Yamada Y. Radiotherapy and radiosurgery for metastatic spine disease: what are the options, indications, and outcomes? Spine (Phila Pa1976). 2009;34(22 Suppl):S78-92.
25. Mizumoto M, Harada H, Asakura H, Hashimoto T, Furutani K, Hashii H, et al. Radiotherapy for patients with metastases to the spinal column: a review of 603 patients at Shizuoka Cancer Center Hospital. Int J Radiat Oncol Biol Phys. 2011;79(1):208-13.
26. Maranzano E, Latini P. Effectiveness of radiation-therapy without surgery in metastatic spinal-cordcompression – final results from a prospective trial. Int J Radiat Oncol. 1995;32(4):959-67.
27. Ghia AJ, Chang EL, Bishop AJ, Pan HY, Boehling NS, Amini B, et al. Single-fraction versus multifraction spinal stereotactic radiosurgery for spinal metastases from renal cell carcinoma:

secondary analysis of phase I/II trials. J Neurosurg Spine. 2016;24(5):829-36.
28. Chang UK, Cho WI, Lee DH, Kim MS, Cho CK, Lee SY, et al. Stereotactic radiosurgery for primary and metastatic sarcomas involving the spine. J Neuro-Oncol. 2012;107(3):551-7.
29. Gerszten PC, Burton SA, Quinn AE, Agarwala SS, Kirkwood JM. Radiosurgery for the treatment of spinal melanoma metastases. Stereotact Funct Neurosurg. 2005;83(5-6):213-21.
30. Bilsky MH, Boland P, Lis E, Raizer JJ, Healey JH. Single-stage posterolateral transpedicle approach for spondylectomy, epidural decompression, and circumferential fusion of spinal metastases. Spine (Phila Pa 1976). 2000;25(17):2240-9; discussion 250.
31. Lovelock DM, Zhang Z, Jackson A, Keam J, Bekelman J, Bilsky M, et al. Correlation of local failure with measures of dose insufficiency in the high-dose single-fraction treatment of bony metastases. Int J Radiat Oncol Biol Phys. 2010;77(4):1282-7.
32. Laufer I, Iorgulescu JB, Chapman T, Lis E, Shi W, Zhang Z, et al. Local disease control for spinal metastases following "separation surgery" and adjuvant hypofractionated or high-dose single-fraction stereotactic J Neurosurg Spine. 2013;18(3):207-14.
33. Altaf F, Weber M, Dea N. Evidence-based review and survey of expert opinion of reconstruction of metastatic spine tumors. Spine. 2016;41(20S):S254-61.
34. Cloyd JM, Acosta FL Jr, Polley MY, Ames CP. En bloc resection for primary and metastatic tumors of the spine: a systematic review of the literature. Neurosurgery. 2010;67(2):435-44.

CHAPTER 14

Percutaneous Thoracolumbar Pedicle Screw Fixation

Barrett S Boody, Glenn S Russo, Greg Anderson

■ INTRODUCTION

Pedicle screws can be used to impart spinal stability in a variety of settings including iatrogenic, infectious, traumatic, or degenerative etiologies. The value of pedicle screws is that they can provide three-column support. By utilizing a percutaneous technique, this stability can be applied with minimal damage to the surrounding soft tissues. As with many spinal techniques, patient selection is critical to obtaining successful outcomes with this procedure. Novice surgeons should begin using percutaneous techniques on less complex anatomy, such as degenerative spondylolisthesis or well-aligned trauma cases. Factors such as morbid obesity, significant spinal deformity such as scoliosis or high-grade isthmic spondylolisthesis, severe osteoporosis, or major spinal instability increase the complexity of the procedure and are best pursued as a surgeon achieves proficiency and comfort with this technique.

■ TECHNIQUE

Preoperative Planning

Preoperative planning is critical for successful procedures and in the case of percutaneous pedicle screw placement, it is essential to identify dysplastic pedicles, lumbosacral dysmorphism, or obese body habitus ahead of time with thorough preoperative planning.

- Review high-quality imaging studies, including preoperative X-rays, computed tomography (CT), and/or magnetic resonance imaging (MRI). Make sure to evaluate for lumbosacral dysmorphism and landmarks to identify the correct level.
  - Be aware that large and/or obese patients with poor preoperative radiographic studies due to their size will also be difficult to visualize with intraoperative imaging.
- On preoperative axial imaging studies, estimate the distance lateral to midline your approach will need to be (especially for obese patients) so that you have a straight "line-of-sight" trajectory from the soft tissue dissection through the channel of the pedicle. Starting too medial or lateral with your dissection may result in struggling with tissue retraction during screw placement and increase difficulty of screw placement.
- If you have to "cheat" with your incision, then do so laterally as this deviation is easier to overcome intraoperatively. Remember that an overly medial-based incision will require that you drop your hand laterally and require you to work against a greater soft tissue burden to achieve proper screw placement. This mistake favors a lateral pedicle breech during screw insertion.
- If you are performing a decompression or interbody fusion through the same incision, you may need to place your incision in a slightly more medial location to facilitate laminectomy or facetectomy. However, this medial approach may make the pedicle screw placement more difficult for the reasons described above. In these cases, make sure the incision is placed optimally for the decompression work, but then undermine and mobilize the skin incision, and release extra fascia as needed to enable the proper screw trajectory.
- Additionally, note the lumbosacral junction anatomy when operating in the lower lumbar area as lumbosacral dysmorphism may exist and should be appreciated as they relate to pedicle screw trajectory, but also may affect the determination of the correct lumbar level. Ensure that counting for the correct level is agreed upon with all available imaging. Be aware that the visualization afforded by fluoroscopy may be inferior as compared to flat plate X-ray, so any difficulty visualizing bony anatomy on fluoroscopy can be encountered especially in the setting of obesity, poor bone quality, or hyperlordosis of the lumbosacral spine [due to the extreme obliquity of the C-arm to achieve a true anteroposterior (AP) image of the sacrum].

SET-UP AND POSITIONING

The key to successful minimally invasive spine (MIS) techniques is maintaining high levels of precision and attention to detail at each step, and this begins with positioning. Because each step is built upon the one before it, errors made early in the procedural process will have significant implications later in the case. For example, suboptimal positioning can lead to poor imaging which could lead to errant screw placement. Therefore, time spent on precise set-up will help speed up the later parts of the procedure.

- Make sure the operative table and attachments are fully radiolucent, such as an open Jackson or Allen table. Placement of the chest pad along the sternum (just below the sternal notch) and the hip pads just below the anterior superior iliac spine allows for decompression of the abdomen which will minimize epidural bleeding during surgery as well as decreased the adipose tissue shadow on the lateral fluoroscopy views. Avoid excessively low placement of the hip and thigh pads as this can sometimes make it difficult to visualize the lumbosacral junction on AP fluoroscopy.
- The surgeon should also ensure that the patient is properly aligned on the bed without any rotation or bending.
- Wide draping allows for appropriately lateral start points for proper pedicle screw, or decompressive trajectory, especially in obese patients.

LOCALIZATION

- After sterile preparation and draping of the surgical site, the C-arm is brought into the surgical field. Identify the midline by palpation of the spinous processes and mark the midline with a surgical marker, as this is a helpful frame of reference for the procedure. If the patient is significantly obese or has a prior laminectomy, an AP fluoroscopy can assist with finding midline.
- The surgical levels are identified using reproducible fluoroscopic landmarks, such as the lumbosacral junction. The lateral view is the most accurate way to initially confirm the operative levels. A spinal needle placed under fluoroscopic guidance on the lateral view can be a useful tool to confirm the correct level and also to help plan out your incision. This will help orient your incision to ensure that the areas of interest can be accessed appropriately. In the case of revision surgeon, existing spinal implants can also be used as helpful surgical landmarks.
- The authors find it useful to mark out the location of the pedicles on a "true" AP image of the vertebra. A true AP image is obtained by aligning the C-arm so that there is perfect overlap of the anterior and posterior margins of the superior endplate (endplate projects as a single radiolucent line). Also, a true AP view will show

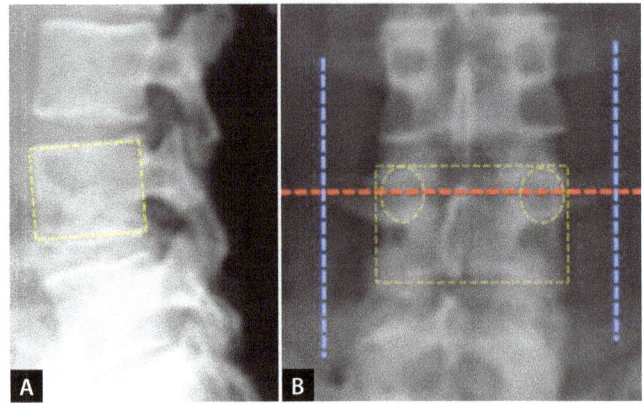

Figs. 1A and B: Lateral (A) and anteroposterior (AP) (B) fluoroscopic images. On the lateral, perfect overlap of the superior and inferior endplates, creating an outline of the vertebral body (yellow dashed line) and pedicles, is obtained. On the AP, the pedicles (yellow dashed circles) are at the upper and outer corners of the vertebra and symmetric in appearance (yellow dashed square). The superior and inferior endplates are overlapped and the spinous process is midline. The red dashed line signifies the proper pedicle screw trajectory and the blue dashed lines are examples of acceptable Wiltse incision placement.
Source: Reprinted with permission: Hartl R., et al. 10-Step-techniques for Minimally Invasive Spine Surgery & Navigation, Thieme: New York. 2021, www.thieme.com.

the pedicles to be located just caudal to the superior endplate and the spinous process to be centered between the pedicles. Do not accept inadequate alignment of the vertebra on fluoroscopic images as this can lead to the inaccurate placement of instrumentation **(Figs. 1A and B)**.

- Using the true AP view, the authors will mark out each vertebral level in the construct prior to making any incisions. A K-wire is placed over the skin and adjusted until it is seen to bisect the mid-portion of the pedicles of a particular level. A transverse line is drawn over the midline of the pedicles.
- The authors prefer to write the vertebral level of each line and the sagittal angle of the C-arm neck to each pedicle line (i.e., L3, +10° of sagittal plane angle on the true AP view) to help facilitate quick transition from one level to the next as the case moves on. Next, vertical lines are drawn over the lateral borders of each pedicle.
- Next, the optimal location of the skin incision(s) must be determined. Generally speaking, the authors use paramedian incisions, positioned about 2 cm lateral to the lateral boarder of the pedicle; however, this can be adjusted based on your preoperative axial images and the size of the patient. In some situations, a single incision can be utilized to reach multiple pedicles due to the lordosis of the spine **(Fig. 2)**. Obese patients will require a more lateral incision to reach the pedicle as their soft tissue envelope is thicker, creating a longer path from the skin to the spine **(Fig. 3)**. In contrast, a very thin patient or when at an upper lumbar instrumentation

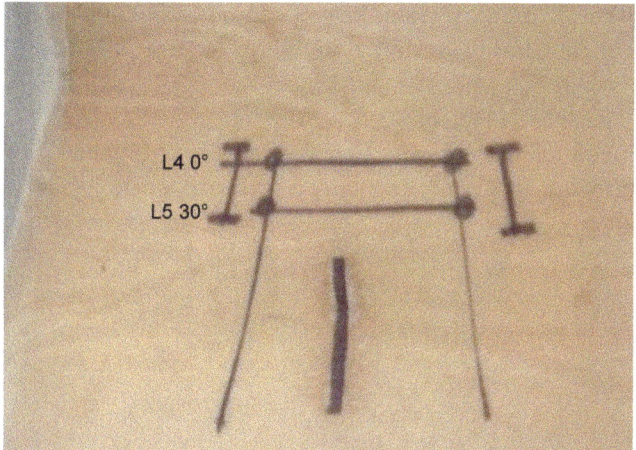

Fig. 2: Clinical example of skin incision localization following fluoroscopic localization. The parasagittal longitudinal Wiltse incisions are marked. Transverse skin markings are made in line with the pedicles (solid circles) and referenced vertebral level and amount of cephalad-caudad angulation needed.
Source: Reprinted with permission: Hartl R., et al. 10-Step-techniques for Minimally Invasive Spine Surgery & Navigation, Thieme: New York. 2021, www.thieme.com.

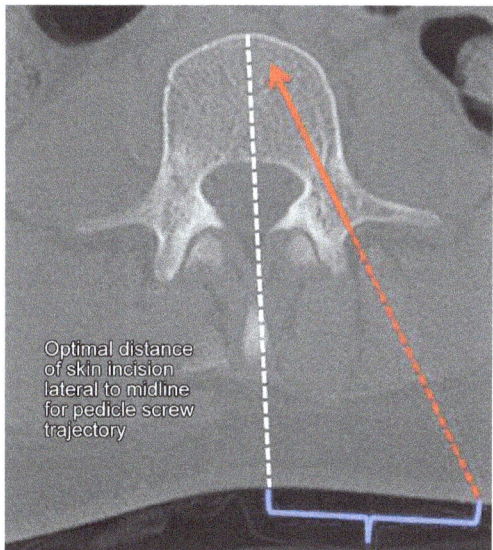

Fig. 3: The medial-lateral distance of the Wiltse incision from midline is proportional to the depth of soft tissue dissection and medial angulation required of the pedicle screw.
Source: Reprinted with permission: Hartl R., et al. 10-Step-techniques for Minimally Invasive Spine Surgery & Navigation, Thieme: New York. 2021, www.thieme.com.

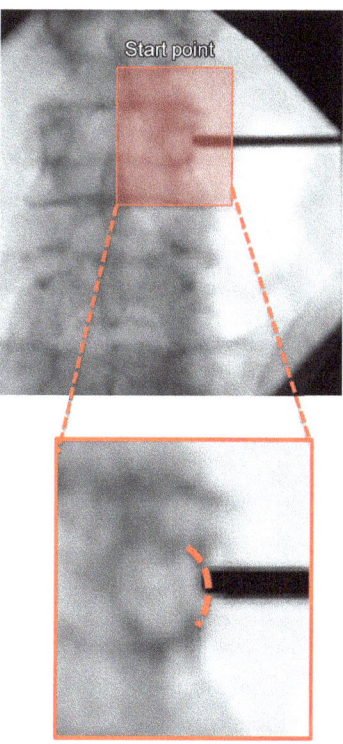

Fig. 4: Left pedicles start at approximately 9 o'clock at lateral border of pedicle. Right pedicles start at approximately 3 o'clock at lateral border of pedicle. Ensure level appropriate medial angulation and proper sagittal trajectory.
Source: Reprinted with permission: Hartl R., et al. 10-Step-techniques for Minimally Invasive Spine Surgery & Navigation, Thieme: New York. 2021, www.thieme.com.

site, one may require a small distance (10 mm) between the incision and the lateral border of the pedicle. Preoperative planning as described above will assist the incision placement.

APPROACH

- After making the skin incision, the two layers of fascia must be incised. Remember that when working lateral, you will encounter both the thicker lumbodorsal fascia and the thinner epimysium covering the erector spinae muscles. It is crucial to adequately release the fascia so that the implants can be placed in the correct trajectory without undue force applied. This may require undercutting of the fascia cephalad and caudad to the skin incision which can be accomplished using curved Mayo scissors.
- Bluntly divide any fascial or muscular bands that will prevent placement of the rods to depth during the later portion of the procedure.
- Palpation will help with the identification of the junction of the transverse process and the facet joint prior to placing the Jamshidi needle.

PEDICLE PREPARATION AND PEDICLE SCREW PLACEMENT

- With the C-arm aligned on the true AP view of a particular level, the Jamshidi needle can be docked at the medial base of the transverse process as medial as possible. The starting point for pedicle entry is generally along the midpoint of the transverse process along the upslope toward the facet joint. The goal is to position the tip of the needle at 9 o'clock (left side) and 3 o'clock (right side) position of the pedicle shadow as seen on the true AP view **(Fig. 4)**. Additionally, the trajectory of the Jamshidi needle should be colinear to the superior vertebral

endplate to maintain a proper cephalocaudal trajectory as it traverses the pedicle.
- If the needle tip is malpositioned, it should be adjusted to achieve this position prior to penetrating the bony surface.
- After the tip has been properly positioned, the cortex of the bone is penetrated with a gentle tap of the mallet on the upper portion of the Jamshidi needle.
  - If the needle slides down the upslope of the facet because of its oblique angle on the bony surface, you can drop your hand laterally and drive the needle through the cortex at the proper start position, then reorient the needle into the appropriate pedicle screw trajectory.
- Next, the position is rechecked fluoroscopically to ensure that the Jamshidi needle remains on target to the pedicle.
- The needle should be held so that the tip is pointing toward the center of the pedicle. By adjusting the amount of angulation of the needle, the needle can be directed toward the center of the pedicle. This allows the surgeon to "steer" the needle into position based on imaging taken during pedicle cannulation.
- After the cortex is breached, so the tip of the Jamshidi needle is only a few millimeters into the bone, use a marking pen to place a line on the needle shaft about 20 mm above the skin edge. This can be helpful in allowing the surgeon to be cognizant of the depth of the needle as it passes into the pedicle. As the needle is inserted into the pedicle, the surgeon will know that the tip of the needle should be at the level of the pedicle/vertebral body junction when the mark reaches the skin edge.
- At approximately 20 mm of depth, the optimal position of the needle tip should still lie within the pedicle shadow about three-fourth of the distance from lateral to medial across the pedicle. Crossing the medial wall prior to the 20 mm of needle advancement would suggest a medial pedicle breach and the needle should be repositioned. Although not required in each case, lateral C-arm imaging is useful to confirm the depth of needle penetration if there are any concerns based on AP images **(Fig. 5)**.
- Assuming the pedicle is safely traversed by the Jamshidi needle, the needle is impacted another 10–15 mm into the bone of the vertebral body. The guidewire is then placed through the needle and advanced further into the bone by several millimeters beyond the tip. The surgeon should be aware of the tactile feedback while advancing these instruments into the bone. A "crunchy" feel of the cancellous bone should be appreciated as the guide wire is advanced beyond the Jamshidi needle. The absence of any resistance to the guide wire suggests malpositioning which should be immediately corrected. Remember that excessive advancement of the guidewire can lead to perforation the anterior cortex, especially in osteoporotic bone with an inherent risk of serious vascular or visceral injury. It can be useful to clamp the guidewires to the drapes to reduce the risk of unintended migration while the remainder of the pedicles cannulated for screw placement.
- Following guidewire placement, some surgeons prefer to tap the pedicles using a cannulated tap **(Fig. 6)**.

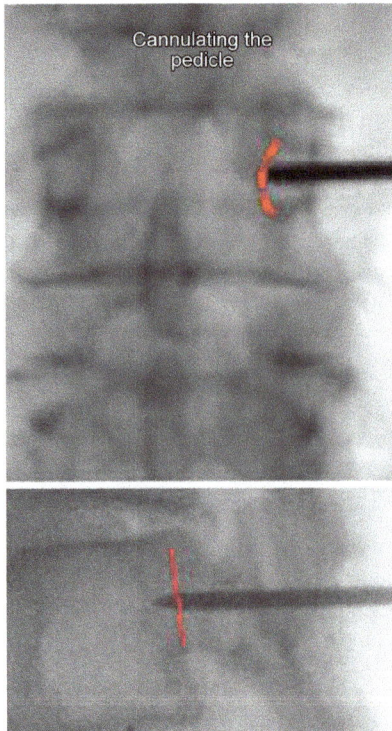

Fig. 5: After advancing the wire approximately 20 mm, check anteroposterior (AP) and lateral imaging. When the guidewire is at the medial border of the pedicle on the AP, the guidewire should be beyond the neurocentric junction on the lateral view.
Source: Reprinted with permission: Hartl R., et al. 10-Step-techniques for Minimally Invasive Spine Surgery & Navigation, Thieme: New York. 2021, www.thieme.com.

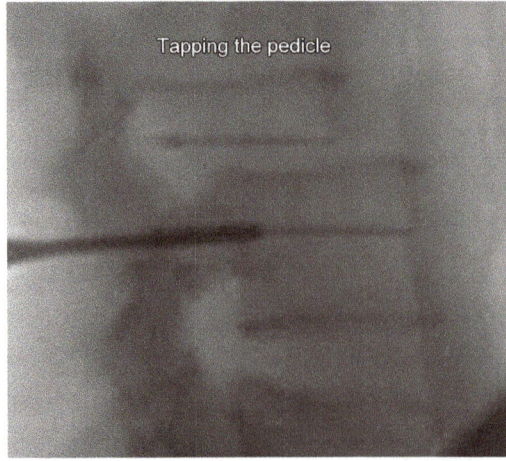

Fig. 6: Tapping of pedicle path using cannulated tap over previously placed guidewire.
Source: Reprinted with permission: Hartl R., et al. 10-Step-techniques for Minimally Invasive Spine Surgery & Navigation, Thieme: New York. 2021, www.thieme.com.

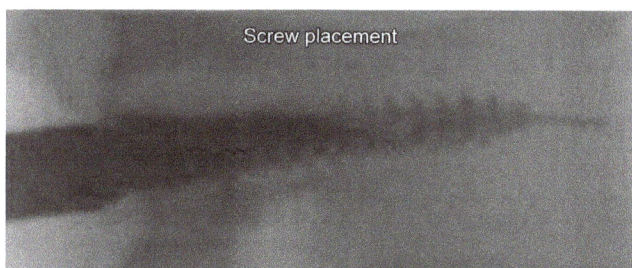

Fig. 7: The pedicle screw is placed over the guidewire. Prior to any further advancement of this pedicle screw, the guidewire should be removed.
Source: Reprinted with permission: Hartl R., et al. 10-Step-techniques for Minimally Invasive Spine Surgery & Navigation, Thieme: New York. 2021, www.thieme.com.

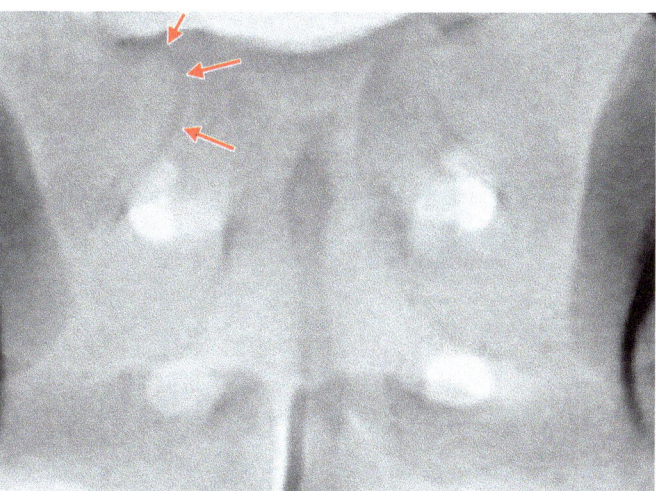

Fig. 8: Anteroposterior view of the S1 pedicle. Red arrows outline the medial border of the pedicle. The medial border of the pedicle resembles an upside-down "fishhook".
Source: Reprinted with permission: Hartl R., et al. 10-Step-techniques for Minimally Invasive Spine Surgery & Navigation, Thieme: New York. 2021, www.thieme.com.

It is important that the guidewires are held and secured manually at all times as surgeon pass instruments over the guidewires to prevent unintended guidewire migration, either advancement or removal. The lateral fluoroscopic view can be helpful to follow the depth of tapping.

- Any amount of axis deviation between the wire and tap or screw can create friction between the two and advance the guidewire, potentially through the anterior cortex. Additionally, the sharp leading edge of the tap or screw can shear and fracture the wire if they are not maintained in a colinear alignment.
- Next, a cannulated pedicle screw can be inserted over the guidewire. Lateral fluoroscopic imaging is helpful to follow the depth of screw placement during this maneuver **(Fig. 7)**. Again, ensure the guidewire is controlled during the screw advancement to prevent inadvertent wire advancement with screw placement. When the pedicle screw has traversed the pedicle, the guidewire can be removed to reduce the risk of wire migration or breakage. These steps are then repeated for all pedicle within the planned construct.
- A slight modification of this technique is used for the S1 pedicle screws. On the true AP view of the sacrum, the S1 pedicles project as an upside down "fishhook" **(Fig. 8)**. The Jamshidi needle tip is docked about 10 mm lateral to the medical edge of the pedicle border and targeted parallel to the sacral ala. The Jamshidi tip should be about three-fourth of the distance between the docking point and the medial wall of the pedicle at the point that 20 mm of needle advancement has been achieved.

PLACEMENT OF RODS

- Minimally invasive spine pedicle screw systems may vary on the exact technique used to place rods, however, most systems have some form of measurement device to determine the appropriate rod length.
- The rods of the appropriate size are selected and contoured as needed.
- The rods are inserted. Depending on the system, the rods can be placed through the incision or via a separate stab incision using a targeting handle to guide the rod into proper position. After the rods have been successfully passed, set screws are placed in each screw to capture the rod securely.
  - Prior to final tightening of set screws, you should confirm sufficient rod length, with rod visualized beyond the proximal and distal screw heads either fluoroscopically or visually.
- Elongated reduction tabs or reduction instruments may be helpful to set the rods within the pedicle screws. Be mindful that excessive reduction force to reduce the rod may compromise screw purchase by pulling the screw out of the vertebral bone.
- Final fluoroscopic imaging is routinely used to confirm adequate rod length, alignment, and capture of each of the implants in the construct.

COMPLICATIONS

There is a similar complication profile between open and percutaneously placed implants. However, in addition, it should be noted that potentially preventable complications of percutaneous pedicle screw placement may result from a wide array of technical or judgment errors during the procedure. Careful attention to detail and use of a structured technique can help to reduce the incidence of these types of complications. Important steps include preoperative planning, proper incision placement, the acquisition of precisely aligned images, adherence to optimal starting points and trajectories during pedicle preparation, and the use of confirmatory imaging for each critical process.

CHAPTER 15

Thoracolumbar Osteotomies: Posterior Column, Pedicle Subtraction, and Vertebral Column Resection

Daniel R Rubio, Sean M Rider, Munish C Gupta

CONSIDERATIONS

Patient selection is key: Decision to pursue spinal osteotomies requires careful patient selection.
- Benefit must be balanced by the increased risk incurred using osteotomy techniques, specifically, the potential for neurologic injury, increased blood loss, greater operative time, and increased risk of infection.[1]
- Risks can be mitigated with improved surgeon comfort with the different osteotomy techniques, careful surgical dissection and decompression, and the use of an experienced anesthesia team comfortable with complex hemodynamic monitoring.

Evaluation of deformity magnitude and flexibility:
- Detailed physical examination:
  - Evaluation of standing and walking coronal and sagittal balance
  - Evaluation of hip and knee contractures—sequelae of long-standing attempt to compensate for sagittal imbalance
  - Supine examination to assess for flexibility of kyphosis, i.e., "can the patient lay flat on the table?"
- Imaging:
  - Routine use of standing radiographs to assess sagittal and coronal balance
  - Supine radiographs to assess flexibility of kyphosis
- In relatively smaller or more flexible deformities, posterior-based apical releases (release of interspinous ligament, ligamentum flavum, and facet capsule) may result in adequate correction.
  - The apical release adds little time and risk to spinal deformity surgery, and, as such, is the first tool utilized by the deformity surgeon.
- In larger or more rigid deformities, the addition of anterior releases or posterior-based osteotomies renders the spine more amenable to correction.

- The progression of spine osteotomies should occur in a step-wise manner from Schwab Grade 1 to 6 according to the *Schwab Anatomical Classification of Spinal Osteotomies*[2] (**Fig. 1**).

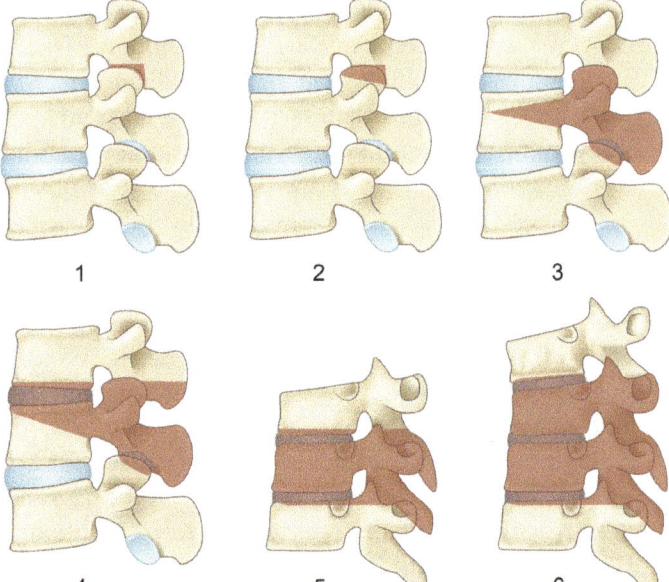

Fig. 1: Schwab anatomical classification of spinal osteotomy. (1) Grade 1, partial facet joint resection. Resection of the inferior facet and facet capsule. (2) Grade 2, complete facet joint capsule. Resection of both the inferior and superior facet, facet capsule, and ligamentum flavum. (3) Grade 3, pedicle and partial body resection. Wedge resection of the vertebral body through the resection of posterior elements and pedicles without resection of neighboring intervertebral disks. (4) Grade 4, pedicle, partial body, and disk resection. Wider wedge resection of the vertebral body through the resection of posterior elements and pedicles with resection of neighboring endplate and intervertebral disks. (5) Grade 5, complete vertebra and disk resection. Complete resection of the vertebral body and both neighboring intervertebral disks. (6) Grade 6, multiple adjacent vertebrae and disk resections. Resection of at least one complete vertebra and partial or complete resection of a second vertebra.

CHAPTER 15: Thoracolumbar Osteotomies: Posterior Column, Pedicle Subtraction, and Vertebral Column Resection

Set-up/instrumentation:
- *Set-up:*
  - Neuromonitoring is required in all cases, including motor evoked potentials (MEPs), somatosensory evoked potentials (SSEPs), and electromyography (EMG) monitoring.
  - Gardner-Wells tongs routine practice in all instrumented cases at our institution: 15 pounds of traction utilized to suspend head throughout the case.
  - Foley catheter and arterial line placed for complex hemodynamic monitoring: Mean arterial pressure (MAP) goal on exposure around 70–80 to minimize blood loss during exposure.
- *Instrumentation:*
  - Leksell rongeurs, standard and narrow
  - Pituitary rongeurs, variable sizes
  - Combination of elevators—Woodson, Freer
  - Penfield dissectors
  - Cobb elevators, variable sizes
  - Curved and straight osteotomes, variable sizes
  - Right-angle impactor.

POSITIONING/APPROACH

- Four poster-type open Jackson table with abdomen free to decrease blood loss and facilitate lumbar lordosis
  - ProAxis table, which allows for extension of both chest and lower extremities through a mid-table hinge, can be used to facilitate correction—especially in pedicle subtraction osteotomies and vertebral column resections (VCRs).
- Meticulous subperiosteal dissection and confirmation of levels by intraoperative radiograph
- *Inferior facetectomy performed half-inch straight osteotome:* Wedge-shaped resection with apex directed cranial and lateral.
- *Apical soft tissue release performed as initial release in all circumstances:*
  - The interspinous ligament released with Leksell rongeur down to the base of the spinous process, which usually exposes a midline raphe in the ligamentum flavum.
  - A Freer or Woodson elevator is inserted in the raphe between the ligamentum flavum and the epidural fat/thecal sac to develop a plane for resection.
  - Kerrison rongeurs are used resect the ligamentum flavum from medial-to-lateral out to the superior articular process (SAP).

POSTERIOR COLUMN OSTEOTOMY
Indications
- Kyphotic deformity that fails to correct to <40–50° in extension
- Scoliotic deformity with Cobb angle >70–75° that does not correct to <40° on bending.
- May be used in significant rotational deformity to facilitate correction, especially in thoracic spine and thoracolumbar junction
  - If osteotomy is performed at level with significant rotational deformity, the resection should be greater on the side of the convexity to avoid introducing coronal plane derangement with osteotomy closure.[3]
- Most effective in the setting of a large disk space (>5 mm of disk height) without bridging osteophytes
  - The fulcrum for the osteotomy is the posterior longitudinal ligament (PLL), so the correction is dependent on both amount of posterior column resection and the amount of anterior opening that can be achieved.
- *Rule of thumb:* Each millimeter of bone resection translates in to approximately 1° of correction.
  - Routinely, 1–1.2 cm of bone is resected which equates to theoretical correction of 10–15° per level.[4]
  - Realistically, each posterior column osteotomy (PCO) can obtain 5–10° of correction per level; and, therefore, to obtain corrections >10°, multiple segmental osteotomies may be required.

Technique
- After the apical soft tissue release, a Freer or Woodson elevator is used to create a plane between the SAP and the underlying neural elements.
- SAP is resected from medial-to-lateral using a Kerrison rongeur through the foramen:
  - Typically, the width of the resection is 7–10 mm and is chevron-shaped with apex pointed caudally.
  - Symmetric resection is important to prevent introduction of coronal plane deformity with osteotomy closure.
- Epidural bleeding is controlled with hemostatic agents and bipolar cautery.
- After osteotomy is performed, transpedicular fixation is achieved and rods are placed.
- The osteotomy is closed either passively by lordosis induced by Jackson table and/or cantilever bending and compression with the rods in place.
  - It is important to check for neural compression both in the canal and foramen after osteotomy closure, especially in the setting of preexisting spinal or neuroforaminal stenosis as shortening the posterior column can decrease surface area in the canal and neuroforamen, respectively.
    - If spinal stenosis is present, the osteotomy can be widened centrally by undercutting the lamina above and below the osteotomy.
    - If neuroforaminal stenosis is present, the osteotomy can be widened laterally by removing the SAP to increase the size of the foramen for the cranial nerve root.

- Set screws are then tightened to maintain the correction.
- Prior to skin closure, intraoperative radiograph is used to check coronal and sagittal balance.

■ PEDICLE SUBTRACTION OSTEOTOMY

Indications

- Fixed sagittal imbalance secondary to regional lumbar hypolordosis and patients who have a circumferential fusion of multiple vertebrae, which prevents the use of PCO for deformity correction
- Most patients considered for pedicle subtraction osteotomy (PSO) require at least 30° of additional lordosis and/or have a large sagittal vertical axis (SVA > 12 cm)
  - This technique allows for 30–40° of focal lumbar lordosis to be achieved.[5]
- Can be used in biplanar correction through asymmetric wedge resection
- Can be combined with multiple segmental PCO of the thoracic/thoracolumbar spine to facilitate correction, especially for rigid global kyphotic deformities
- In planning the level of the osteotomy, given the amount of dural retraction required by the technique, the procedure is usually performed below the level of the conus (L2 or below).

Technique

- After the apical soft tissue release, with or without segmental PCO, transpedicular fixation points above and below the osteotomy are placed to allow for the placement of temporary rods.
- Prior to beginning the osteotomy, epidural bleeding is controlled with hemostatic agents and cottonoids.
- The osteotomy begins with wide decompression at the level of the osteotomy.
  - A complete laminectomy is performed extending laterally out through the pars interarticularis.
  - *The decompression is extended to the level cranial and caudal:* The level of the pedicle superior and inferior to the osteotomy level.
- The pedicle at the level of the osteotomy is skeletonized.
  - A plane between superior and inferior articular processes (IAPs) and the underlying neuroelements is created with a Freer or Woodson elevator.
  - The superior and IAPs are resected with a combination of Kerrison and Leksell rongeurs, exposing the cranial and caudal nerve roots.
  - A plane is created between the transverse process and the underlying soft tissue and nerve root with a Freer or Woodson elevator.
  - The transverse process is resected with a Kerrison or Leksell rongeur.
- A plane is created between the lateral border of the skeletonized pedicle and psoas musculature using a Cobb elevator.
  - If segmental vessels are encountered, hemostasis is obtained with bipolar cautery and hemostatic agents.
  - This soft tissue plane is maintained using sponges and retractors throughout the osteotomy.
- Prior to resection of the pedicle, the cranial and caudal nerve roots are identified and protected.
- A high-speed burr is used to start to decancellate the pedicle and the lateral aspect of the vertebral body.
  - This creates a void for the placement of straight and angled curettes to further decancellate the pedicle and lateral vertebral body.
- The lateral cortical wall of the pedicle is then removed using a Leksell rongeur creating a path to further decancellate the vertebral body with straight and angled curettes.
- The lateral cortical wall of the vertebral body is removed using a Leksell rongeur.
  - The anterior vertebral body is left intact during the decancellation, which is the fulcrum for the osteotomy closure.
- The medial cortical wall of the pedicle is then removed using a Leksell and pituitary rongeur to the level of the posterior vertebral body.
  - The thecal sac is protected with a Freer elevator positioned between the pedicle and dura.
  - The complete resection of the pedicle creates a "super-foramen" that houses the cranial and caudal nerve roots.
- A temporary rod is placed on the resected side and secured with set screws.
- The resection of the contralateral pedicle and lateral wall of the vertebral body is then performed is similar fashion.
- A plane is then created between the posterior vertebral body and the dura using a Freer or Woodson elevator.
- The posterior wall of the vertebral body is then impacted with a right-angle impactor into the void of the decancellated vertebral body.
  - The impacted posterior wall of the vertebral body is removed with a pituitary rongeur while protecting the thecal sac.
- A second temporary rod is placed and secured with set screws.
- After the osteotomy is complete, it is closed in a controlled manner under neuromonitoring.
  - Set screws are loosened during correction to allow for compression across the closing-wedge.
  - During closure, the canal and "super-foramen" are checked for undue compression.
  - Closure can be facilitated with the following maneuvers:
    - ProAxis table—extension of chest and lower extremities

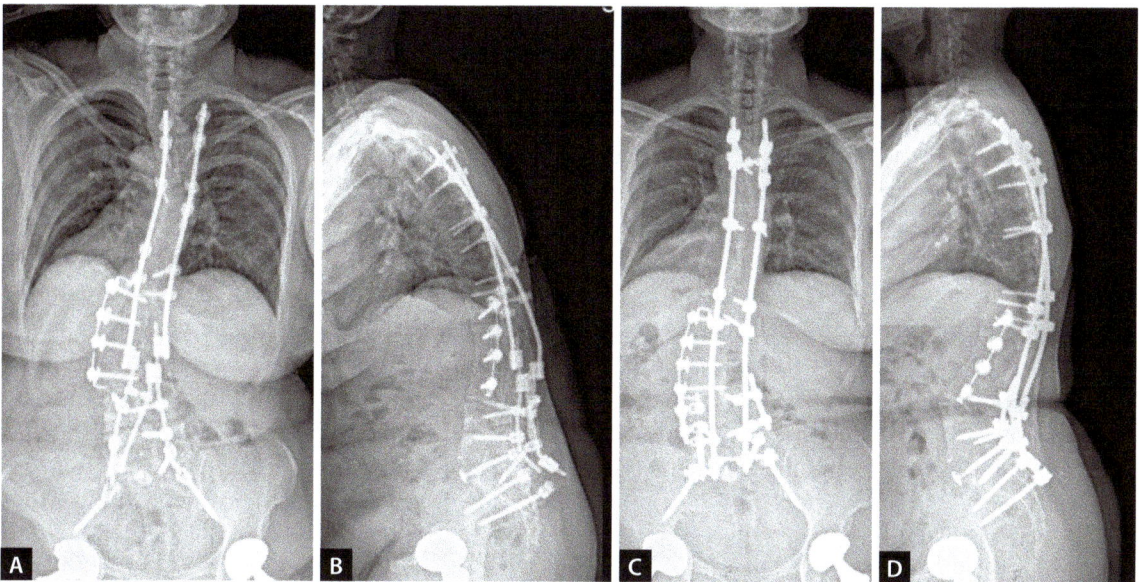

Figs. 2A to D: Pedicle subtraction osteotomy for iatrogenic flatback deformity. (A and B) The preoperative standing anteroposterior (AP) and lateral scoliosis radiographs, respectively, of a 49-year-old female with iatrogenic flatback deformity with significant positive sagittal balance. (C and D) The 1-year postoperative standing AP and lateral scoliosis radiographs, respectively, status-post removal of instrumentation T5-ilium with revision instrumented posterior spinal fusion T3-ilium and L4 pedicle subtraction osteotomy.

- Cantilever bending using a lordotically contoured rod
- Compression across a single set of pedicle screws bridging the osteotomy site
- After closure of the osteotomy, a segmental rod is secured across the osteotomy site extending one vertebral level cranial and caudal.
  - The use of segmental rods decreases rates of rod failure and pseudoarthrosis.[6,7]
- The remaining pedicle screws are attached to a longer rod creating the final four-rod satellite construct.
- The correction is confirmed with intraoperative radiograph prior to skin closure **(Figs. 2A to D)**.

VERTEBRAL COLUMN RESECTION

Indications

Severe rigid spinal deformity (Cobb angles >100°): This technique allows for approximately 60% coronal correction and 45–50° of focal lordosis to be achieved.[8]

Technique

- After the apical soft tissue release, with or without segmental PCO, transpedicular fixation points above and below the osteotomy are placed to allow for the placement of temporary rods.
- Epidural bleeding is controlled with hemostatic agents and cottonoids prior to starting the osteotomy.
- A short-segment temporary rod is secured unilaterally spanning multiple levels cranial and caudal to the level of the osteotomy.
- The osteotomy begins on the side opposite of the temporary rod and starts with a wide decompression of the neural elements.
  - A complete laminectomy is performed at the osteotomy level and the cranial and caudal level.
- A plane is created between the SAP and the underlying with neuroelements with a Woodson or Freer elevator, this is done similarly with the IAP.
  - The SAP and IAP at the level of the osteotomy are resected with a combination of a Leksell and Kerrison rongeurs, exposing the exiting cranial and caudal nerve roots.
    - In cases of scoliosis, the concave resection is done before the convex resection.
    - In cases of kyphosis, either side can be approached first.
- The pedicle at the level of the osteotomy is skeletonized.
  - In the lumbar spine:
    - A plane is created between the transverse process and the underlying soft tissue and nerve root with a Freer or Woodson elevator.
    - The transverse process is resected with a Kerrison or Leksell rongeur.
  - *In the thoracic spine:*
    - The transverse process is resected with a Leksell rongeur exposing the underlying rib head.
    - The rib head of the vertebral body to be resected is removed.
      - A Freer elevator is used to create a plane between the rib and the underlying parietal pleura.

- The rib head is detached from the rest of the rib with a Kerrison rongeur.
  - The rib head is then resected with a Leksell rongeur.
- The rib of the vertebral body caudal to the resected level is removed in a similar fashion.
  - This rib also articulates with the vertebral body and disk to be resected.
- A Cobb elevator is then used to develop a plane between the lateral vertebral body and the psoas muscle (or parietal pleura, if thoracic level) cautiously until the anterior vertebral body is palpable.
  - If segmental vessels are encountered, hemostasis is achieved with bipolar electrocautery, hemostatic agents, and sponges.
- The pedicle is decancellated with a high-speed burr.
- The cranial and caudal nerve roots are identified prior to further resection of the pedicle.
- The lateral pedicle wall and the lateral vertebral body are resected with a Leksell rongeur and a high-speed burr creating a path to decancellate the vertebral body.
- The vertebral body is then decancellated with straight and curved curettes extending in to the cranial and caudal intervertebral disks.
- The cranial and caudal intervertebral disks are removed piecemeal with pituitary rongeurs.
- Next the anterior vertebral body is removed piecemeal using curved curettes, Kerrison, and pituitary rongeurs with care to preserve the soft tissues to vertebral body.
- Attention is then turned to resection of the medial wall of the pedicle.
  - A Freer elevator is placed between medial pedicle wall and the dura, and the medial pedicle wall is resected down to the level of the posterior wall of the vertebral body with Leksell and pituitary rongeurs.
- A temporary rod is then placed on the resected side and secured with set screws.
- The contralateral temporary rod is then removed and the resection of the pedicle, lateral, and anterior vertebral body is performed in similar fashion.
- When the osteotomy is near-complete, a plane is developed between the dura and posterior vertebral body and posterior intervertebral disk with a Freer or Woodson elevator.
- The posterior wall of the vertebral body is then impacted into the void created with decancellation of the vertebral body.
  - Placement of two temporary rods is preferred before the resection of the posterior wall, when possible.
- The impacted posterior vertebral body and remaining intervertebral disks are removed piecemeal with curettes and a pituitary rongeur while protecting the dura.
- Prior to osteotomy closure, a final check of the neural elements is done to ensure there is no undue compression or tethering.
- Osteotomy closure is done in a controlled manner using the following techniques:
  - Manual manipulation
  - Cantilever bending
  - Compression across the osteotomy site

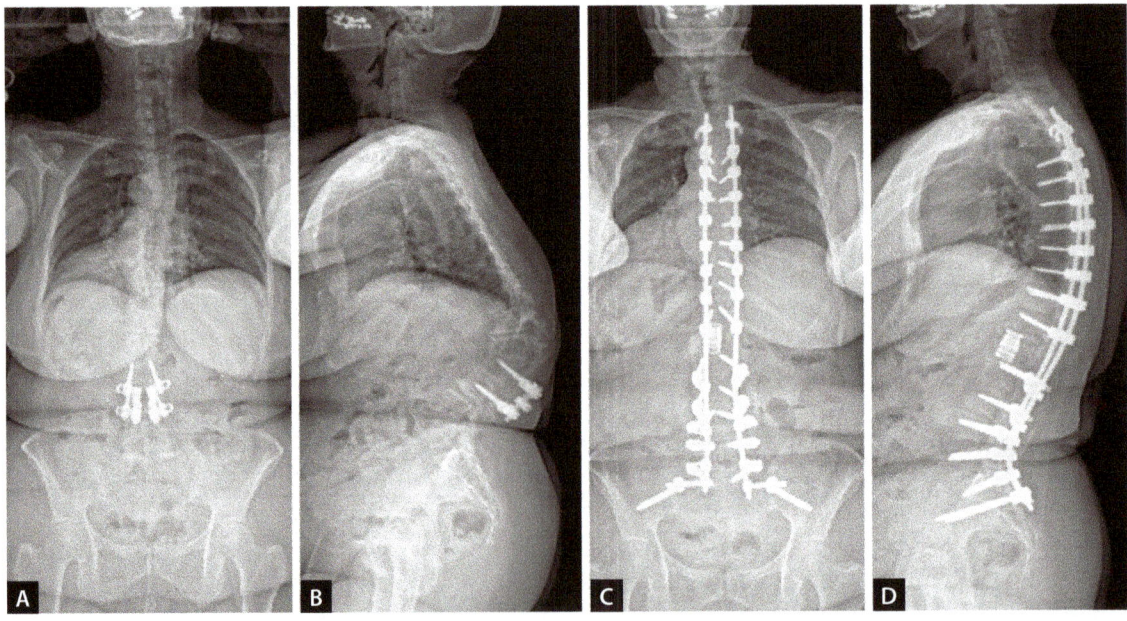

Figs. 3A to D: Vertebral column resection for significant thoracolumbar kyphosis. (A and B) The preoperative anteroposterior (AP) and lateral scoliosis radiographs, respectively, of a 69-year-old female with significant focal thoracolumbar kyphosis. (C and D) The AP and lateral scoliosis radiographs, respectively, obtained at 1-year postoperatively after T2-ilium instrumented posterior spinal fusion with L1 vertebral column resection with placement of expandable cage and T3–T12 posterior column osteotomies.

- The initial temporary rods are gradually exchanged with contoured rods that facilitate the achievement of regional alignment.
- During osteotomy closure, the patient is monitored with neuromonitoring and direct inspection of the neural elements for unacceptable compression.
- *Anterior column support options:*
  - If anterior gap is <5 cm, cancellous grafting or interbody device
  - If anterior gap is >5 cm, interbody device may be required.
- After anterior column reconstruction, the pedicle screws holding the segmental rod are secured with set screws.
- An allograft rib or femoral segment can be used to cover the gap between the lamina at the level of the resection to protect the exposed neural elements as well as to optimize fusion.
- This can be secured with fiber-wire spanning the segmental rods at the level of the resection.
- Intraoperative radiograph is used to confirm adequate correction and balance is obtained **(Figs. 3A to D)**.

REFERENCES

1. Bridwell KH, Lewis SJ, Edwards C, Lenke LG, Iffrig TM, Berra A, et al. Complications and outcomes of pedicle subtraction osteotomies for fixed sagittal imbalance. Spine (Phila Pa 1976). 2003;28(18):2093-101.
2. Schwab F, Blondel B, Chay E, Demakakos J, Lenke L, Tropiano P, et al. The comprehensive anatomical spinal osteotomy classification. Neurosurgery. 2014;74(1):112-20; discussion 20.
3. Bridwell KH, Lenke LG, Lewis SJ. Treatment of spinal stenosis and fixed sagittal imbalance. Clin Orthop Relat Res. 2001;(384):35-44.
4. Diab MG, Franzone JM, Vitale MG. The role of posterior spinal osteotomies in pediatric spinal deformity surgery: indications and operative technique. J Pediatr Orthop. 2011;31(1 Suppl):S88-98.
5. Boachie-Adjei O, Ferguson JA, Pigeon RG, Peskin MR. Transpedicular lumbar wedge resection osteotomy for fixed sagittal imbalance: surgical technique and early results. Spine (Phila Pa 1976). 2006;31(4):485-92.
6. Gupta S, Eksi MS, Ames CP, Deviren V, Durbin-Johnson B, Smith JS, et al. A Novel 4-rod technique offers potential to reduce rod breakage and pseudarthrosis in pedicle subtraction osteotomies for adult spinal deformity correction. Oper Neurosurg (Hagerstown). 2018;14(4):449-56.
7. Gupta S, Gupta MC. The nuances of pedicle subtraction osteotomies. Neurosurg Clin N Am. 2018;29(3):355-63.
8. Suk SI, Kim JH, Kim WJ, Lee SM, Chung ER, Nah KH. Posterior vertebral column resection for severe spinal deformities. Spine (Phila Pa 1976). 2002;27(21):2374-82.

CHAPTER 16

Thoracolumbar Instrumentation

Ron Lehman

■ INTRODUCTION

The goal of thoracolumbar instrumentation is to stabilize the spine to ensure appropriate alignment and rotation, prevent worsening deformity, and restore patient function while facilitating bony fusion. Indications for thoracolumbar instrumentation and fusion include trauma, degenerative conditions, deformity, and tumor. Over the last 120 years, new techniques and technology have been developed to improve thoracolumbar instrumentation. The transpedicular screw is arguably one of the most important advances for spinal fusion.[1] In contrast to plates or hooks, this allowed for a three-column fixation which provides a stiffer construct to facilitate earlier fusion, greater pullout strength, and more powerful deformity correction. To this day, spine surgeons continue to research better and safer ways to stabilize the spine.

■ RELEVANT ANATOMY

The proximity of neural structures and the variability in anatomy can make thoracolumbar instrumentation challenging. Especially in the case of spinal deformity, there can be abnormal pedicles and closer proximity to the spinal cord, nerves, as well as vital structures. For instance, if a pedicle screw is placed beyond the anterior cortical margin of the vertebral body, it may endanger superior intercostal vessels, esophagus, azygos vein, inferior vena cava, thoracic duct, lungs, sympathetic chain, etc. Therefore, it is essential to have a solid understanding of the relevant anatomy for every patient.

■ THORACIC PEDICLE ANATOMICAL CONSIDERATIONS

- *Pedicle diameter:* The smallest transverse diameter is commonly at the level from T4 to T6 with a mean isthmus diameter of 2.5-4.5 mm.[2-4] The medial pedicle wall (MPW) width is two to three times thicker than the lateral pedicle wall.[5] The MPW serves as a "buttress" that can provide a path for the trajectory of the pedicle screw.
- *Pedicle length:* The length generally increases caudally. T1-T3: 26-34 mm, T4-T6: 34-44 mm, and T7-T12: 36-50 mm. The distance from the dorsal cortex to the pedicle isthmus has been reported to range from 10.7 to 13.6 mm depending on the level of the thoracic spine. This is the basis for keeping the pedicle gearshift turned laterally for the first 15 mm, followed by turning medially to enter the vertebral body.[6]
- *Transverse pedicle angulation (TPA):* T12 pedicle is typically neutral, but moving cranially the pedicles converge approximately 25° at T1.[7-9]
- *Sagittal pedicle angulation (SPA):* The SPA is typically between 5 and 15° in the cephalocaudal direction from anterior to posterior throughout all thoracic levels.[8,9]
- *Proximity to neural structures:* Ugur et al. found the dural sac to be juxtaposed to the medial pedicle with mean distance being 0.0-1.4 mm.[10] Liljenqvist reported that the spinal cord is <1 mm from the MPW in adolescent scoliosis. Thoracic nerve roots have been found to be from 0.8 to 6.0 mm from the inferior pedicle depending on vertebral level.[11]

■ LUMBAR PEDICLE ANATOMICAL CONSIDERATIONS

- *Pedicle diameter:* The pedicle width is significantly larger than that of the thoracic pedicle. It is reported that the medial to lateral width increases caudally with L1 about 6-9 mm and L5 12-21 mm.[12,13]
- *Pedicle length:* Pedicle length gradually decreases as moving caudally with L1 at 47-55 mm and L5 is at 43-52 mm.
- *TPA:* The degree of medial angulation from midline increases from L1 to L5. At L1 it is about 6.5-14.5° and at L5 it is about 19-44°.[4,14]

- *SPA:* Generally, the degree of cephalad angulation decreases from L1 (−13 to +15°) to L5 (−8 to +8).[4,14-16]
- *Proximity to neural structures:* The average distance from the lumbar pedicle to the dural sac medially is 1.3-1.6 mm.[17] The mean pedicle-superior nerve root distance is 1.10-1.06 mm. The mean pedicle-inferior nerve root distance is 4.12-5.52. In another study, the results indicated that the average distance from the lumbar pedicle to the adjacent nerve roots superiorly, inferiorly, and to the dural sac medially at all levels ranged from 2.9 to 6.2 mm, 0.8 to 2.8 mm, and 0.9 to 2.1 mm, respectively.[17,18]

INSTRUMENTS SUGGESTED

- Open bottom Jackson Table, or similar (Wilson frame or regular bed with gel rolls is not recommended)
- *Electrocautery:* Monopolar and bipolar
- Straight and angled retractors
- High-speed bur with AM8 bit
- Curved pedicle probe (Gearshift)
- Ball-tipped sounder/feeler probe
- Pedicle tract taps
- Polyaxial pedicle screws (commercially available from many companies)
- Titanium or cobalt chromium rods (5.5-6.0 mm in diameter, material depending on indication).

A NOTE ON HEMOSTASIS

Throughout surgery, it is important to be cognizant of blood loss. Studies show the degree of blood loss to be related to higher rates of complications.[19-22] During the approach, actively cauterize areas of bleeding. Use bone wax and hemostatic agents liberally. Consider intravenous infusion of tranexamic acid. Remember to avoid using a Bovie when near any neural structure. Instead consider using a bipolar device which uses lower energy and thereby a lower risk of neural injury.

TECHNIQUE

Positioning

- Patient will lie supine. Apply Gardner-Wells tongs or utilize a prone view face mask to allow a more neutral physiologic position, and allow anesthesia to access the face and tube if needed. Position bed in slight reverse Trendelenburg. Place arms up even if going up to T2, but place arms are down if going up to C2.
- Confirm adequate padding on any bony prominences.
- Confirm with anesthesia, that perioperative antibiotics and antifibrinolytics have been administered.

Prepping and Draping

- Shave any hair on patient's back. Apply povidone ointment widely (upper neck, along bilateral curves of flank, bottom butt crack), and 10 × 10 drapes. Prepare with sterile gloves and chloraprep sticks × 2. Drape widely.
- Mark vertical incision line, bilateral rib cage, iliac crest, and horizontal hash marks.

Incision and Exposure

- Use a 10 blade to make an incision through skin/dermis to subcutaneous fat.
- Angle Bovie away from the skin when near the cranial or caudal apex of incision to avoid thermal injury to skin. Remember to proactively Bovie areas of bleeding. At the most proximal and distal incisions, place a Weitlander to hold retraction.
- During exposure remember to avoid working self into a hole. Aim to work evenly along spinous processes taking care to obtain adequate hemostasis.
- Once fascia is opened, begin exposing bony spine and switch to Cobb/Bovie when convenient. Use Cobb to carry down and perform a subperiosteal dissection of spinous process and medial lamina. Do not get near any facet until levels are confirmed. May place a perforating towel clamp into each spinous process, place a Penfield 4 into the facet joint, and then shoot a lateral X-ray to confirm levels.
- After confirming appropriate levels, aim for meticulous exposure of posterior elements. With lamina exposed move directly lateral along pars to transverse processes bilaterally. Make sure to remain subperiosteal to reduce bleeding. This is important for anatomic placement of screws and for bony harvest and fusion.
- After bony spine is exposed, use curettes to scrape off all the char from bone. This is to clean the bone for fusion and better visualization of anatomy.
- Prior to facetectomies, make sure to add topical vancomycin powder and change gloves.

Facetectomies

- Thoroughly clean off soft tissue from facet joints. Use half an inch osteotome and mallet to remove inferior 3-5 mm of inferior facet bilaterally at each level to harvest autograft bone and expose starting points. Scrape off the cartilage on top of superior facet to enhance intra-articular arthrodesis.
- Tamponade any bleeding with Raytec sponges usually into the exposed superior facet.
- Do same for lumbar facets. Work from L5 to L1. Remove spinous processes too and use as autograft for later. Bone wax for hemostasis
- If working on thoracic levels, make sure to cover lumbar spine with 1-2 lap sponges.

A NOTE ON PEDICLE FIXATION

Achieving solid and safe fixation with pedicle screws relies on numerous factors, notably bone quality, screw design, and location in bone. To date, several approaches to obtaining stable fixation using augmentations with allograft, various screw designs, polymethyl methacrylate (PMMA), etc., have been described.[23-27] Identifying optimal starting points and trajectories can also enhance bone-screw purchase to achieve necessary construct integrity.

Thoracic Pedicle Fixation Principles

- *Identify starting point:*
  - *Medial to lateral starting point:*
    - *Ventral lamina and the superior facet rule:*
      - The ventral lamina is formed at the confluence of the roof of the spinal canal and the MPW **(Fig. 1)**. A recent study shows this to be a reproducible structure. In about 85% of studied specimens, the ventral lamina is medial to the midline of the superior articular facet (SAF). The remaining 15% of the time, the ventral lamina may be lateral to the midline of the SAF at a mean distance of 0.52 mm. Furthermore, a starting point of 2 mm lateral to the midline of the SAF is associated with only a 0.43% chance placing a screw medial to the pedicle or into the spinal canal. Based on this anatomic relationship of the ventral lamina and pedicle with the SAF, the ideal starting point for the thoracic screw insertion should be 2-3 mm lateral to the midline of the SAF. Using the superior facet rule allows reliable placement safely in the center of the pedicle and avoid having to adjust the starting point depending on the level of thoracic vertebrae[28] **(Fig. 2)**.
  - *Cephalocaudal starting point:* The ideal cephalocaudal starting point and degree of sagittal inclination remains unknown. As described by Kim et al., the cephalocaudal starting point is at the bisected transverse process for the most caudal (T12) and the most cephalad (T1-3) vertebrae. Toward the midthoracic region (T7-T9), the starting point tends to be more cephalad relative to the transverse process (e.g., proximal edge transverse process or junction of transverse process and SAF).[29]
  - *Ventral starting point:* A recently published modification to the "freehand" technique has demonstrated utility in creating a more ventral starting point at the depth of the base of the SAF in the dorsal-ventral axis. The authors of this study suggest using a large rongeur to aggressively remove the dorsal transverse process bone down to the depth of the SAF prior to creating a pilot hole. The main advantages of this is fourfold:[30]
    - By creating a starting point closer to the pedicle entrance, the maximal insertional arc (MIA), as defined as Dhawan et al. as a measure of tolerance for accurate screw placement,[31] increases by 51% when compared to the conventional dorsal starting point.[30]
    - Allows for more medial angulation of screws for improved triangulation
    - Creates an even surface on which to start the pilot hole and seat the screw head
    - Allows harvesting of more autograft bone for arthrodesis
- *Identify trajectory:*
  - There are two popular methods of pedicle screw trajectory: (1) Anatomical trajectory (AT) and (2) straight-forward (SF) technique **(Fig. 3)**.
  - In the AT, the screws are angled about 22° in the cephalocaudal direction along the sagittal plane (may use superior or inferior endplate of vertebral body as

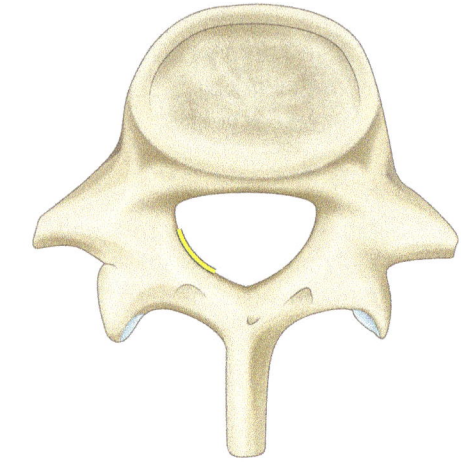

Fig. 1: *Ventral lamina (yellow line),* which is the confluence of the roof of the spinal canal and the medial pedicle wall.

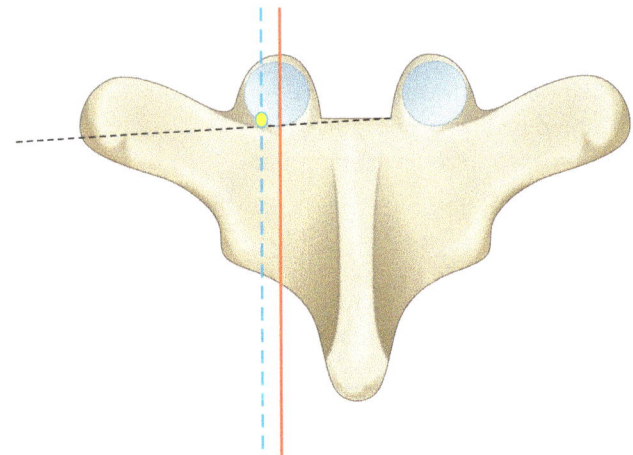

Fig. 2: *Thoracic pedicle medial to lateral starting point.* Red line is the midline of the superior articular facet (SAF). Blue dotted line is 2 mm lateral to the SAF midline.

a reference) and parallel to the anatomical axis of the pedicle. In the superior to inferior dimension, the starting point is typically (when above T10) 3–5 mm cephalad to the junction of the laminar and superior articular process. In the mediolateral dimension, the starting point is centered on the facet joint with the initial orientation being perpendicular to the dorsal cortical surface of the SAF. The starting point for the AT is the same at each thoracic level.

- *SF technique:* The screws are aligned parallel to the superior endplate of the vertebral body in the sagittal plane. Unlike the AT, the starting point for the SF technique varies slightly at each level based on posterior spine anatomy. The thought behind the SF technique is that it will engage more superior cortex of the pedicle and the compact cancellous bone along superior endplate. In theory, there is a higher density of subchondral juxta-endplate bone than in the center of the vertebral body. At the midthoracic spine, the starting point occurs at the junction of the proximal edge of the transverse process where it meets the lamina and the superior facet, medial to the lateral aspect of the pars region.
- *A comparison of approaches:* The main advantage of the anatomic trajectory is that it allows for multiaxial or variable angle screw (VAS) which may allow for easier seating of rod. Although this trajectory may allow for a longer screw, it requires violation of the suprajacent facet and may not allow for sufficient derotation correction. The SF technique may allow for either fixed head or VAS. Fixed head allows for derotation and improved deformity correction. However, the starting point varies by level and may be more difficult to seat rods with fixed heads. When comparing the fixation strength between the two techniques, the pull-out strength for the SF technique was 27% higher than that for anatomic trajectory.

■ Do not countersink or "hub" the pedicle screw in the thoracic spine. Recent literature suggests that this will lead to a decrease in pull out strength compared to the conventional insertion techniques and a predisposition toward iatrogenic fracture of the dorsal lamina, pedicle, and SAF during insertion of screw.[32]

Lumbar Pedicle Fixation Principles

Similar to thoracic pedicle fixation, the first and most important step in successful pedicle screw placement is meticulous exposure of the posterior elements. Once the transverse processes are exposed and facet joints are thoroughly cleaned of soft tissue, use an osteotome to remove the inferior 3–5 mm of the inferior facet and scrape cartilage on top of the superior facet to enhance intra-articular arthrodesis.

■ *Identify starting point:*
- Various entry points of the lumbar pedicle screw have been described. Typically, the ideal starting point of the pedicle screw is traditionally described as the confluence of any of the four lines: (1) Pars interarticularis, (2) mammillary process, (3) lateral border of the SAF, and (4) mid-transverse process **(Fig. 4)**. As per the literature:
  - *Su et al. (Margel's technique):* Junction of the lateral border of superior articular process and the bisector of the transverse process was able to achieve 93.5% accuracy.[33]
  - *Silbermann et al. (Roy-Camille method):* Intersection between midlines of facet joint and transverse process was able to achieve 94.1% accuracy.[34]
  - *Beck et al. (Du and Chao method):* Junction of the mammillary process, inferior aspect of transverse process, and pars interarticularis was able to achieve 96.8% accuracy.[35]
  - *Karapinar et al. (Levin and Edward method):* Intersection of the transverse process with the junction of the middle and lateral one-third of the

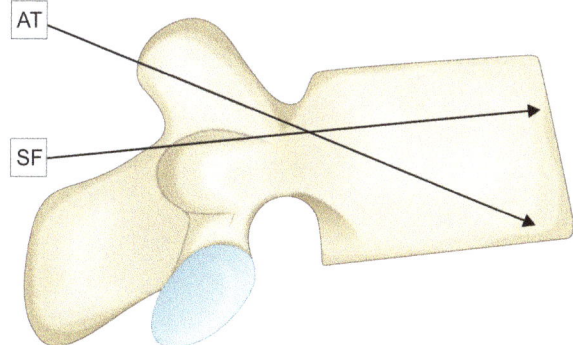

Fig. 3: *Thoracic pedicle trajectory.* Anatomical trajectory (AT) and straight-forward (SF) technique.

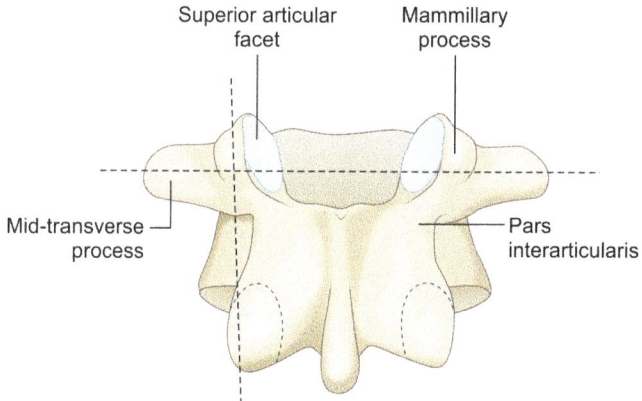

Fig. 4: *Lumbar pedicle starting point.* The ideal starting point of the pedicle screw is traditionally described as the confluence of any of the four lines: (1) Pars interarticularis, (2) mammillary process, (3) lateral border of the superior articular facet, and (4) mid-transverse process.

corresponding superior articular process was able to achieve 97.7% accuracy.[11]

- These techniques use the transverse process and facet joint as important anatomical landmarks to identify the ideal starting point. However, facet orientations may change with degenerative disease which can obscure the facet joint edge and may distort the SAF making it difficult to identify reliable landmarks. Oh et al. uses the junction of the proximal edge of transverse and lamina. He described an entry point of the lumbar pedicle screw which is at the junction of the proximal edge of transverse process and lamina, where it meets the lamina and the superior facet, just lateral to the midportion of the base of the superior process. Authors with this approach yielded an accuracy of 98.6%.[36]

- For the lower lumbar vertebra, surgeons tend to lateralize starting point to avoid medial wall breaches and account for the increasing axial angular trajectory.[12,37] Weinstein et al. recommends a more lateral starting point at the "nape of the neck" which is defined as the lateral and inferior corner of the SAF. Hou et al. advocated that the starting point should move laterally with caudal progression with L5 starting at a point lateral to one-third of the facet width. Su et al. suggest using the mid-lateral pars (MLP) which consists of dense cortical bone at the most medial aspect of the lateral pars. Su et al. suggest vertical line should be 2.9 mm lateral to the MLP at L3 and L4, and 1.5 mm lateral for type 1 L5.[38] This approach does not require violation of the facet joint of the most superiorly instrumented level.

- *Identify trajectory:* As explained above, the transverse and sagittal pedicle angles gradually increase for the former and decrease for the latter from cephalad to caudal. The cranial-caudal angulation should navigate down the isthmus of pedicle into vertebral body. Ideally it should be parallel to the superior end plate.

A NOTE ON CORTICAL BONE TRAJECTORY

Cortical bone trajectory (CBT) has been described as an alternative to the more conventional transpedicular screw placement.[39] In CBT, screw insertion projects along a lateral path in the transverse plane and along a caudocephalad path in the sagittal plane. In contrast to the transpedicular approach, CBT does not penetrate the vertebral body trabecular bone but obtains purchase in the dense cortical bone. The starting point is defined at the junction of the center of the SAF and a line 1 mm inferior to the inferior border of the transverse process of the lumbar vertebra. In both the axial and sagittal planes, the trajectory connects the starting point to the midpoint of the pedicle to the most anterior part of the track. CBT may be less invasive due to the more medial starting point which translates to less muscular dissection and retraction. A laterally directed trajectory in the transverse plane may reduce risk of neurovascular injury. However, CBT requires a smaller and narrower screw which may increase risk of implant failure.[40] Currently, the literature provides promising preliminary data but remains limited due to relatively smaller sample sizes, nonrandomized study designs, and heterogeneity in terms of surgical technique, screw parameters, and follow-up durations **(Figs. 5A and B)**.

Gear Shift Probing

A thoracic gearshift (2 mm blunt-tipped, slightly-curved pedicle finder) is placed into the base of the pedicle searching for a cancellous "soft spot." The amount of ventral pressure in the thoracic is slightly higher that what is needed when inserting the lumbar gear shift probe. Note that the pedicle is quite small in the thoracic spine so allow the pedicle

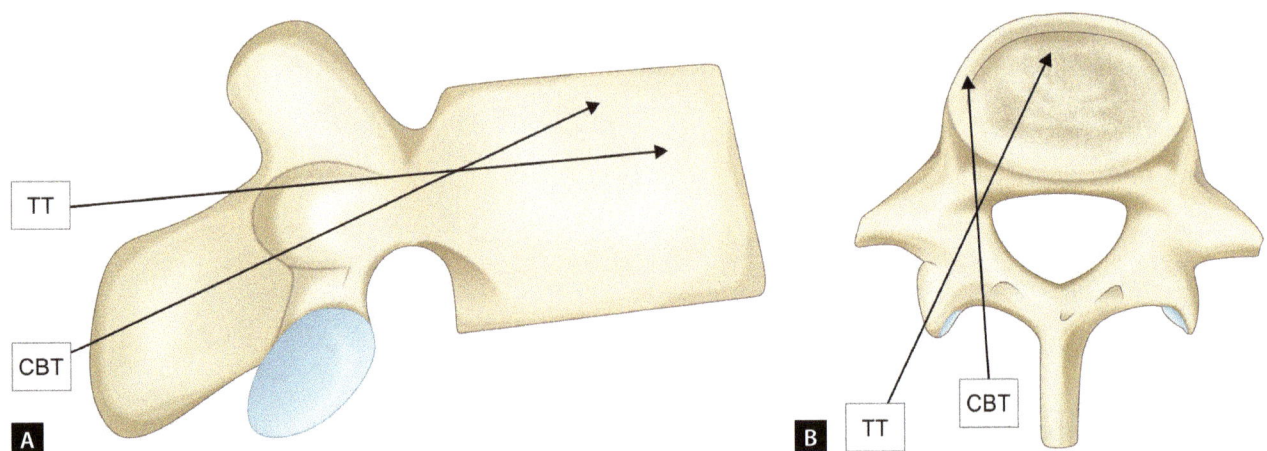

Figs. 5A and B: Cortical bone trajectory (CBT). In both the sagittal (A) and the axial (B) planes, the trajectory connects the starting point (the junction of the center of the superior articular facet and a line 1 mm inferior to the inferior border of the transverse process) to the midpoint of the pedicle to the most anterior part of the track.

finder to "fall" into the pedicle. Initially the tip is pointed laterally to avoid medial wall perforation. After inserting 15–20 mm, remove gearshift and turn tip medially. Then advance pedicle finder about 30–40 mm for the lower thoracic region, 25–30 mm in the mid thoracic region, and 20–25 mm for the proximal thoracic region in adolescents and most adults.[41] Then rotate the finder 180° to make room for the screw.

Palpation of Pedicle Length Measurement

- Use a flexible ball-tipped pedicle sounding or palpating device to palpate the five distinct borders (floor and four walls) and ensure no breech.
- If bleeding through pedicle, ensure only blood is coming out and not cerebrospinal fluid. If excessive bleeding and/or pulsatile bleeding, this may indicate epidural bleeding secondary to medial wall perforation.
- If breech is made, this is the opportunity to redirect screw. Place bone wax into pedicle hole to halt any bleeding.
- With a sounder at base of anticipated tract, mark the length of the tract with a hemostat and measure it.
- Typical screws are 7.5 × 45–50 in mid to lower lumbar spine, 7.0 × 45 in upper lumbar spine, 6.5 × 40–45 in mid to lower thoracic spine, and 6.0–6.5 × 35–40 in the upper thoracic spine. These can be tailored on preoperative imaging depending on how small pedicles are. The author's preference is to avoid going below a 6.0 and would rather go in/out/in with a large screw grabbing the vertebral body, which in his experience is a stronger screw than a tiny 4.5 diameter screw in a tiny pedicle.

Tap, Re-palpate, and Screw Placement

- Under tap with 0.5 mm less than the intended diameter of screw. If difficult, then use next smaller tap.
- Re-palpate tract after tap and re-measure tract.
- Then place screw slowly down pedicle to allow for viscoelastic expansion.
- If pedicle is quite small or when more than one pass has been made, may consider using K-wire to tap. However, make sure that bony floor exists so as to avoid advancing beyond the anterior or lateral cortex.

Confirm Placement of Screw by Imaging and Electromyograph/Neuromonitoring

- Remove all retractors, pack the wound with laps, drape to cover wound, push lights out of way, then un-scrub.
- On X-ray or intraoperative computed tomography (CT) scan, look for medial breaches, trajectories, and if screws are too long.
- If no screw needs to be replaced, then start stimming screws.
- Keep track of which level has the lowest stim and any that are in the single digits.
- Electromyograph (EMG) stimulations are performed with real-time monitoring of thoracic nerve root recordings from rectus abdominus musculature. T6–T12 innervate the recuts abdominus muscles. A triggered EMG < 6.0 mA coupled with a threshold value 65% or more decreased from the "average" of all other T6–T12 screws should serve as a red flag to suspect for medial wall breach.

Rodding

- Place Bovie at upper instrumented vertebrae (UIV) to lower instrumented vertebrae (LIV) and mark the rod. Cut the rod. Using a French bender, dial in the lordosis and kyphosis. Then place in rod and start locking them down.
- Rodding strategy, theory, and nuances may be found in another chapter.
- X-rays again—make sure on lateral that the UIV and distal or LIV are in view, on anteroposterior (AP), make sure shoulders/clavicle are in view to assess balance.
- After X-rays, change gloves again and start to tighten set plugs.

CLOSURE

- Lay down 2 g of vancomycin powder in muscle.
- Place deep drain.
- At the proximal and distal apices, place a cruciate stitch.
- Close fascia with 1 Vicryl in cruciate figure of 8's to include the muscle. After fascial closure, place a superficial drain. Dermal stiches are normal interrupted 2-0 Vicryls. Make sure not to stab the drain. Use cutting 3-0 Vicryl stitch as the subcuticular.
- Prineo on top, wax paper, and tegaderms over incision so the dermabond does not stick to anything. Gauze and tegaderms for the drain. No stitches needed for drains.

A NOTE ON NAVIGATION AND ROBOTIC SURGERY

One of the major challenges in spine surgery is overcoming the inherent lack of direct visualization of relevant anatomical landmarks, especially in case of complex deformity. Meticulous surgical dissection can provide adequate exposure of only the posterior spinal anatomy and requires extensive disruption of soft tissue, longer operative time, and higher blood loss. Computer-assisted navigation (CAN) and robotic surgery attempt to mitigate these challenges. CAN has been shown to increase accuracy rate in pedicle screw placement. Options include two-dimensional (2D) fluoroscopy-based navigation, three-dimensional (3D) fluoroscopy-based navigation, and preoperative and intraoperative CT/magnetic resonance imaging (MRI)-based navigation.[42-44]

Robot-assisted platforms are currently at the leading edge of innovation in spine surgery. This emerging technology is attractive to both surgeons and patients for a number of potential reasons. These include (1) increased accuracy of pedicle screw placement versus historical freehand techniques, (2) minimally invasive applications (small incisions and less dissection, retraction, bleeding, and infection), (3) decreased radiation exposure to the operator versus traditional fluoroscopically-assisted techniques, and (4) reduced human error including fatigue, tremor, and precise repetition. Robotic technology has only been recently introduced in spine surgery, but current literature is already demonstrating promise.[45-49]

REFERENCES

1. Boucher HH. A method of spinal fusion. J Bone Joint Surg Br. 1959;41-B(2):248-59.
2. Kretzer RM, Chaput C, Sciubba DM, Garonzik IM, Jallo GI, McAfee PC, et al. A computed tomography-based morphometric study of thoracic pedicle anatomy in a random United States trauma population. J Neurosurg Spine. 2011;14(2):235-43.
3. Liljenqvist UR, Allkemper T, Hackenberg L, Link TM, Steinbeck J, Halm HF. Analysis of vertebral morphology in idiopathic scoliosis with use of magnetic resonance imaging and multiplanar reconstruction. J Bone Joint Surg Am. 2002;84(3):359-68.
4. Zindrick MR, Wiltse LL, Doornik A, Widell EH, Knight GW, Patwardhan AG, et al. Analysis of the morphometric characteristics of the thoracic and lumbar pedicles. Spine. 1987;12(2):160-6.
5. Kothe R, O'Holleran JD, Liu W, Panjabi MM. Internal architecture of the thoracic pedicle. An anatomic study. Spine. 1996;21(3):264-70.
6. Rampersaud YR, Simon DA, Foley KT. Accuracy requirements for image-guided spinal pedicle screw placement. Spine. 2001;26(4):352-9.
7. Vaccaro AR, Rizzolo SJ, Allardyce TJ, Ramsey M, Salvo J, Balderston RA, et al. Placement of pedicle screws in the thoracic spine. Part I: Morphometric analysis of the thoracic vertebrae. J Bone Joint Surg Am. 1995;77(8):1193-9.
8. Lehman RA Jr, Polly DW Jr, Kuklo TR, Cunningham B, Kirk KL, Belmont PJ Jr. Straight-forward versus anatomic trajectory technique of thoracic pedicle screw fixation: a biomechanical analysis. Spine. 2003;28(18):2058-65.
9. McCormack BM, Benzel EC, Adams MS, Baldwin NG, Rupp FW, Maher DJ. Anatomy of the thoracic pedicle. Neurosurgery. 1995;37(2):303-8.
10. Ugur HC, Attar A, Uz A, Tekdemir I, Egemen N, Genç Y. Thoracic pedicle: surgical anatomic evaluation and relations. J Spinal Disord. 2001;14(1):39-45.
11. Karapinar L, Erel N, Ozturk H, Altay T, Kaya A. Pedicle screw placement with a free hand technique in thoracolumbar spine: is it safe? J Spinal Disord Tech. 2008;21(1):63-7.
12. Hou S, Hu R, Shi Y. Pedicle morphology of the lower thoracic and lumbar spine in a Chinese population. Spine. 1993;18(13):1850-5.
13. Kim NH, Lee HM, Chung IH, Kim HJ, Kim SJ. Morphometric study of the pedicles of thoracic and lumbar vertebrae in Koreans. Spine. 1994;19(12):1390-4.
14. Li B, Jiang B, Fu Z, Zhang D, Wang T. Accurate determination of isthmus of lumbar pedicle: a morphometric study using reformatted computed tomographic images. Spine. 2004;29(21):2438-44.
15. Robertson PA, Stewart NR. The radiologic anatomy of the lumbar and lumbosacral pedicles. Spine. 2000;25(6):709-15.
16. Ebraheim NA, Rollins JR Jr, Xu R, Yeasting RA. Projection of the lumbar pedicle and its morphometric analysis. Spine. 1996;21(11):1296-300.
17. Soyuncu Y, Yildirim FB, Sekban H, Ozdemir H, Akyildiz F, Sindel M. Anatomic evaluation and relationship between the lumbar pedicle and adjacent neural structures: an anatomic study. J Spinal Disord Tech. 2005;18(3):243-6.
18. Attar A, Ugur HC, Uz A, Tekdemir I, Egemen N, Genc Y. Lumbar pedicle: surgical anatomic evaluation and relationships. Eur Spine J. 2001;10(1):10-5.
19. Huang YH, Ou CY. Significant blood loss in lumbar fusion surgery for degenerative spine. World Neurosurg. 2015;84(3):780-5.
20. Yao R, Zhou H, Choma TJ, Kwon BK, Street J. Surgical site infection in spine surgery: Who is at risk? Global Spine J. 2018;8(4 Suppl):5s-30s.
21. Seicean A, Alan N, Seicean S, Neuhauser D, Weil RJ. The effect of blood transfusion on short-term, perioperative outcomes in elective spine surgery. J Clin Neurosci. 2014;21(9):1579-85.
22. Theusinger OM, Spahn DR. Perioperative blood conservation strategies for major spine surgery. Best Pract Res Clin Anaesth. 2016;30(1):41-52.
23. Sanden B, Olerud C, Johansson C, Larsson S. Improved bone-screw interface with hydroxyapatite coating: an in vivo study of loaded pedicle screws in sheep. Spine. 2001;26(24):2673-8.
24. Fini M, Giavaresi G, Greggi T, Martini L, Aldini NN, Parisini P, et al. Biological assessment of the bone-screw interface after insertion of uncoated and hydroxyapatite-coated pedicular screws in the osteopenic sheep. J Biomed Mater Res A. 2003;66(1):176-83.
25. Pfeifer BA, Krag MH, Johnson C. Repair of failed transpedicle screw fixation. A biomechanical study comparing polymethylmethacrylate, milled bone, and matchstick bone reconstruction. Spine. 1994;19(3):350-3.
26. Renner SM, Lim TH, Kim WJ, Katolik L, An HS, Andersson GB. Augmentation of pedicle screw fixation strength using an injectable calcium phosphate cement as a function of injection timing and method. Spine. 2004;29(11):E212-6.
27. Cook SD, Barbera J, Rubi M, Salkeld SL, Whitecloud TS 3rd. Lumbosacral fixation using expandable pedicle screws. An alternative in reoperation and osteoporosis. Spine J. 2001;1(2):109-14.
28. Lehman RA Jr, Kang DG, Lenke LG, Gaume RE, Paik H. The ventral lamina and superior facet rule: a morphometric analysis for an ideal thoracic pedicle screw starting point. Spine J. 2014;14(1):137-44.
29. Kim YJ, Lenke LG, Bridwell KH, Cho YS, Riew KD. Free hand pedicle screw placement in the thoracic spine: is it safe? Spine. 2004;29(3):333-42; discussion 42.
30. Lin JD, Wei C, Shillingford JN, Beauchamp EC, Tan LA, Kim YJ, et al. Evaluation of a more ventral starting point for thoracic pedicle screws: higher maximal insertional arc and

more medial and safer screw angulation. J Neurosurg Spine. 2018;30(3):337-43.
31. Dhawan A, Klemme WR, Polly DW Jr. Thoracic pedicle screws: comparison of start points and trajectories. Spine. 2008;33(24):2675-81.
32. Paik H, Dmitriev AE, Lehman RA Jr, Gaume RE, Ambati DV, Kang DG, et al. The biomechanical effect of pedicle screw hubbing on pullout resistance in the thoracic spine. Spine J. 2012;12(5):417-24.
33. Su P, Zhang W, Peng Y, Liang A, Du K, Huang D. Use of computed tomographic reconstruction to establish the ideal entry point for pedicle screws in idiopathic scoliosis. Eur Spine J. 2012;21(1):23-30.
34. Silbermann J, Riese F, Allam Y, Reichert T, Koeppert H, Gutberlet M. Computer tomography assessment of pedicle screw placement in lumbar and sacral spine: comparison between free-hand and O-arm based navigation techniques. Eur Spine J. 2011;20(6):875-81.
35. Beck M, Mittlmeier T, Gierer P, Harms C, Gradl G. Benefit and accuracy of intraoperative 3D-imaging after pedicle screw placement: a prospective study in stabilizing thoracolumbar fractures. Eur Spine J. 2009;18(10):1469-77.
36. Oh CH, Yoon SH, Kim YJ, Hyun D, Park HC. Technical report of free hand pedicle screw placement using the entry points with junction of proximal edge of transverse process and lamina in lumbar spine: Analysis of 2601 consecutive screws. Korean J Spine. 2013;10(1):7-13.
37. Weinstein JN, Spratt KF, Spengler D, Brick C, Reid S. Spinal pedicle fixation: reliability and validity of roentgenogram-based assessment and surgical factors on successful screw placement. Spine. 1988;13(9):1012-8.
38. Su BW, Kim PD, Cha TD, Lee J, April EW, Weidenbaum M, et al. An anatomical study of the mid-lateral pars relative to the pedicle footprint in the lower lumbar spine. Spine. 2009;34(13):1355-62.
39. Santoni BG, Hynes RA, McGilvray KC, Rodriguez-Canessa G, Lyons AS, Henson MA, et al. Cortical bone trajectory for lumbar pedicle screws. Spine J. 2009;9(5):366-73.
40. Phan K, Hogan J, Maharaj M, Mobbs RJ. Cortical bone trajectory for lumbar pedicle screw placement: A review of published reports. Orthop Surg. 2015;7(3):213-21.
41. Zindrick MR, Knight GW, Sartori MJ, Carnevale TJ, Patwardhan AG, Lorenz MA, et al. Pedicle morphology of the immature thoracolumbar spine. Spine. 2000;25(21):2726-35.
42. Bydon M, Xu R, Amin AG, Macki M, Kaloostian P, Sciubba DM, et al. Safety and efficacy of pedicle screw placement using intraoperative computed tomography: consecutive series of 1148 pedicle screws. J Neurosurg Spine. 2014;21(3):320-8.
43. Cleary K, Clifford M, Stoianovici D, Freedman M, Mun SK, Watson V. Technology improvements for image-guided and minimally invasive spine procedures. IEEE Trans Inf Tech Biomed. 2002;6(4):249-61.
44. Sonntag VK. Navigation and MRI during surgery: spine advances. World Neurosurg. 2012;78(1-2):76-7.
45. Devito DP, Kaplan L, Dietl R, Pfeiffer M, Horne D, Silberstein B, et al. Clinical acceptance and accuracy assessment of spinal implants guided with SpineAssist surgical robot: retrospective study. Spine. 2010;35(24):2109-15.
46. Ringel F, Stuer C, Reinke A, Preuss A, Behr M, Auer F, et al. Accuracy of robot-assisted placement of lumbar and sacral pedicle screws: a prospective randomized comparison to conventional freehand screw implantation. Spine. 2012;37(8):E496-501.
47. Roser F, Tatagiba M, Maier G. Spinal robotics: current applications and future perspectives. Neurosurgery. 2013;72 Suppl 1:12-8.
48. Stuer C, Ringel F, Stoffel M, Reinke A, Behr M, Meyer B. Robotic technology in spine surgery: current applications and future developments. Acta Neurochir Suppl. 2011;109:241-5.
49. Overley SC, Cho SK, Mehta AI, Arnold PM. Navigation and robotics in spinal surgery: Where are we now? Neurosurgery. 2017;80(3s):S86-S99.

CHAPTER 17

Sacral and Pelvic Instrumentation

Barrett S Boody, Glenn S Russo, Joseph D Smucker

■ INDICATIONS

- Sacral pedicle screws are most commonly indicated as part of a fusion construct when:
  - The L5–S1 level has been iatrogenically destabilized [i.e., transforaminal lumbar interbody fusion (TLIF)]
  - The L5–S1 level exhibits instability (degenerative spondylolisthesis, isthmic spondylolisthesis, facet fractures, and lateral listhesis)
  - There is a clinical need for coronal realignment in the coronal plane and/or to provide indirect decompression with foraminal stenosis.
- A comprehensive discussion of the indications for sacral pedicle screws is beyond the scope of this chapter.
  - It is a point of contention as to whether this screw is truly a "pedicle" screw. While the morphology of the sacrum exhibits a pedicle-like passage or connection between the ala and the body of S1, it does not share the tight cortical window of the lumbar pedicles and therefore screws may not have strong cortical engagement in S1.
  - Techniques have been described to improve the pullout strength of the S1 screws, but S1 screws are limited by their predominantly cancellous trajectories.
- With an understanding of these limitations, pelvic instrumentation is utilized to provide improved fixation in lumbosacral fusions. Either S2-alar-iliac (S2AI) or iliac screws may be utilized to achieve similar improvements in strength of fixation, however multiple studies have shown reduced wound complications and screw prominence with S2AI techniques.
  - The most common indication to utilize pelvic instrumentation is for fusions extending from the sacrum to L2 or cephalad.
  - However, in certain situations of osteopenia or osteoporosis, trauma, coronal or sagittal imbalance, or suboptimal S1 screw fixation, pelvic screws can be considered for shorter constructs.
  - Additionally, pelvic screws can be utilized as a bail-out for a failed S1 screw.

■ SET UP/INSTRUMENTATION

- Open Jackson frame
- *Pedicle screws and iliac bolt system of choice:* Make sure to have cross connectors available
- C-arm fluoroscopy
- Intraoperative computed tomography (CT) and navigation system (optional)
- Neuromonitoring with triggered electromyography (EMG) screw stimulation (optional).

■ TECHNIQUE

Sacral Screws

- The starting point for sacral screws is at the confluence of the lateral aspect of the facet and sacral ala, approximately 3 mm cephalad from the inferior aspect of the facet. The cranial/caudal trajectory is determined by intraoperative fluoroscopy with commonly approximately 20-30° medial trajectory.
  - Due to facet hypertrophy and lumbosacral dysmorphism, we believe the S1 pedicle screw exhibits more variability in start points and trajectory than the lumbar pedicle screws. Therefore, when placing free-hand S1 screws, we commonly use the medial canal access afforded by the laminectomy to palpate the medial and superior borders of the pedicle and optimize our starting point and trajectory of the screws.
  - The trajectory can be optimized using intraoperative lateral fluoroscopy to obtain the "tricortical" screw, oriented toward the intersection of the S1 endplate and anterior sacral wall. Engaging the tip of the screw between the S1 endplate and the anterior sacral wall

improves cortical purchase and pullout strength of the screw.
- With obese patients, high pelvic incidences, and high degrees of lumbar lordosis, obtaining the proper medial angulation, can be extremely challenging with open approaches. It is important to have adequate exposure and soft tissue excursion before starting the S1 pedicle screw. Lateral breaches can be dangerous at S1, potentially contacting and injuring vasculature or L5 nerve roots passing over the sacral ala.
- A curved awl is advanced through the starting point, initially with the tip directed lateral for the first 15 mm to avoid medial breaches. The remainder of the trajectory, the awl is redirected medial to avoid lateral breaches.
- The trajectory is palpated with a ball tip probe to detect breaches.
- The trajectory is tapped with a 1 mm undersized tap and probed again for breaches.
- The screw is placed in line with the trajectory.
- The screw can be stimulated then to determine nerve root contact with the screw.
  - Whereas for lumbar screws, medial and inferior breaches contact the exiting nerve only, sacral screws have the potential to contact both L5 and S1. The S1 nerve can be contacted with medial and inferior breaches, but the L5 nerve can be contacted with anterior/lateral breaches. With low voltage stimulated triggered EMGs, ask the neuromonitoring technician which muscle group is demonstrating the response.

PERCUTANEOUS S1 PEDICLE SCREWS

- A slight modification of the percutaneous pedicle screw technique described previously is utilized for fluoroscopic percutaneous pedicles screw placement.
  - On the true anteroposterior (AP) view of S1, the pedicles will appear as an "upside-down fish hook." This is outlining the cortical border of the medial and inferior walls of the pedicle. As it is not a "true" pedicle, the ovoid shape seen in the lumbar vertebrae will not be seen **(Fig. 1)**.
  - The Wiltse plane is created and the Jamshidi needle is started approximately 10 mm lateral to the medial aspect of the pedicle (upside down fish hook) and directed approximately 20–30° medial and in-line with the S1 endplate cranial-caudal.
  - The Jamshidi needle is advanced approximately 20 mm and AP fluoroscopy is taken. The tip of the needle should be approximately three-fourth of the distance from the starting point to the medial aspect of the pedicle at this point. If the tip is at or beyond the medial pedicle at this depth, it must be redirected lateral.
  - After confirmation on AP view at 20 mm that the Jamshidi needle is medial to the pedicle, it is advanced

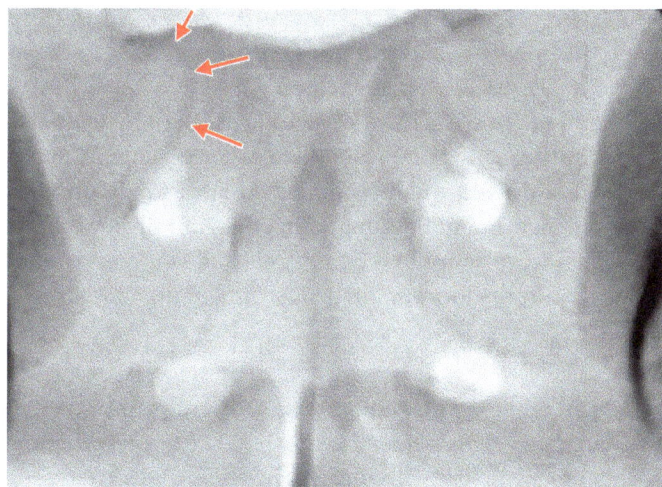

Fig. 1: A true anteroposterior view of the sacrum. The red arrows outline the medial cortical wall of the pedicle. Notice how the medial cortical trajectory resembles an upside-down fish hook. This is a helpful radiographic finding for safe percutaneous placement of S1 pedicle screws.

another 10–15 mm and a guidewire is placed. Ensure cancellous bone is felt with the guidewire to ensure there is not a ventral breach. You can take a lateral X-ray here to confirm your depth as well if desired.
- The pathway is tapped over the guidewire approximately 20–25 mm (just beyond the pedicle) and the screw is subsequently placed.
  - Make sure to remove the guidewire as the screw traverses the pedicle. Leaving the guidewire in during the final seating of the pedicle screw risks shearing off the guidewire tip.

NAVIGATED S1 PEDICLE SCREWS

- A note on navigated S1 pedicle screws. Navigation can be used with an iliac percutaneous pin/reference array to perform percutaneous S1 screw placement as well as using an open technique.
  - Percutaneous techniques proceed similar to the fluoroscopic technique but may not require the use of a guidewire. Be careful using guidewires for navigated techniques as the navigation cannot determine where the guidewire is at any given time. Additionally, make sure to confirm accuracy of the navigation system frequently as you are entirely relying on navigation accuracy for screw placement. We recommend obtaining a second intraoperative spin following screw placement or using triggered EMG screw stimulation and/or fluoroscopic confirmation of screw placement following final screw placement.
  - Placing the array on the sacral spinous process, directed caudally toward the camera, will help facilitate the correct angulation for safe S1 screw placement by staying out of the planned navigated trajectory.

- Open techniques can have the same limitations from soft tissue interference with your trajectory. It is critical that navigated S1 screws have direct, unencumbered line-of-sight passage of instruments during screw placement. Excessive retraction of soft tissues with the instruments creates small amounts of instrument bending/deflection, but the navigation software cannot recognize this and will inaccurately report the location of the instrument tip.

S2AI SCREWS

- We recommend placement of the S1 screws prior to S2AI placement. This allows for the S2AI screw placement to be directly in line with the S1 screw, allowing an easy rod placement.
- Identify the S1 and S2 foramen and the cephalad/caudad start point will be between these foramen. The S2AI screw medial/lateral start point is just lateral to the starting point for the S1 screw. Due to the high degree of lateral angulation, this places the tulip of the screw in line with the S1 pedicle screw.
  - The critical landmark to identify here is the S2 foramen. As long as your starting point is lateral to this, there is no risk of canal intrusion or nerve injury. Lumbosacral dysmorphism may require you to start higher or lower than planned, but as long as you are lateral to the S2 foramen, you will traverse sacral ala with your screw path.
  - More caudad start points will help to get the screw trajectory within the "tear drop" (the confluence of the inner and outer iliac tables and the sacral notch). Higher start points may traverse the narrower, cephalad aspect of the teardrop and result in shorter screws.
- Use the awl to advance approximately 25–30 mm in a direction roughly 30° caudal and 30° inferior, toward the ipsilateral greater trochanter of the hip. Stop before traversing the sacroiliac (SI) joint.
- Take an AP fluoroscopic image of the ipsilateral hemipelvis. Ensure your trajectory is aiming just above the sciatic notch. Once you traverse the SI joint, you will not be able to redirect your trajectory **(Figs. 2A and B)**.
- You may require a mallet to traverse the SI joint, but advance the awl further beyond this by hand. The goal to is advance the awl at least 80 mm total distance.
  - Ventral breaches can risk injuring the external iliac artery and vein and inferior breaches risk injury to the superior gluteal artery, whereas dorsal breaches are benign.
  - If you find that your depth is less than what you anticipated and are stuck at hard cortical bone, use the teardrop view to visualize the trajectory. The fluoroscopy machine is oriented approximately 30° caudal and toward the floor from the direct lateral position. An easy way to communicate this to your X-ray technician is to line up the X-ray beam with your awl and make slight adjustments from there. Using the teardrop view can be a helpful way to make small adjustments or determine if you need to withdraw and make a new pass through the SI joint **(Figs. 2A and B)**.

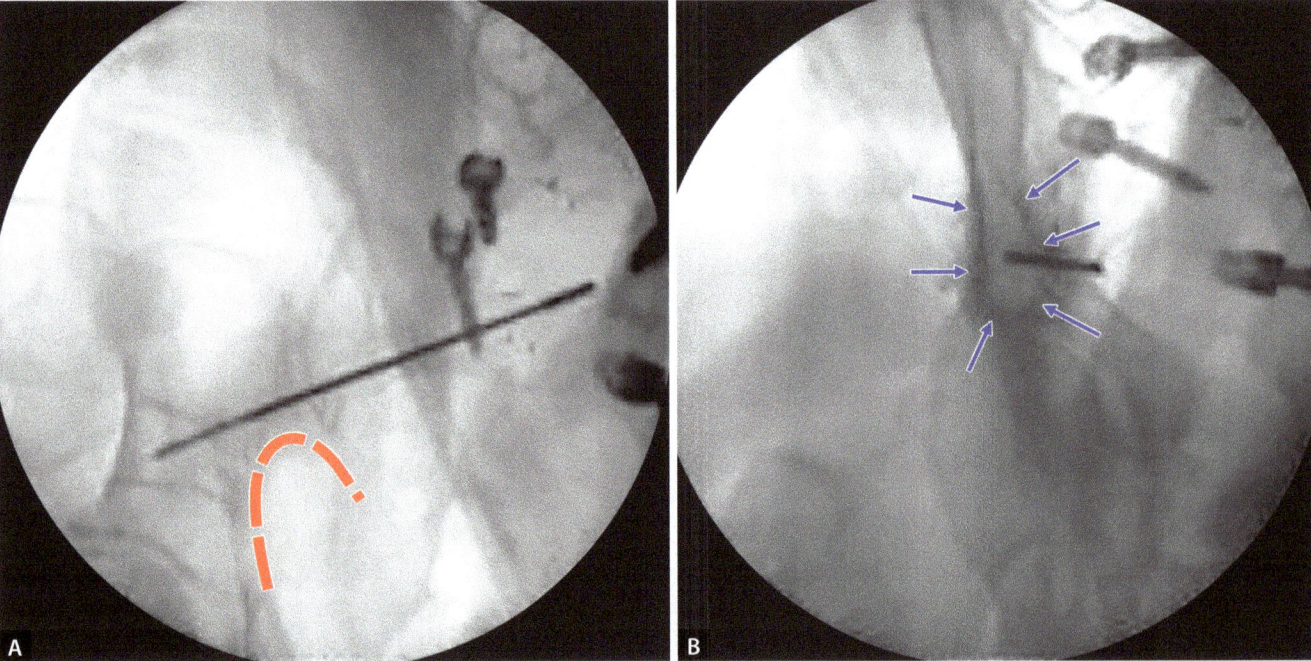

Figs. 2A and B: Anteroposterior and "teardrop" fluoroscopic views. (A) The sciatic notch is visualized by the red dashed line. Make sure to say cephalad to this to prevent iatrogenic vascular injury; (B) The the teardrop view is visualized and outlined with blue arrows. This represents the corridor available for safe pelvic screw placement, either using S2AI or iliac trajectories.

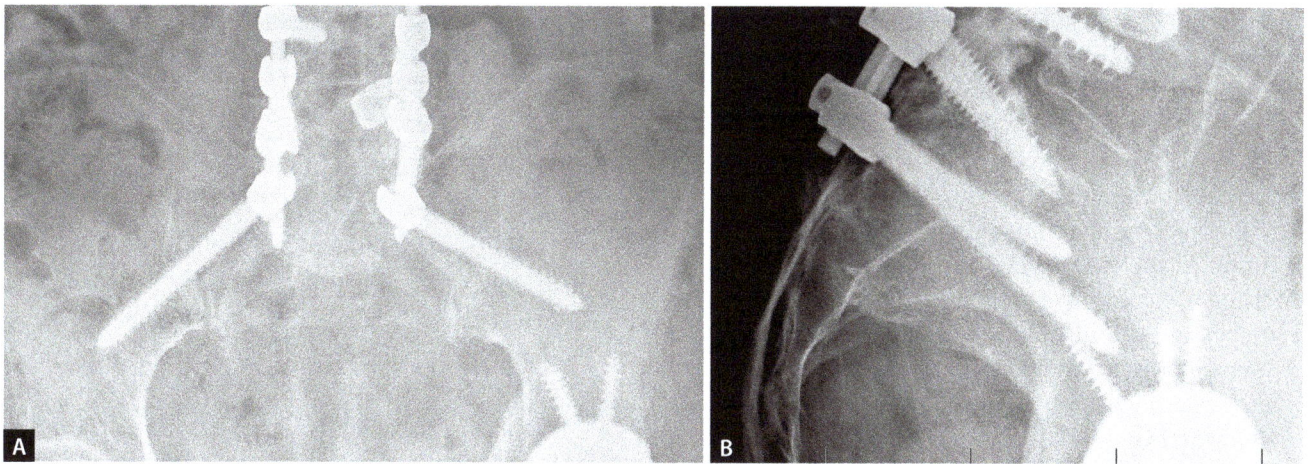

Figs. 3A and B: (A) Anteroposterior and (B) lateral views of S2AI screws. Notice the in-line placement of the S1 and S2AI screws, facilitating straightforward rod placement and low profile of hardware with respect to soft tissues.

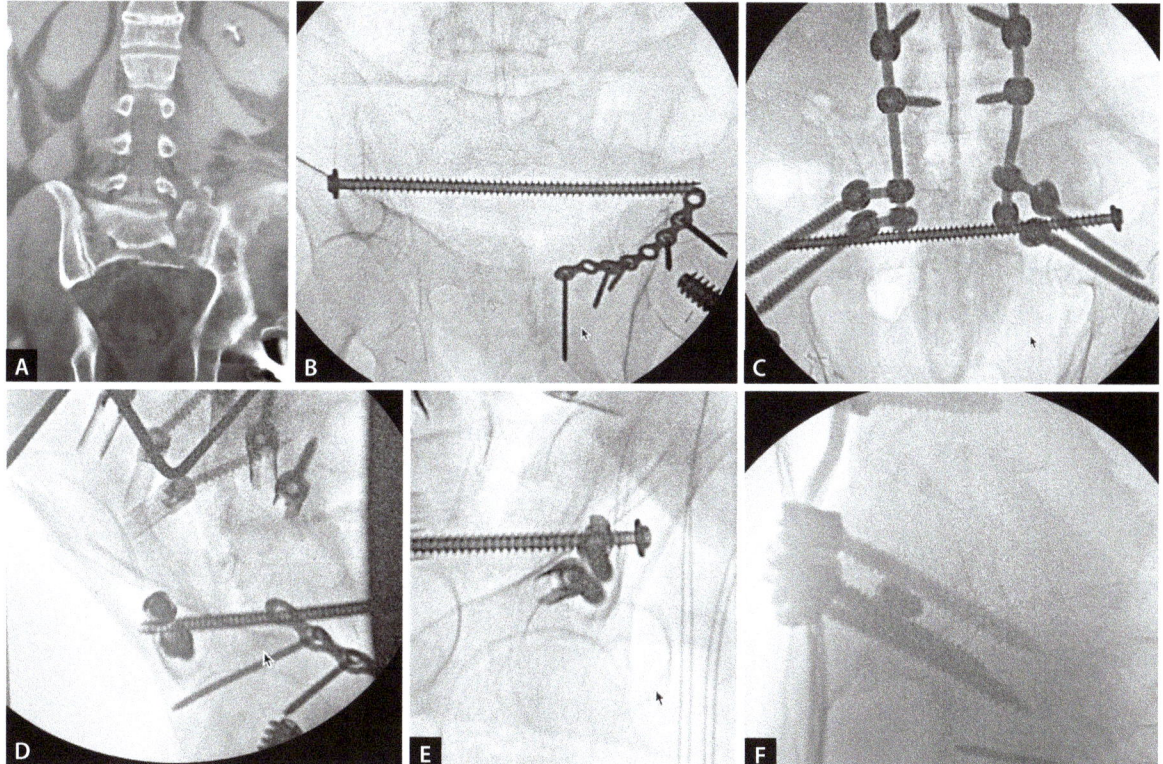

Figs. 4A to F: (A) Comminuted S1 fracture with resultant lumbopelvic dissociation. Patient underwent; (B) Trans-sacral screw placement; (C) As we were unable to perform S2AI screws, iliac screws were placed around the trans-sacral screw; (D and E) Utilizing the tear drop views; (F) Lateral of final construct.

- Once you have advanced the awl to the desired depth (at least 80 mm), use a ball tip probe to detect breaches and measure the length of the screw on the ball tip probe using a hemostat.
- Tap the trajectory using a 1 mm undersized tap. We recommend using a T-handle attachment to generate the force needed to tap. Probe again to detect breaches. Finally, the screw is placed. The T-handle is again helpful to generate the force needed for screw placement **(Figs. 3A and B)**.
- For challenging anatomy, suboptimal X-ray imaging, or lumbosacral dysmorphism, consider converting to iliac screw placement rather than placing a suboptimal or dangerous S2AI screw placement.

ILIAC SCREWS

- Iliac screws require less X-ray imaging, but can be more prominent, leading to wound breakdown and prominence of hardware. Additionally, the screws require offset connectors. However, advantages of this technique is that it can be used when S2AI screws are not appropriate (trauma, tumor, infection) and also that they can be safely performed without intraoperative imaging **(Figs. 4A to F)**.

- To minimize hardware prominence, the posterior superior iliac spine (PSIS) is identified as the start point and approximately a 2 cm width of the PSIS is resected to a depth of approximately 2 cm. This allows for the screw head to be seated beneath the iliac crest, reducing hardware prominence.
- Another technique to mitigate the risk of wound issues is to place the iliac screws through a separate fascial incision. Connectors can be placed deep to the muscle by elevating the muscle between the screws and the primary incision. While this can be cumbersome, it helps preserve a robust soft tissue envelope and decrease the risk of wound complications.
- The awl is inserted within the cancellous bone and directed toward the ipsilateral greater trochanter of the hip, approximately 30° toward the floor and caudally.
- Fluoroscopy can be used if there is concern for breach or suboptimal distance of awl placement prior to feeling a hard, cortical endpoint.
- The path is confirmed with a ball tip probe to detect breaches, tapped with a 1 mm undersized tap, and confirmed again with a ball-tip probe.
- The screw is placed and fluoroscopy is used to confirm placement. Offset connectors are used to connect the iliac screw to the S1 screw/rod construct.

NAVIGATED S2AI SCREWS

- *A few comments on navigation for S2AI screws:*
  - Make sure to obtain a wide field of imaging view to ensure visualization of the pelvic during screw placement. An imaging dataset that is more caudal than that traditionally obtained for navigated S1 fixation will be required in this technique.
  - After starting awl advancement, project the image out 60 mm to visualize the teardrop on the coronal imaging. Decrease the distance of the projection as you advance the screw.
  - Once you traverse the SI joint, the hard iliac cortical bone can deflect the awl tip. Therefore, ensure you have a safe trajectory before you pass the SI joint as the accuracy can be diminished once you traverse this. Rely on tactile feedback with the awl and augment with fluoroscopy if needed for confirmation.

CHAPTER 18

Transforaminal Lumbar Interbody Fusion

Barrett S Boody, Glenn S Russo, Jeffrey Rihn

■ INTRODUCTION

The transforaminal lumbar interbody fusion (TLIF) technique is a versatile and useful tool for the modern spine surgeon to have in their repertoire as it allows for posterior access to the interbody space in the lumbar spine. The TLIF allows for direct foraminal decompression with removal of the ipsilateral facet, indirect decompression through discectomy and distraction through the disk space using a prosthetic cage, as well as increased fusion area through decortication of the vertebral endplates and bone grafting of the intervertebral space. While most commonly utilized in degenerative conditions, the TLIF has a wide spectrum of applications, such as deformity correction, treatment of osteodiscitis, and management of multiply recurrent disk herniations.

■ INSTRUMENTS/SET-UP

- Open Jackson with hips extended on a flat top plate
- Standard laminectomy trays
- Posterior lumbar pedicle screws and rod systems (per surgeon preference)
- Osteotomes
- Lamina spreader
- Interbody shavers and dilators
- *Interbody curettes and pituitaries:* These will commonly be provided by the manufacturer. They have varied lengths and offsets as compared to many standard instruments.
- *Interbody cages (per surgeon preference):*
  - Options include polyetheretherketone (PEEK), titanium, carbon fiber, or structural allograft
  - PEEK and titanium cages may have expandable options.
- Fluoroscopy.

■ APPROACH

- We utilize a standard open approach using an extensile posterior midline incision localized at the levels of interest.
- The lamina and transverse process of the cephalad and caudad levels to be fused are exposed using a standard subperiosteal approach and deep retractors are placed.
- Level identification is critical, as facetectomy is an irreversible step and obligates fusion at the level excision. It is the authors' practice to use a Kocher clamp on the spinous process of interest, to reconfirm the level selection, a bayoneted forceps can also be placed over and around the exposed transverse process and on the lateral radiograph will be in line with the concordant pedicle. We tend to find the more ventral the placed instrument for level identification (spinous process versus transverse process), the more accurate the localization will be.

■ FACETECTOMY

- The interspinous ligament is removed at the fusion level with a rongeur.
  - Take care not to remove excessive bone from the spinous processes, as the disk space distraction is performed with a lamina spreader placed between spinous processes.
- With regard to planning of the facetectomy, we choose to perform the procedure on the side of more significant clinical symptoms (radiculopathy). However, since both foramen and lateral recesses will be decompressed, the surgeon can choose the side for facetectomy per their preference.
  - For coronal deformity correction, the facetectomy is placed on the side of disk wedging for correction of the deformity with cage placement.

- For sagittal deformity, a posterior column osteotomy can be performed in addition to increasing disk space height through the TLIF. Make sure to well decompress the contralateral foramen to avoid creating new foraminal stenosis with the application of compression and lordosis at the operative level.
- Next, the inferior articular process (IAP) is removed. This can be done with a burr or osteotome, with the latter being the authors' preference.
  - First, a cephalad trajectory with the osteotome beginning at the junction of the IAP with the lamina is used, separating the medial lamina from the IAP to the level of the pars. Ensure the trajectory is not directed too deep; to the level of the cauda equina or traversing nerves.
    - Do not pass cephalad to the level of the pars, as cephalad to this point you may no longer be protected ventrally by the ligamentum flavum.
  - Next, the osteotome is pointed lateral, separating the IAP from the cephalad pars. This will commonly then separate the IAP from the lamina. However, if there is an arthritic facet, the IAP fragment may be densely adhered to the superior articular process (SAP). A rongeur, osteotome, or Cobb may be used to disconnect the IAP from the SAP if needed.
- Next, a lamina spreader is placed in the interspinous region between the spinous processes and gently distracted. Place the handle away from the side of the facetectomy.
- The SAP will now be removed. First use a forward angle curette to identify a plane between the ligamentum flavum and the ventral surface of the SAP.
  - If there is severe lateral recess stenosis and this plane is difficult to open, the ligamentum flavum can be removed in the midline and progressively removed laterally until the SAP is reached. We commonly leave the ligamentum flavum if able, as it protects the traversing nerve and dural sac during interbody work.
- A Kerrison rongeur is used to resect enough medial SAP until a Woodson elevator can be used to palpate the medial and ventral surface of the caudad pedicle.
  - This is a critical step, as incorrectly identifying and protecting the pedicle may result in a pedicle fracture during SAP resection, requiring caudad extension of fusion to potentially asymptomatic levels.
- After the medial and cephalad aspects of the pedicle are identified, the Woodson elevator is placed out into the foramen above (cephalad to) the pedicle. This serves as a guide for the SAP osteotomy because an osteotomy directed over the Woodson will assuredly avoid the pedicle and subsequent fracture. With a twist, the osteotome is then used to separate the SAP. A rongeur can then be used to remove the fragment. This will expose Kambin's triangle, through which the disk access and preparation will be performed.
  - At this point in the case, significant bleeding may be encountered initially. A large facet artery may be adherent to the SAP and start bleeding during removal. Additionally, multiple epidural venous bleeders will be encountered overlaying the disk space.
  - Use bipolar cautery and Floseal with patties to control the bleeding. While patties are placed in Kambin's triangle, use a Kerrison rongeur to finish resection any residual bone. Ensure that there is no bony tether out laterally.

Disk space preparation and cage placement:
- Once bleeding is controlled, identify the traversing and exiting nerve roots. Safe and early identification prevents iatrogenic injury to these structures.
- Bluntly expose the intervertebral disk using a Woodson elevator or Penfield 4. Use a nerve root retractor to protect the traversing nerve root. Minimal retraction of the traversing nerve root should be necessary for disk space access.
- Perform the annulotomy with an 11 or 15 blade on a long handle, making a box-shaped defect.
- The authors prefer to use an "opening" or small wedge-shaped distractor to gain initial access to the disk space. Then, the smallest available disk space shaver is inserted into the disk space and rotated to free disk material. Multiple trajectories should be used with each size shaver, angling medially and laterally. The shavers can be increased successively until cortical contact is achieved. Be mindful not to engage the endplate and create any cortical defects. Pituitary rongeurs can be used intermittently to remove disk material. The largest shaver used is a good predictor of the height of the interbody cage to be used.
  - As the shavers are progressively enlarged, continue to provide incremental distraction through the lamina spread to maximize disk space working height.
  - We recommend avoiding using the shaver for endplate decortication because we feel that the shavers can be too aggressive and can subside the endplates when used in this fashion.
- Next, curettes are used to complete disk removal and perform endplate decortication. Again, be mindful to avoid creating defects in the bony endplate. Remove the endplate cartilage and disk with pituitaries.
  - Following use of the shavers, you may need to increase the size of the annulotomy to allow for curettes and cages to be placed through it. Kerrison rongeurs can be used to remove overhanging annulus, posterior osteophytes, to enlarge the size of the annulotomy in the cephalocaudal and medial-lateral direction.

- Various types of curettes are available for discectomy and decortication. Angled curettes are helpful for accessing the contralateral dorsal aspect of the disk space, which tend to be the most difficult areas to access.
- Make sure to spend sufficient time on disk preparation and double check your work. This is a crucial time to ensure you have removed sufficient disk material for your cage placement and bone grafting.
- Following a thorough discectomy and endplate decortication, you may trial cage sizes or use the last shaver size for the final implant height.
- Morcelized IAP/SAP and allograft are then placed into the disk space. Use an up-biting pituitary to advance the bone graft into the contralateral and ventral aspects of the disk space. Avoid overpacking the disk space, as this can impair proper cage placement.
  - After placement of bone graft, you can consider using an undersized trial cage to create a pathway for your cage through the bone graft.
- The final implant cage is packed with autograft bone on the back table and brought onto the field. The traversing nerve is protected with a nerve root retractor. The cage is then gently malleted through the annulotomy into the disk space.
  - Depending on your cage length, the implant is usually countersunk 5 mm with the initial inserter. A secondary inserter can be used to advance the implant as needed.
  - For standard interbody fusion procedures, we commonly place the cage midline at the ventral aspect of the disk space. For foraminal stenosis, you can consider preferentially placing the cage toward the side of stenosis to increase the indirect decompression.
- Hemostasis in Kambin's triangle is achieved again with Floseal and patties as well as bipolar cautery.

DECOMPRESSION

After cage placement, the laminar spreader is removed and posterior lumbar decompression is performed bilaterally if necessary.

- Ensure adequate decompression of the contralateral lateral recess and foramen, as changes in alignment or lordosis can potentially create symptomatic stenosis of previously asymptomatic contralateral pathology.

SCREW PLACEMENT AND POSTEROLATERAL BONE GRAFTING

- We use an open pedicle screw placement technique following decompression, using direct palpation of the pedicle with Woodson elevators to confirm screw trajectory.
- We decorticate the contralateral transverse process and lateral facet for supplemental posterolateral fusion. Local autograft and allograft is placed in the contralateral posterolateral recess for fusion purposes following decortication.
- We do not routinely place bone graft in the ipsilateral posterolateral recess to avoid compression of the exiting nerve root or cauda equina from migrated bone graft.

CLOSURE

- Meticulous hemostasis is critical following TLIF procedures to avoid postoperative epidural hematoma formation.
- We commonly place subfascial drains, although this is controversial in the literature in regards to efficacy of preventing symptomatic epidural hematoma.
- Standard layered closure is performed.

AFTERCARE

- We encourage same day physical therapy after lumbar fusion procedures to facilitate early mobilization.
- Drains are removed when output is below 30 cc per 8-hour shift.
- Anticoagulation is performed on a case-by-case basis, but commonly utilizes heparin 5,000 units subcutaneously q8hrs starting postoperative day 1. Sequential compression device (SCD) and thromboembolic deterrent (TED) hose are continued postoperatively.

CHAPTER 19

Technical Pearls in the Management of Adult Scoliosis

Lawrence Lenke, James D Lin

■ INTRODUCTION

- Surgical treatment of adult scoliosis is complex.
- Setting up a consistent workflow is key, due to potential for many pitfalls in a "long" operation.
- Constant vigilance regarding safety, efficiency, and sterility are keys to success.
- *Four tenants of posterior-only treatment:*
  1. Pedicle screws "stabilize"
  2. Posterior osteotomies to "loosen"
  3. Transforaminal lumbar interbody fusions (TLIFs) at base for "support"
  4. Prone positioning and rods for "correction"
- Three-column osteotomies are rarely needed in a primary case.

■ CLASSIFICATION/PREOPERATIVE EVALUATION

- *Classification:*
  - *Adult degenerative scoliosis:* Many classification systems [Schwab, Scoliosis Research Society (SRS), etc.]
  - *Adult idiopathic scoliosis (AdIS):*
    - AdIS classification (Lin/Lenke, 2020 Spine Deformity)
    - Three-component classification helps communicate radiographic findings:
      1. *Curve type:* 1-6, maintained from Lenke classification
         - Structural coronal plane when >35° residual curve on supine X-rays
      2. *Lumbosacral modifier:*
         - Nonstructural/structural (NS/S)
           - Structural if supine X-ray lumbosacral curve >20°
      3. *Global alignment modifier:*
         - Aligned
         - *Sag malalign:* Sagittal vertical axis (SVA) > 40 mm
         - *Cor malalign:* Coronal vertical axis (CVA) > 40 mm
         - *Comb malalign:* SVA and CVA > 40 mm
    - *Example: 3/S/Sag Malalign*
  - *Clinical application:*
    - Radiographic categorization of adult idiopathic curves.
    - Guides preoperative radiographic assessment, but must also evaluate patient age, bone quality, symptoms, magnetic resonance imaging (MRI) findings.
    - Structural curves should be considered for inclusion in arthrodesis.
    - Consider fusion/instrumentation to include S1/ilium in the setting of global malalignment.
- *Preoperative planning:*
  - Upper instrumented vertebra (UIV)/lower instrumented vertebra (LIV):
    - In adult scoliosis without global malalignment and focal stenosis/symptoms, consider short segment decompression and fusion rather than deformity correction.
    - *Proximal thoracic UIV:* Often T2-4, final choice dependent on picking neutral to lordotic segment will consider C7 or T1 in rare cases, especially with a proximal thoracic hyperkyphosis and osteoporosis.
    - *Distal thoracic UIV:* Often T10, but UIV choice based on pathology (do not end on a bad disk), alignment (nonkyphotic segment), and presence of "protective" osteophytes on computed tomography (CT) at UIV/UIV+1 disk will consider T9-T12 as UIV.
    - *LIV:* Most often S1/ilium in adult deformities unless young adult with nonstructural lumbosacral curve and no lumbosacral pathology.

- *L5 versus S1:* Controversial if no L5–S1 pathology, but patients over 50 years old with long construct (proximal thoracic UIV) likely more reliable result with fusion/instrumentation to S1/ilium.
- *Fractional curve:* If large and stiff fractional curve or coronal malalignment, consider "kickstand" screw-rod construct.
- *Leg length discrepancy:*
  - If <1 cm, treat "as is."
  - If >1 cm, consider shoe lift preoperative to balance pelvis.
- *Bone mineral density (BMD):*
  - If osteoporotic, delay elective surgery with treatment of BMD
  - Can resume bisphosphonates at 4 months postoperation
- *Alignment goals:*
  - Whole body EOS films to assess global alignment
  - Rule of thumb: Age ~ SVA in mm
- *Proximal junctional kyphosis (PJK) prevention:*
  - Most important, get the alignment right (avoid over/under correction)
  - Many adjunctive techniques available, proximal tethers seem most beneficial
- Adult degenerative scoliosis versus AdIS: Adult degenerative scoliosis typically has more central/lateral recess stenosis, AdIS has more deformity (but may have fractional lumbosacral curve stenosis).

INSTRUMENTS SUGGESTED

- Open Jackson frame
- Intraoperative neuromonitoring
- Smoke evacuator
- *Retractors:* Short/medium/long Weitlanders, Cerebellars, Gelpi, and Adson Beckman
- *Basic instruments:* Osteotomes, Kerrison rongeurs, Leksell rongeurs, large curettes, AM8 burr, Woodson probe, and Penfields
- Thoracolumbar pedicle screws placed free hand with regular thoracic and "baby" (1 mm tip) Lenke blunt curved gearshifts
- Long cassette coronal and sagittal plane intraoperative radiographs.

PERIOPERATIVE MEDICATIONS

- *Tranexamic acid:*
  - Low dose (10 mg/kg bolus—1 mg/kg/hr infusion)—well studied
  - High dose (50 mg/kg bolus—5 mg/kg/hr infusion)—our preference, limited but growing evidence
- *Antibiotics:* Intravenous (IV) cefazolin and gentamycin
- *Intrawound antibiotics:* Vancomycin power 2 g after exposure, and 2 g prior to closing along with tobramycin 2.4 g.

POSITIONING/DRAPING

- Position the patient prone on a radiolucent table.
- Prone positioning is ideal for most deformity surgery. It induces lordosis in lumbar spine, and allows for "single position" spinal deformity surgery.
- Chest pads one hand breadth distal to axilla, top of hip pads at anterior superior iliac spine (ASIS).
  - If more lordosis is needed, place top of hip pads more distal to ASIS.
- *Draping:* Sterility is key to infection prevention.
  - Use skin staples liberally around drape edges to prevent migration during case, particularly at distal aspect of wound.

EXPOSURE

- Meticulous subperiosteal dissection and hemostasis are critical for controlling blood loss.
  - Set electrocautery to 65/65.
  - Make sure skin bleeders are controlled and wound is dry.
  - 1 cc/min of skin bleeding over 5 hours is equivalent to the loss of one unit packed red blood cell (PRBC).
  - Maintain mean arterial pressure (MAP) 65–75 mm Hg during exposure.
- Relax retractors when not in active use to prevent muscle necrosis.
- Work in sections of spine: Lumbosacral, then lumbar, then mid-distal thoracic then finally proximal thoracic.

FACETECTOMIES/DECOMPRESSION/POSTERIOR COLUMN OSTEOTOMIES/OSTEOTOMIES

- *Facetectomies:*
  - Four reasons to perform inferior facetectomies at all levels (except most cephalad level in older patients): Source of autograft, exposes anatomic landmarks for freehand screw placement, promotes fusion, and loosens the spine.
  - *Technique:*
    - ½" straight osteotome and mallet
    - Caudal to cephalad cut starting at the medial facet/lamina junction
    - Dorsal to ventral cut just distal to the caudal aspect of the transverse process (TP):
      - Take care to not violate the superior articular facet (SAF) in thoracic spine with the second cut to avoid canal penetration.

SECTION 2: Thoracolumbar

- *Posterior column osteotomies (PCO):*
  - This is the "workhorse" osteotomy for majority of patients, as three-column osteotomies are rarely needed in primary idiopathic spinal deformity cases.
  - PCOs loosen spine and can also help visualize lateral dura and medial pedicle wall for freehand pedicle screw placement, particularly in apical regions.
  - *Technique:*
    - Remove spinous process with large Leksell and superficial layer of ligamentum flavum.
    - Use small Leksell to find midline raphe in ligamentum.
    - Insert Woodson probe through midline raphe directed laterally to develop plane between ligamentum flavum and dura.
    - Kerrison #2 or 3 biting laterally remove SAF to lateral extent of foramen.
    - Floseal and gelfoam with cottonoids for hemostasis.
  - *Technique (if fusion mass):*
    - Fusion mass PCOs are a powerful technique to loosen the spine in the setting of a previous posterior fusion, if the anterior disk spaces are unfused.
    - Thin the fusion mass with large Leksell rongeur based on preoperative CT anatomy, creating a chevron shape (apex distal) from foramen to foramen **(Fig. 1)**.
    - Use side-cutting matchstick burr (such as AM8) to thin fusion mass and enter spinal canal centrally, taking care to avoid dural injury.
    - Woodson probe to develop plane between bone and dura
    - Kerrison #2 or 3 biting laterally to complete PCO to lateral extent of foramen **(Fig. 2)**.
    - Consider carefully placing laminar spreader to "loosen" up osteotomy site in the lumbar spine with slow posterior distraction of osteotomized residual lamina/pedicles.
- *Lumbar decompression:*
  - In general, we prefer to perform an interlaminar decompression rather than a full laminectomy to maintain bone for fusion, as most stenosis is at the disk/ligament level/subarticular levels. A full laminectomy should be performed as needed if any residual stenosis remains after decompression or when alerted by neuromonitoring of a potential localized stenotic region.
  - *Technique:*
    - The inferior facet has been removed through facetectomies at this point.
    - Remove spinous processes for bone graft.
    - Insert small laminar spreader between lamina and distract.
    - Use large Leksell to thin ligamentum flavum and identify midline raphe.

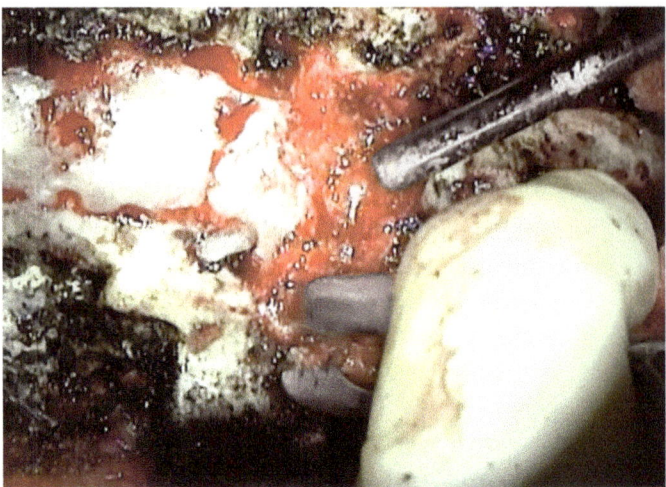

Fig. 1: Leksell rongeur to create V shaped trough in fusion mass.

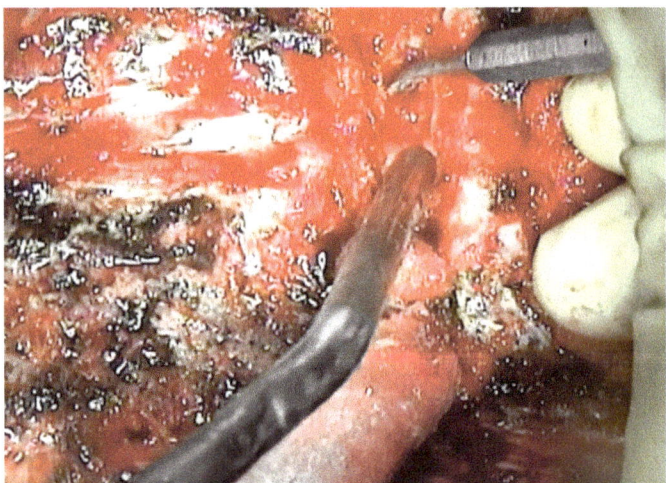

Fig. 2: Woodson elevator to palpate from foramen to foramen, ensuring completion of posterior column osteotomy.

- Woodson probe into midline raphe to develop plane between ligamentum flavum and dura.
- Kerrison #2 or 3 biting laterally to remove SAF out to foramen.
  - Your assistant can use the Woodson to gently depress the dura to help prevent durotomy.
- Decompress lateral recess until pedicle is palpated.

INSTRUMENTATION

- All screws can be placed freehand based on anatomic landmarks.
- We place TLIFs from L4 to S1 for anterior column support and decrease risk of pseudarthrosis.
- *Juxtapedicular screw technique:*
  - In the setting of idiopathic scoliosis, small cortical pedicles (type C and D) are common in the concavity of the curve.
  - We instrument these pedicles using a freehand "juxtapedicular" or "in-out-in" technique **(Figs. 3A and B)**.

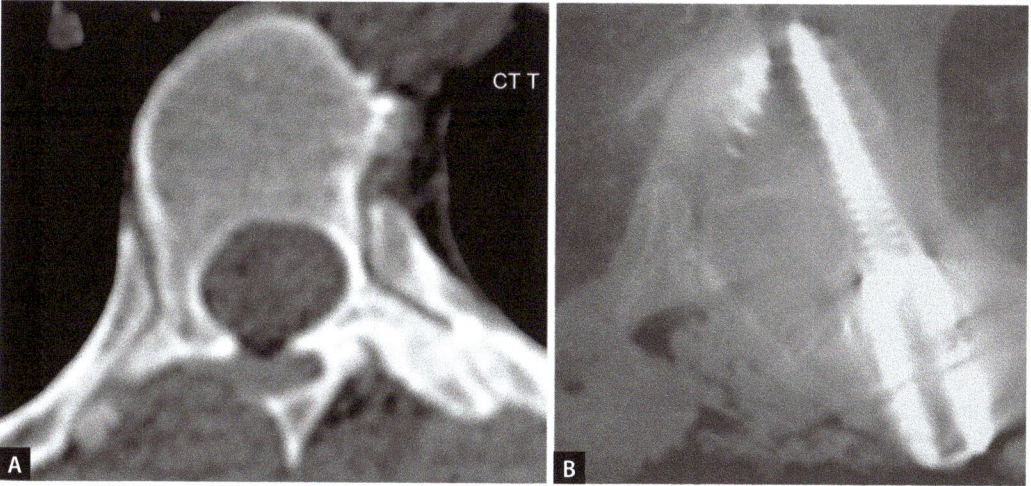

Figs. 3A and B: Preoperative computed tomography (CT) versus intraoperative CT spin showing juxtapedicular screw placement in type D pedicle.

- The technique is slightly modified compared to standard freehand placement of pedicle screws.
- Starting points are 1 mm more lateral: In-line with the lateral edge of the SAF in the thoracic spine and 1 mm lateral to the ascending pars in the lumbar spine.
- A matchstick burr is used to enter the lateral juxtapedicular space, and a 1 mm gearshift directed medially is used to enter the vertebral body at the pedicle-body junction approximately 20 mm deep to TP.
- The screw tract is palpated using a ball-tip probe, ensuring a bony floor.
- A k-wire is inserted into the screw tract, again ensuring the bony floor, and the tract is tapped with a cannulated tap to avoid inadvertently developing a second lateral tract.
- The tract is palpated again and a noncannulated screw is inserted by hand.

- *Kickstand screw-rod construct:*
  - The kickstand screw-rod construct is a powerful technique to correct lumbosacral fractional curves or coronal malalignment. A laterally based iliac screw provides a long lever arm for powerful construct-to-ilium distraction.
  - The iliac crest is exposed proximally and laterally until the most proximal aspect (as it turns laterally/horizontal), approximately 6 cm lateral to midline.
  - A large Cobb elevator is used to expose several centimeters of the outer table of the ilium to provide a guide for the trajectory of the kickstand screw.
  - A long gearshift is used to develop the screw path, which should follow the visualized lateral border of the ilium. The trajectory is approximately 10° laterally and approximately 30° from horizontal toward the floor in the cephalocaudal direction.
  - The tract is palpated to ensure bony walls.

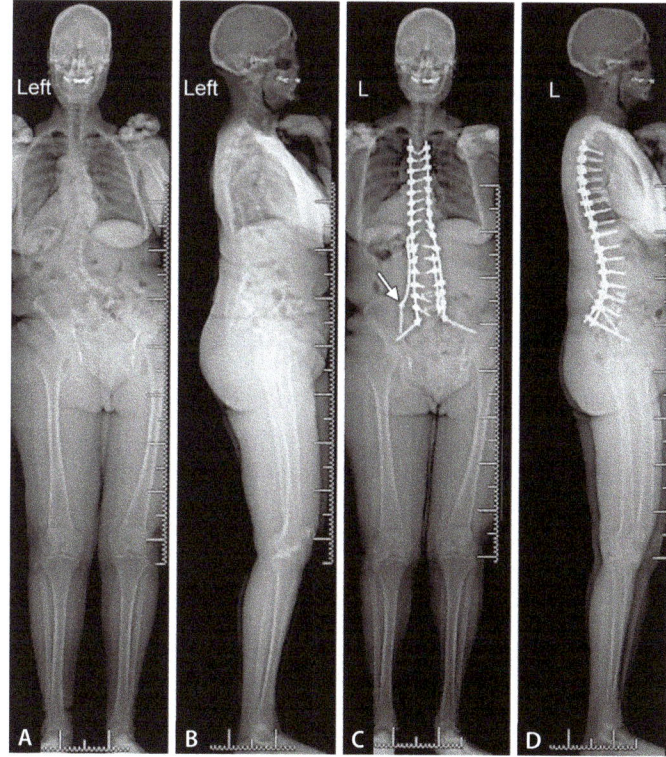

Figs. 4A to D: Patient with adult idiopathic scoliosis (AdIS) (6/S/Cor Malalign) treated T4–S1/ilium fusion, kickstand screw rod construct, TLIF L4–S1.

  - The tract is undertapped, and a large screw, typically 7.5–8.5 and 70–80 mm in length, can be inserted.
  - A kickstand rod is attached to main construct at the thoracolumbar junction with a side–side connector. Set screws are loosened in the ipsilateral lumbar spine distal to the connector, and powerful "construct-to-ilium" distraction can be performed to correct stiff fractional curves **(Figs. 4A to D)**.
- *Pearls:*
  - Perform PCOs prior to screw placement which allows visualization of lateral dura and palpation of medial

pedicle wall which can be helpful in dysplastic cortical pedicles.
- Low threshold to perform laminotomy to directly visualize or palpate medial pedicle wall if neuromonitoring picks up screw breach.
- If screw is lateral, recannulate, and then tap over a K wire, to prevent screw falling into original tract.
- Tactile feel during screw purchase is critical.

DEFORMITY CORRECTION

- *Pearls:*
  - Do not over correct.
  - *Rule of thumb:* SVA goal (in mm) should be patient's age.
- *Strategy:*
  - We generally think about deformity correction from caudal to cephalad when fusing to sacrum/pelvis; cephalad to caudad when not.
  - We will generally use a 6.0 mm cobalt chrome rod as the first correcting rod, and a 6.0/5.5 mm cobalt chrome transition rod as the second rod, with the transition at the distal thoracic spine.
  - Long-cassette anteroposterior (AP) and lateral X-rays are obtained after rod placement/deformity correction to confirm appropriate coronal and sagittal alignment.
- *Lumbosacral curve:*
  - In general, the first rod that is placed is on the convexity of the lumbosacral curve.
    - This allows compression of the convexity to induce lordosis while horizontalizing L4 and L5 vertebrae.
  - The contralateral rod is then placed with concave lumbosacral curve distraction performed by careful screw distraction.
- *Lumbar curve:*
  - The concavity of the lumbar curve is typically contralateral to the lumbosacral curve.
  - The initial rod, which is secured through the lumbosacral curve, is loosely captured through reduction tabs through the lumbar curve. Final seating of the rod can be achieved through the reduction towers.
  - Cantilever and compression are applied through the second contralateral rod through the convex apex of the mid lumbar curve.
- *Thoracic curve:*
  - The rods are in-situ contoured into the appropriate sagittal plane using the straight in-situ benders.
  - The rod should lay into the screwheads with minimal force, particularly at the cephalad aspect of the construct, to prevent PJK.
  - Any residual coronal deformity can be corrected with in-situ coronal benders.
  - We rarely perform significant kyphosis correction or perform cantilever maneuvers in the thoracic spine, in a primary adult scoliosis as most sagittal plane correction can be obtained in the lumbar spine; however, we will produce thoracic kyphosis with reduction screws/towers when correcting a thoracic hypokyphotic/lordotic malalignment.
- *De-rotation:*
  - For adult spinal deformity with fusions to the ilium, formal derotation is rarely needed as goals of surgery are curve correction, global alignment, and neural decompression.
  - In young adults with thoracic/thoracolumbar/lumbar curves, we perform derotation of the curve apex.

ARTHRODESIS

- Decorticate all available bone surfaces.
- Significant autograft is available through facetectomies and PCOs.
- We use about 100 cc of autograft, 100 cc of morselized fresh frozen allograft, and two large kits or bone morphogenetic protein (BMP) for a T10–S1/Ilium fusion.

CLOSURE

- Long cassette AP and lateral X-rays are obtained after rod placement and any "tweaking" performed before closure.
- We perform watertight fascial closure with #1 Vicryl in a figure-of-8 fashion, followed by 2-0 Vicryl deep dermal interrupted stitches, and a running 3-0 Vicryl for epidermal closure, followed by skin mesh/glue.
- We place one deep hemovac drain and one superficial hemovac drain on 3:1 suction (3 hours off and 1 hour on suction to encourage noncompressive hematoma formation in wound without excessive blood loss from continual evacuation).

POSTOPERATIVE CARE

- No brace is given routinely unless poor BMD.
- Outpatient physical therapy (PT) can be started at 2 weeks to 2 months depending on overall recovery and motivation.
- Clear for unrestricted activity at 4–6 months depending on age and bone density.

CHAPTER 20

Anterior Lumbar Interbody Fusion Technique

Barrett S Boody, Glenn S Russo, Mark Kurd

INDICATIONS

- The anterior lumbar approach can be an extremely useful technique providing wide exposure to the lumbar disk space and allow for the ability to perform circumferential anterior releases, place large interbody cages, achieve significant alignment correction, obtain indirect neural decompression, and maximize the opportunity to obtain fusion.
- The anterior lumbar interbody fusion (ALIF) can be used as a standalone technique or as an augment to the posterior approach. It is a powerful tool for correction of lumbar scoliosis, reduction of significant degenerative or isthmic spondylolisthesis, and comprehensive debridement and grafting of osteodiscitis.
- ALIF is an alternative to posterior-based interbody fusion techniques [transforaminal lumbar interbody fusion (TLIF) and posterior lumbar interbody fusion (PLIF)]. Of the interbody fusion techniques, there is no clearly superior choice with regard to clinical outcomes, sagittal and coronal correction, and fusion rate. However, ALIF should be considered when there is a need for significant deformity correction, maximized fusion rate, or revision of a posterior-based cage.

CONTRAINDICATIONS

- While there are no absolute contraindications to ALIF, multiple patient-related factors can make the approach and instrumentation more challenging:
    - Prior abdominal surgeries, history of abdominal/pelvic radiation, and obesity can make the approach and exposure of the disk space more challenging.
    - Transperitoneal approaches may be utilized in a revision setting but often require an experienced access surgeon.
- The magnetic resonance imaging (MRI) should be scrutinized preoperatively for the location of the major vessels. When the aorta and/or inferior vena cava (IVC) is draped and flattened across the disk space, mobilization of the vasculature can be challenging.

INSTRUMENTATION/SET-UP

- Flat Jackson table [allows for unencumbered anteroposterior (AP) and lateral fluoroscopy]
- Access surgeon—typically a vascular or general surgeon
- C-arm
- Disk preparation instruments with long handles (long handle 10 blade, Cobb, Kerrison, curettes, pituitaries, and trials)
- Intradiscal distraction shims or vice grip distractors
- *Implants—commonly either a prosthetic cage or femoral ring allograft:* Some surgeons may use an additional anterior plate or select prosthetic cages with integrated screw systems. Others utilize an interference screw construct with or without a washer. We commonly avoid anterior instrumentation for the rare but potentially catastrophic risk of vascular injury with plate loosening. Additionally, anterior instrumentation can make a revision approach to that level even more challenging due to scarring of the vasculature to the plate.
- Bone graft options to supplement implant—commonly demineralized bone matrix and/or bone morphogenic protein.
- Vascular instruments—discuss with your access surgeon the preferences for retraction, vessel ligation, and vessel repair instruments that they will require. We recommend having multiple peanut-type instruments for clearing soft tissue off the disks to avoid inadvertent vascular injuries. One precaution practiced but the authors is the having a 4-0 Prolene and two sponge sticks readily available on the back table in case of a vascular injury.
    - As spine surgeons, we rarely encounter significant bleeding that cannot be ultimately stopped by pressure or electrocautery. A special note should be made for anterior abdominal work as injuries even

to the segmental arteries and veins can cause rapid, catastrophic bleeding that cautery will rarely control and, in fact, can exacerbate. Commonly segmental artery injuries require identification of the injury, exposure of the artery, and ligation with clips or silk ties. If you are not well trained for this, hold direct pressure with the sponge stick and alert your access surgeon. Similarly, for suspected aorta, IVC, or iliac injuries, do not attempt repair; hold pressure and alert your access surgeon.

■ TECHNIQUE

Approach and Positioning

- The patient is positioned supine, a Foley is placed to decompress the bladder, and the entirety of the abdomen is prepped and draped extending from the xiphoid process to the pubic symphysis. This facilitates rapid extension of the incision in the event of a vascular injury (**Figs. 1 and 2**).
- The approach is commonly performed by vascular or general surgeon. We commonly defer the type of incision and selection of vascular retraction system to the specific surgeon with whom we work. For L5–S1 approaches, we commonly utilize a Pfannenstiel approach. Conversely, for more cephalad approaches, a midline, longitudinal approach is used.
- We commonly use a left-sided retroperitoneal approach to the L2–S1 disks (**Fig. 3**). From L2 to L5, the left-sided approach allows improved disk space access and retraction on the more resilient aorta versus the thinner-walled IVC. Working above L2–L3 disk levels with the supine position is difficult due to difficulty mobilizing the kidney and renal vasculature.
  - For approaches above L2, we utilize a right lateral decubitus position with a direct left lateral approach to the thoracolumbar area.
- Following exposure, the disk is cleared of soft tissue using a peanut (**Figs. 4 and 5**).

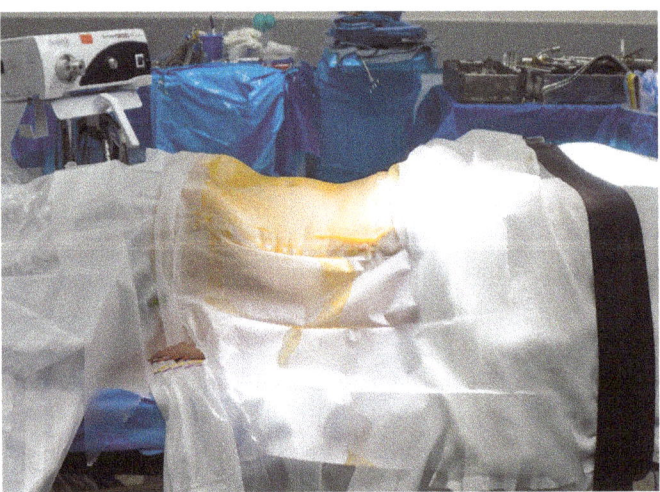

Fig. 1: Patient positioned supine on flat Jackson table with the abdomen widely prepped.

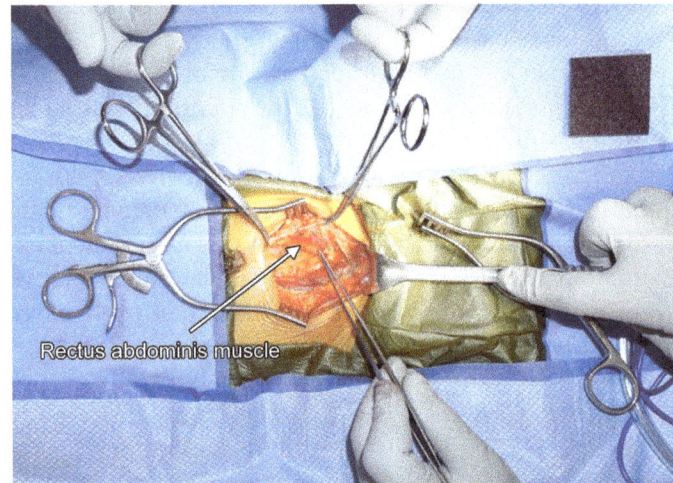

Fig. 3: The rectus abdominis is split midline along the raphe and the left retroperitoneal plane is developed beneath the muscular dissection.

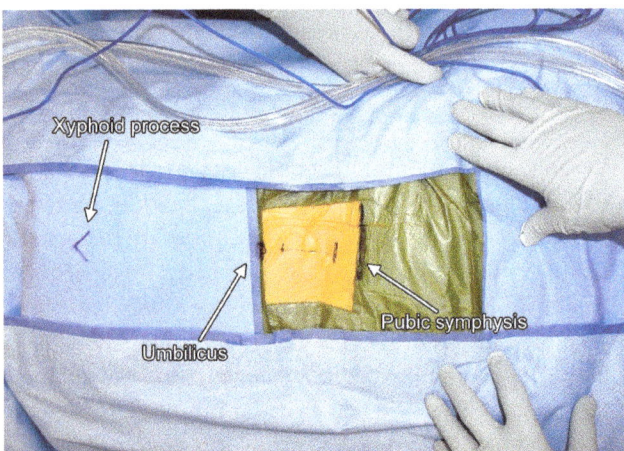

Fig. 2: Surgical drape application for L5–S1 disk space access. The umbilicus and pubic symphysis are observed within the draped surgical field.

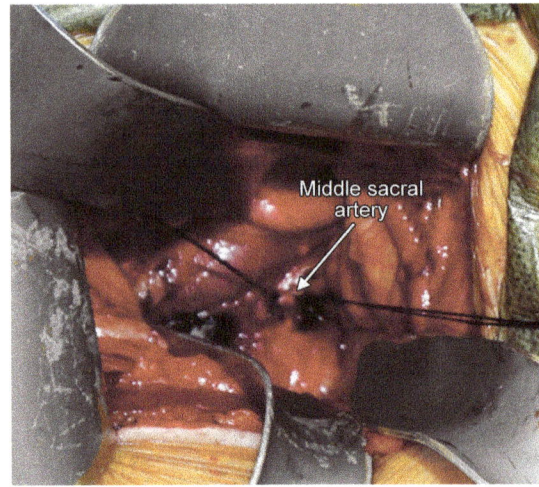

Fig. 4: Intraoperative view of the L5–S1 disk space. The middle sacral artery was ligated to allow access to the L5–S1 disk space.

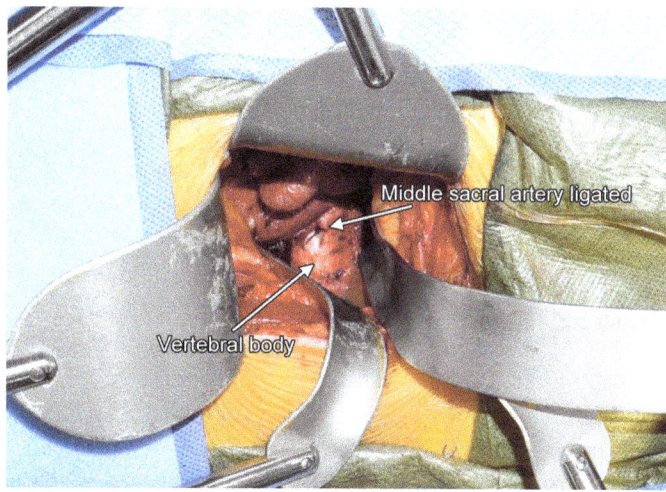

Fig. 5: After ligation of the middle sacral artery, the retractors are adjusted to expose the L5–S1 disk space.

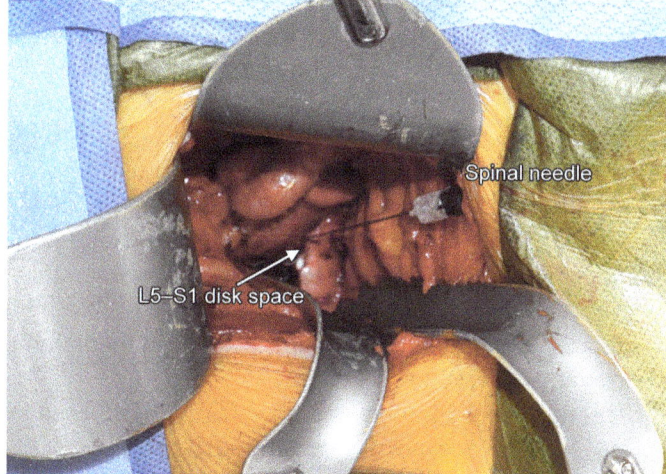

Fig. 6: A needle is placed within the L5–S1 disk space to confirm the operative level using lateral fluoroscopy.

- Using a peanut for dissection minimizes the risk of damaging a vessel during disk exposure.
- Retractors are placed. Be aware throughout the case that thin-walled venous structures may creep underneath retractors into the surgical field.
- Prolonged retraction on the vasculature may cause limb ischemia. We commonly use a pulse oximeter placed on the great toe of the left foot to monitor for blood flow to the lower extremities during the case. Adjust the retractors if diminishing pulse oximeter readings are observed.
- The disk is localized with placement of a spinal needle and a lateral fluoroscopic image **(Fig. 6)**.

Discectomy

- The annulus is incised sharply with a 10 blade in a box shape. We make every effort to cut in a controlled fashion away from the vessels.
  - The size of the annulotomy is based on the purpose of the approach. For coronal and/or sagittal realignment, a more extensive lateral release can be necessary. This can be performed either sharply or with Kerrison rongeurs.
- Next a sharp Cobb is used to develop the interface between the subchondral cartilage and the bone and advanced posteriorly along the endplate. This is done for the entirety of the superior and inferior endplates. This allows for large sections of disk to be quickly and efficiently removed.
  - Use two hands with the Cobb instrument and avoid plunging. Commonly, Cobb instruments have depth markings on the shaft. We avoid using them any deeper than 25–30 mm depending on patient size.
- The disk is removed with a pituitary rongeur from the disk space.
- Enlarge the annular opening with a Kerrison rongeur, removing overhanging anterior osteophytes on the cephalad vertebra. This allows for improved access into the disk space for discectomy and subsequent cage placement. Make sure your annulotomy is wide enough at this point to accept the dimensions of your intended graft.
  - Clearly define annular tissue as you take your Kerrison laterally. This can risk an inadvertent vascular injury as you proceed to your lateral borders.
- If you have a collapsed disk space, you may need to initiate some distraction during your discectomy and potentially immediately following annular incision. For tightly collapsed disks, inserting a thin Cobb and rotating it can initiate some distraction and loosen adhesions, but try to avoid excessive force to avoid subsidence of the endplates. Next serial bullet or rotating dilators can be used to provide a slow progression of dilation for disk space access.
  - Inserting a rotating dilator at the side of the disk space can provide some distraction while you perform the contralateral discectomy and vice versa.
- Following discectomy, use curettes to finish removing endplate cartilage and any residual disk for exposure of the subchondral bone of the endplates as well as residual posterior disk. Take care to avoid aggressive decortication to avoid subsidence of your implant. Make sure disk is completely removed both laterally and posteriorly to the annulus.
  - To ensure that the posterior annulus has been released, use the C-arm to confirm that a curved curette can be positioned over the posterior-superior corner of the body.

Trialing and Implant Placement

- Based on either the size of the rotating dilators or visual inspection of the disk, select an initial trial size for insertion.

- Utilize the C-arm for trial insertion. Pay attention to see that the placement of the trial results in concentric distraction of the disk space.
    - If you note that the trial placement creates lordosis without distraction of the posterior intervertebral space, some additional soft tissue release may be required. A concentric distraction is needed to achieve indirect decompression of the neuroforaminal space.
- Insert the trial into the desired position and take a lateral fluoroscopic image. Make sure it is at least flush with the vertebra prior to X-rays in order to minimize unnecessary fluoroscopic images.
    - Avoid excessive malleting/impacting the trial. If you are not able to completely insert the trial with minimal force, you likely have residual posterior disk. Forceful malleting risks vertebral fracture and neurologic injury. Remove the trial and confirm you have cleared enough posterior disk and are able to distract with endplates with a Cobb or rotating distractors prior to using force to impact trials.
    - Lateral fluoroscopy for trial insertion can be helpful in several ways. First, it can identify if you need to remove more posterior disk with trial placement. Posterior cage placement along the posterior border of the vertebral body maximizes indirect decompression. Additionally, fluoroscopy can be helpful to determine implant sizing in regards to width and depth.
- Increase trial height sequentially to achieve good interference fit of the implant. You should note that for isthmic spondylolisthesis, you may excessively distract the disk space without ever achieving interference fit due to the pars defects.
    - In these cases, preoperatively template a desired implant height and consider either using supplemental anterior fixation (integrated cage/screw construct or an anterior plate).
    - If placing posterior instrumentation, consider use of a rotisserie-type patient flip from supine to prone to minimize the chance of cage extrusion.
- After serial trials, select your implant size and add adjuvant bone graft to the implant.
- Insert the cage similarly, under fluoroscopy, to guide into the desired position.

Anterior Fixation

- Most commonly, this is achieved either via integrated cage/screw designs, anterior plating with screws, or screw/washer type fixation.
- For integrated cage/screw systems, an awl is used to prepare the trajectory followed by placement of the screw.
- Make sure the implant is fully seated behind the anterior cortex of both the cephalad and caudad vertebral bodies, especially at L5–S1. This avoids the potential of skiving out the sacrum or fracturing the vertebral body.
- For difficult angles, hinged awls and drivers are available. Take care with using these, as excessive force may cause the instrument to jump out of the tract, potentially injuring viscera or vasculature.
- Most commonly, issues of difficult screw placement arise in L5–S1 isthmic spondylolisthesis, due to the degree of L5 translation and the often-associated high pelvic incidence. You can use fluoroscopy to facilitate safe screw placement with optimal length and trajectory. For the L5 screw, especially if there is continued listhesis of L5, ensure the screw length does not enter the canal with lateral fluoroscopic imaging. Similarly, for large cages or cages placed excessively to one side or the other, ensure the S1 screw does not enter the S1 foramen. We commonly will ensure our cage is midline with fluoroscopy and slightly angle the screws medially to avoid this complication.
- Anterior plates can be placed in a fashion similar to an anterior cervical decompression and fusion (ACDF). We would caution against using these with significant residual anterolisthesis. After the plate is placed, an awl is used to prepare the start point and trajectory for the screw, followed by screw placement. As you are working anterior to the vertebral body, take care to avoid vascular and visceral injury.
- Screw/washer techniques can be used for femoral ring allograft to provide a buttress type effect to prevent graft extrusion during repositioning for posterior instrumentation. For L5–S1 levels, we commonly place the screw in the sacrum. Make sure to countersink your graft so you can start the screw at the superior-anterior corner of the S1 endplate, as this avoids screw breakout or skiving along the anterior sacral slope.

Technical Pearls in the Surgical Management of Thoracic and Lumbar Trauma

CHAPTER 21

Ashley R Strickland, Rohan Gopinath, Samuel Q Li, Jael E Camacho, M Farooq Usmani, Steven C Ludwig

DISCLOSURES

All authors contributed equally to the development of the chapter. Dr Ludwig is a board member for Globus Medical, the American Board of Orthopaedic Surgery, the American Orthopaedic Association, the Cervical Spine Research Society, and the Society for Minimally Invasive Spine Surgery. He is a paid consultant for DePuy Synthes, K2M, and Globus Medical. He receives payment for lectures and travel accommodations from DePuy Synthes and K2M. He receives payment for patents and royalties from DePuy Synthes and Globus Medical. He has stock in Innovative Surgical Designs and the American Society for Investigative Pathology. He receives research support from AO Spine North America Spine Fellowship support, Pacira Pharmaceutical, and AOA Omega Grant. He is a board member of Maryland Development Corporation. He receives royalties from Thieme, Quality Medical Publishers. He is on the governing board of Journal of Spinal Disorders and Techniques, The Spine Journal, and Contemporary Spine Surgery. The authors have no further potential conflicts of interest to disclose.

TABLE 1: The thoracolumbar injury classification and severity score.

Characteristic	Score
Injury morphology:	
• No abnormality	0
• Compression	1
• Burst component	2
• Translation/rotation	3
• Distraction	4
Posterior ligamentous complex integrity:	
• Intact	0
• Indeterminate	2
• Disrupted	3
Neurological status:	
• Intact	0
• Nerve root injury	2
• Complete cord injury	2
• Incomplete cord injury	3
• Cauda equine injury	3
Total score:	
<4 = nonoperative	
>4 = operative management	

INTRODUCTION

- Thoracolumbar spine trauma is common in the setting of blunt trauma.
- The goals of surgery are to prevent neurological injury, provide stability to the spine, and correct post-traumatic deformity.
- Patients with instability due to posterior ligamentous complex (PLC) injury, a neurologic deficit, or a stable burst/compression fracture not amenable for orthosis are candidates for surgery.
- The thoracolumbar injury classification and severity (TLICS) score[1] **(Table 1)** can also assist with surgical decision-making. Patients with a score of 5 or more should be operated.
- Traditional open spine surgery and minimally invasive surgery (MIS) are standard in the treatment of unstable spine fractures, with or without neurologic injury.
  - In polytraumatic patients who are not candidates for orthosis and have a potentially equivocal TLICS score, we implement the use of MIS stabilization based upon concomitant head, chest, abdominal, and extremity injury.

POSTERIOR APPROACH

Indications and Rationale

- For decompression and fusion with instrumentation
- Permits access to all posterior spinal elements, the spinal cord, and intervertebral disks

- Access for reduction, realignment, stabilization, and instrumentation
- Can be easily extended in caudal and cephalad direction
- Can access ilium if autologous bone graft is necessary for spinal fusion.

Table and Positioning

- Position the patient prone on a radiolucent table, such as the open Jackson or Allen table.
  - We recommend the use of a Wilson frame in ankylosed patients with extension-distraction injuries.
- The chest bolsters should be placed cephalad to the xiphoid process and caudal to the axilla and the sternal notch.
- The iliac spine bolsters should be placed two fingerbreadths caudal to the anterior superior iliac spine without obstruction of the patient's abdomen.
- The neck should be in neutral position.
- The shoulders and elbows should be abducted and flexed to approximately 90°, and forward flexed approximately 10° on well-padded arm pads.
- The hips should be slightly flexed and the legs should be well padded in slight flexion at the knee.
  - A hardtop can be used in flexion-type injuries and a sling can be used for extension-distraction injuries.
- At this point, baseline prepositioning motor evoked potentials (MEPs) can be obtained in cases with a spinal cord level thoracic injury. However, they have minimal utility for lumbar level injuries.

Notes:
1. In highly unstable injury, extreme care should be taken during positioning. For the majority of these cases proper positioning will allow for reduction of fracture.
2. After positioning patient and prior to skin preparation, verify that desired fluoroscopic images can be obtained without obstruction. For the upper thoracic spine, Mayfield tongs and the arms tucked down the side of patient body allow for optimal radiographical visualization.

Draping

- Four clear drapes should be applied wide to the expected site of incision.
- The iliac crest should be incorporated if harvest of autograft is expected.
- After sterile preparation of the surgical site, four sterile towels should be draped around the surgical site and two U-drapes should outline the expected operative field.

Incision

- Use bony landmarks to help guide incision location and length.
- The spinous processes are palpable superficially.
- The gluteal cleft and C7–T1 spinous processes delineate the midline.
- A line drawn across the highest points of the iliac crest typically corresponds to the L4–L5 interspace.
- Fluoroscopic localization with a radiopaque surgical instrument such as a Freer elevator may be utilized to approximate incision location.
- The length of the incision should extend one spinous process above and below the level(s) of anticipated instrumented levels.
- Your skin incision should be directly midline over the spinous processes. To achieve hemostasis, tissue may be infiltrated with 1:500,000 epinephrine solution.

Note: Radiographic visualization of injury should dictate the level for incision. However, in patients with ankylosed spine or when fracture is not as evident, count from down from T1 or up from T12 using the ribs. For the lumbar spine, count down from T12 or up from L5/S1.

Dissection

- Deepen the incision through subcutaneous fat and down to fascia.
- Once at the level of the fascia, we recommend use of a Cobb elevator in order to expose the fascial edges to facilitate reapproximation.
- The dissection is deepened down to the spinous process with electrocautery.
- Subperiosteal dissection with a Cobb elevator and electrocautery device should be used to elevate the paraspinal muscles.
- Dissection of the thoracic spine should proceed in a caudal to cephalad order.
- Conversely, dissection of the lumbar spine should proceed from a cephalad to caudal fashion.

Note: When working with an assistant surgeon, attending can work top to bottom, while assistant works bottom to top.

- Further dissection with a Cobb elevator and electrocautery device laterally along the laminae, facet joints, and transverse processes can be utilized if exposure is necessary.

Caution: Avoid unintentional violation of facet joints at uninvolved levels in order to prevent unnecessary iatrogenic damage to the adjacent uninvolved structures.

Retractors and Retractor Placement

- Use self-retaining retractors such as Weitlaner's, Cerebellar's, or Gelpi's to maintain tissue tension. For larger patients, hinged self-retractors can be used.

- The retractors should be oriented so the finger loops are at the most cephalad and caudal ends with the prongs aimed toward each other.

Localization and Fluoroscopy
- Fluoroscopic localization with a lateral radiograph may be utilized with a spinal needle inserted into the spinous process, or with a towel clamp on the spinous process to determine vertebral level. Counting up from S1 to localize the injury level.
- Unique bony surface anatomy can help with localization as well.

Hemostasis
- Branches of the segmental vessels coming off the aorta and supplying the paraspinal muscles will be encountered during lateral dissection of the transverse process as they appear between the transverse processes.
- Venous bleeders are usually encountered next to the pars interarticularis and just lateral to the facet joint.
- Vigorous cautery of these vessels is necessary for visualization of the surgical field and hemostasis. However, caution should be taken near the intertransverse membranes as exiting nerves can be at risk of injury. More bleeding will be encountered in the thoracic spine due to more muscular attachments to the thoracic spinous processes. Therefore, an optimal subperiosteal dissection and hemostasis during dissection minimizes slow continuous oozing throughout case.
- A bipolar cautery is recommended to achieve hemostasis near nerve roots.
- Thrombin-soaked gelfoam or cotton patties can be generously used to help achieve hemostasis.
- Infiltration of the paraspinal muscles before dissection with 1:500,000 dilution of epinephrine saline with an 18G spinal needle can be helpful to diminish muscle bleeding.

Note: If not contraindicated, the use of antifibrinolytic medication such as tranexamic acid (TXA) can aid in minimizing blood loss. A single bolus can be given for short cases.

ANTERIOR APPROACH

Indications and Rationale
- Incomplete neurologic injury with spinal canal compromise
- The following radiological and clinical features:[2]
  - Retropulsed fragment with clinically and radiographically significant canal compromise
  - Significant anterior column comminution requiring reconstruction to preserve spinal stability and to avoid a multilevel posterior-only procedure
  - Notes:
    1. If patient comes with significant chest or abdominal injuries requiring exploration, we would consider an extracavitary approach over an anterior approach.
    2. In patients with osteoporosis, we would avoid an anterior-only approach and will perform an anterior-posterior combined approach.
- Beware that if considering a standalone anterior-based procedure, the integrity of the posterior elements, including bony and ligamentous structures, needs to be present.
  - Consider initial posterior stabilization (either open or MIS approach) prior to anterior approach if posterior structures are injured, especially in dislocated, translational, or rotational injuries.
- *The approach is based on the level of the injury:*
  - Thoracotomy—above T11
  - Transdiaphragmatic or thoracoabdominal—T12–L1
  - Retroperitoneal—below L2.

Table and Positioning
- For a lateral approach, place the patient in lateral decubitus with left side for T6 and below.
  - It avoids required mobilization of the liver and injury to the inferior vena cava (IVC).
  - Can consider right-sided approach for mid-thoracic anterior approach
- Consider placing a bean bag below umbilicus and posterior spine on a radiolucent table.
- Consider break in table, centered at the level of the fracture to increase opening between ribs and pelvis.
  - If unable to use a breaking table, consider placing a 3-L pressure infuser bag at the waist to achieve the same operative window.

Caution: There is risk for spinal cord injury when positioning patients this way. When positioning, obtain multiple planes of fluoroscopic images to assure positioning has corrected deformity. This maneuver can also place nerves on stretch, so make sure to undo break prior to instrumentation.

- Flex the hips and knees, and pad the bony prominences (axillary roll and upper arms sandwiched between pillows or arm holder).

Thoracotomy
- *Incision:*
  - Use fluoroscopy to guide the placement of the incision. Centered over the injured vertebral level, we typically extend incision one to two levels above planned rib resection. Oblique incision that follows from posterosuperior to anteroinferior.
- Dissect through skin and subcutaneous tissues.
- Divide latissimus dorsi and serratus anterior muscles in line with incision.

- Enter the pleural space and intercostal space.
  - A Doyen or a Woodson can be used.
  - Care is taken inferior to the rib at the location of the neurovascular (NV) bundle. Blood vessels can be ligated, preserving the nerve.
- *Rib resection:*
  - Allows for use of bone graft and provides larger exposure.
  - Subperiosteal dissection of the desired rib should be performed away from the underlying NV bundle.
  - Using rib cutters, you can take off rib anteriorly and as far posterior as the costotransverse joint.
  - Excise the external oblique, internal oblique, and transversalis muscles.
- Incise the pleura, but ensure underlying lung is not injured.
  - If injured, typically placement of a chest tube is sufficient management.
- Use rib spreaders to open the space.
- Mobilize and retract the lung anteriorly with moist lap pad in combination with a malleable retractor. An Allison lung retractor is an alternative to using malleable retractor cover with a lap pad.
- Consider single-lung ventilation during this step to assist with lung mobilization and visualization of spine. Discuss with anesthesia the need for a dual-lumen endotracheal tube to allow for single-lung ventilation during the procedure. Identify the desired level for decompression and instrumentation.
  - Segmental arteries from the aorta can be ligated for access.
  - A chest tube is typically placed while thoracotomy is open prior to closure to ensure optimal location.

Caution: Baseline monitoring of somatosensory evoked potentials (SSEPs) and MEPs prior to starting and during the case assists in assessing the neurologic status of the patient. Pre- and postpositioning MEPs can also be obtained to assess for the possibility of any neurological damage during positioning.

Transdiaphragmatic or Thoracoabdominal

- *Incision:*
  - Fluoroscopically guided
  - Usually at the inferior border of 12th rib
  - Oblique incision as described above for the thoracotomy incision
- Dissect through skin, subcutaneous tissues, and abdominal muscles as mentioned before.
- Enter the retroperitoneal space using blunt dissection to retract the peritoneal contents anteriorly.
- Keep the diaphragm superior to dissection.
  - Use deep retractors. Finochietto rib retractor can be placed between the superior rib and the iliac crest.

Caution: The ureter is attached to the posterior peritoneum and can be injured during mobilization.
- Dissect down to the crus of the diaphragm.
- Release the diaphragm posteriorly at the crus and laterally at the medial and lateral arcuate ligaments.
  - Avoid central release of the diaphragm, in order to avoid denervation.
  - Make sure to allow a 1–1.5 cm cuff to be retained for repair.
- Identify the desired level for decompression and instrumentation.
  - Segmental arteries from the aorta can be ligated for access.

Caution: Baseline monitoring of SSEPs and MEPs prior to starting and during the case assists in assessing the neurologic status of the patient.

Retroperitoneal

- *Incision:*
  - Fluoroscopically guided
  - Centered at the desired level
  - Oblique incision and similar superficial dissection as previously described in the transdiaphragmatic approach
- Enter the retroperitoneal space as previously described and retract the peritoneal contents anteriorly.
  - Retractors can be placed between the 12th rib and the iliac crest.
- Expose the quadratus lumborum and psoas major muscles.
- After localizing the desired level, under fluoroscopy, two methods are utilized to access the anterior portion of the vertebral body:
  - Incise the fascia overlying the psoas muscle. Perform a posterior Cobb dissection of the psoas muscles off the disk spaces first, and then the vertebral body with ligation of the segmental vessels at the midbody.
  - Posterior dissection of the psoas muscle with identification of the pedicle and neuroforamen with a Penfield to identify the posterior wall of the vertebral body.
    - Dissect along the superior endplate of the index level to identify the pedicle and then gradually work inferiorly to identify the posterior vertebral body in order to avoid injuring the exiting nerves.

Note: The psoas muscle can be large and challenging to dissect, if necessary may perform a transpsoas approach with neuromonitoring and care to dissect through the anterior 20% of the muscle width. We recommend monitoring the four heads for the quads in order to assess for femoral nerve function.

ANTERIOR-POSTERIOR APPROACH

Indications[3]

- Thoracolumbar injuries causing canal compromise with incomplete neurologic deficits and severe disruption of the posterior elements (PLC or posterior bony structures)
- Provides better biomechanical stability and improved fusion rates.

Positioning and Approach

- The combined approach can be performed either in a staged procedure or sequentially.
- Start with posterior approach with patient in prone position if patient requires a reduction of a dislocated segment.
- After completing posterior decompression and stabilization, the anterior column is approached.
- Position in lateral decubitus, as described above.
- Perform anterior decompression and stabilization.

INSTRUMENTATION

Posterior Instrumentation: Pedicle Screws

- *Free-hand technique:*
  - *Starting point:*
    - In the lumbar spine, the starting point is on the mammillary process at the midpoint of the transverse process, and always lateral to the pars interarticularis.[4]
    - In the thoracic spine, the starting point is the center of a triangle formed by the lower border of the superior articular process, medial border of the transverse process, and the upper border of the pars interarticularis.[5]
    - Consider lateral "in-out-in" technique for narrow pedicles to avoid medial breach in the thoracic spine.
  - Use a burr or rongeur to create a cortical starting hole at the approximate insertion point.
  - Next, a pedicle probe is used to develop a path through the cancellous bone of the pedicle.
    - Sagittal trajectory should always be 90° orientation to the pars interarticularis.
    - Coronal trajectory starts at 10-15° angled medially in the thoracic spine and decreased to 0° at the T11-T12 level. It then angles medially again at the upper lumbar spine increasing down into the sacrum.
  - Once the probe has proceeded 15-20 mm, it can be angled slightly medial since it has crossed the spinal canal.
  - A pedicle sounding probe can be inserted to insure no cortical breach in any of the medial, lateral, cephalad, or caudal directions.
  - For nonself-tapping screws, a tap is inserted along the path of the pedicle screw prior to inserting the screw.
    - Tapping can be an optional step and usually dependent on surgeons preference. However, we tap all percutaneously placed screws.
  - Direct palpation of the probed pathway should be performed in order to delineate any critical breaches.
- *Fluoroscopy-guided technique:*
  - Allows a surgeon to view the trajectory of a pedicle screw in real time
  - Use a C-arm to take anteroposterior (AP) and lateral images parallel to the superior endplate of the desired level.
  - After the starting point is identified, images in the AP and lateral planes are used to follow the trajectory of the screw path and avoid unwanted breaches.
- *Stereotactic placement technique:*[6]
  - This method requires obtaining a preoperative computed tomography (CT) scan.
    - Using the CT images, easily identified anatomic landmarks (fiducial points) are identified and saved.
  - In the operating room, a camera is set up in a manner to provide an unobstructed view of the surgical field.
  - After the standard posterior exposure, a reference array is secured to a skeletal point (spinous process or iliac crest) and a probe is used to identify each of the preselected fiducial points.
    - This step ensures the computer-generated model correlates to the patient's anatomy in the operating room.
  - Next, the above steps for pedicle screw insertion are carried out with guidance on starting point and trajectory narrated by the computer guidance.
- *Percutaneous or MIS technique:*
  - Techniques for percutaneous pedicle screw placement have been described elsewhere in this book (*see* Chapter 14).
  - Four different methods have been described for percutaneous placement of pedicle screws:[7]
    - *True AP targeting:*
      - Obtained when the anterior and posterior margins are superimposed, and only a single superior endplate shadow is seen
    - Magerl or Owl eye technique
    - Biplanar fluoroscopy
    - Image-guided navigation
  - Our preferred method is the true AP targeting method.[8]
- *Rod placement:*
  - Prior to insertion, each rod is contoured to the appropriate lordosis and kyphosis.
    - Rod contour should be slightly kyphotic from T1 to T10, neutral from T11 to L1, and lordotic from L1-sacrum.
    - Lateral radiographs or fluoroscopic images can aid with rod contouring.

- The set screws are inserted lightly on either the cranial or caudal aspect prior to any reduction maneuver.
- In-situ bending can be performed to obtain additional sagittal correction of the kyphotic deformity.
- Compression and distraction may be performed to assist in correcting the spinal deformity.
- After the rods are in appropriate position, the set screws are tightened.

- *Cement augmentation:*
  - Can be utilized in patients with inadequate bone quality
  - We typically use the injection through cannulated screw technique, although prefilling methods with vertebro- or kyphoplasty can also be performed.

DECOMPRESSION

Indications

- Patients with incomplete neurologic injury and root level neurological symptoms
- Canal compromise, even severe, is not in itself an indication for decompression in the neurologically intact patient. Bony fragments typically resorb.
- For patients with complete neurological injury, there is no compelling evidence they may require a decompression. Although, we still will perform a decompression.
- Can be performed through MIS decompressive techniques and/or indirectly through fracture reduction.

The method of decompression is typically dictated by the injury pattern and the location of the stenosis.

Note: When faced with a cerebrospinal fluid (CSF) leak, attempt direct repair when possible. However, if nonrepairable dura, apply a dural patch in addition to dural sealant.

Posterior Approach (Figs. 1A to E)

- Utilized to perform laminectomy, transpedicular decompression, and extracavitary corpectomy

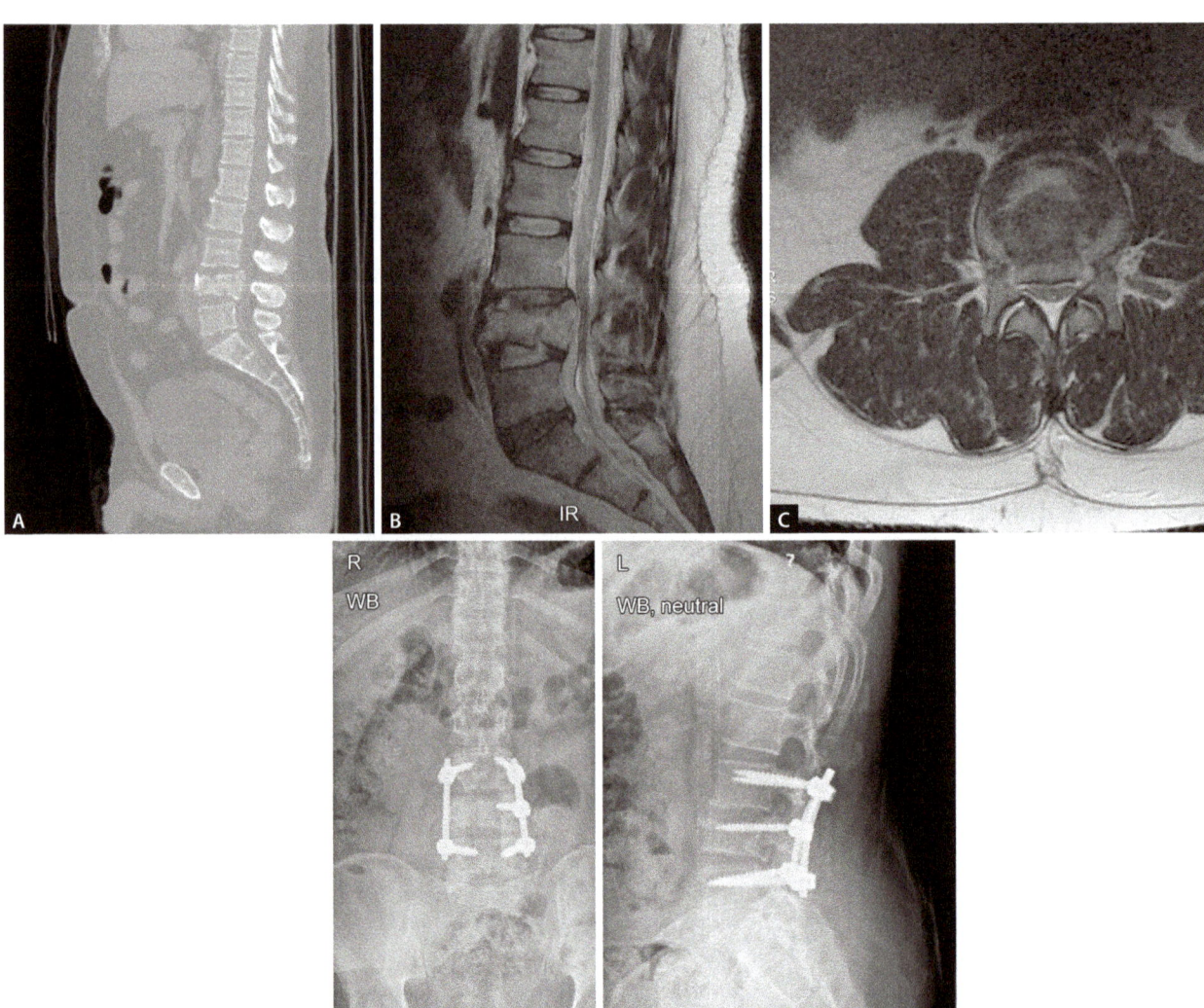

Figs. 1A to E: (A) Sagittal CT scan of L4 burst fracture; (B) Sagittal T2-weighted MRI view of L4 burst fracture with spinal canal compromise and epidural hematoma causing an incomplete neurological injury; (C) Axial T2 weighted MRI of L4 fracture with severe canal compromise causing central compression; (D) Postoperative anteroposterior X-ray showing L3–L5 decompression and instrumented fusion; (E) Postoperative lateral X-ray of posterior L3–L5 instrumented fusion.

- Laminectomy is indicated for patients with posterior compressive pathology (i.e., displaced lamina fracture or infolded ligamentum flavum).
  - Also, used to decompress anterior canal compromise in the lower lumbar spine, or to provide access for decompression of a compromised nerve root.
- Transpedicular or extracavitary approach allows for anterior decompression of the spine by posterior approach. Transpedicular decompression is most safely utilized at the nerve root level, as the thecal sac can be safely retracted in order to visualize the anterior compressive structures. Extracavitary approaches allow for circumferential decompression of the neurological structures with the ability to perform anterior column reconstruction.

Caution: A split fracture of the lamina is often present in patients with an incomplete neurologic deficit. The thecal sac and/or nerve roots may be entrapped in this defect, placing them at increased risk for injury during the decompressive and exposure portion of the procedure.

Anterior Approach (Figs. 2 and 3)

- Indications for anterior decompression include fractures with incomplete neurological deficit and anterior canal compromise, traumatic disk herniation, and ventral epidural hematoma. Additionally, injuries that have significant anterior column deficiency that require reconstruction may be indicated for an anterior approach.
- Anterior decompression is accomplished with either partial or complete corpectomy, with bone graft, and cage placement. Additional anterior instrumentation may be placed to restore the stability to the injured spine.

Indirect Decompression

- Indirect decompression can be utilized to achieve canal decompression in thoracolumbar injuries with an intact posterior longitudinal ligament (PLL). This technique relies on using the PLL to translate retropulsed fragments out of the canal using distraction.

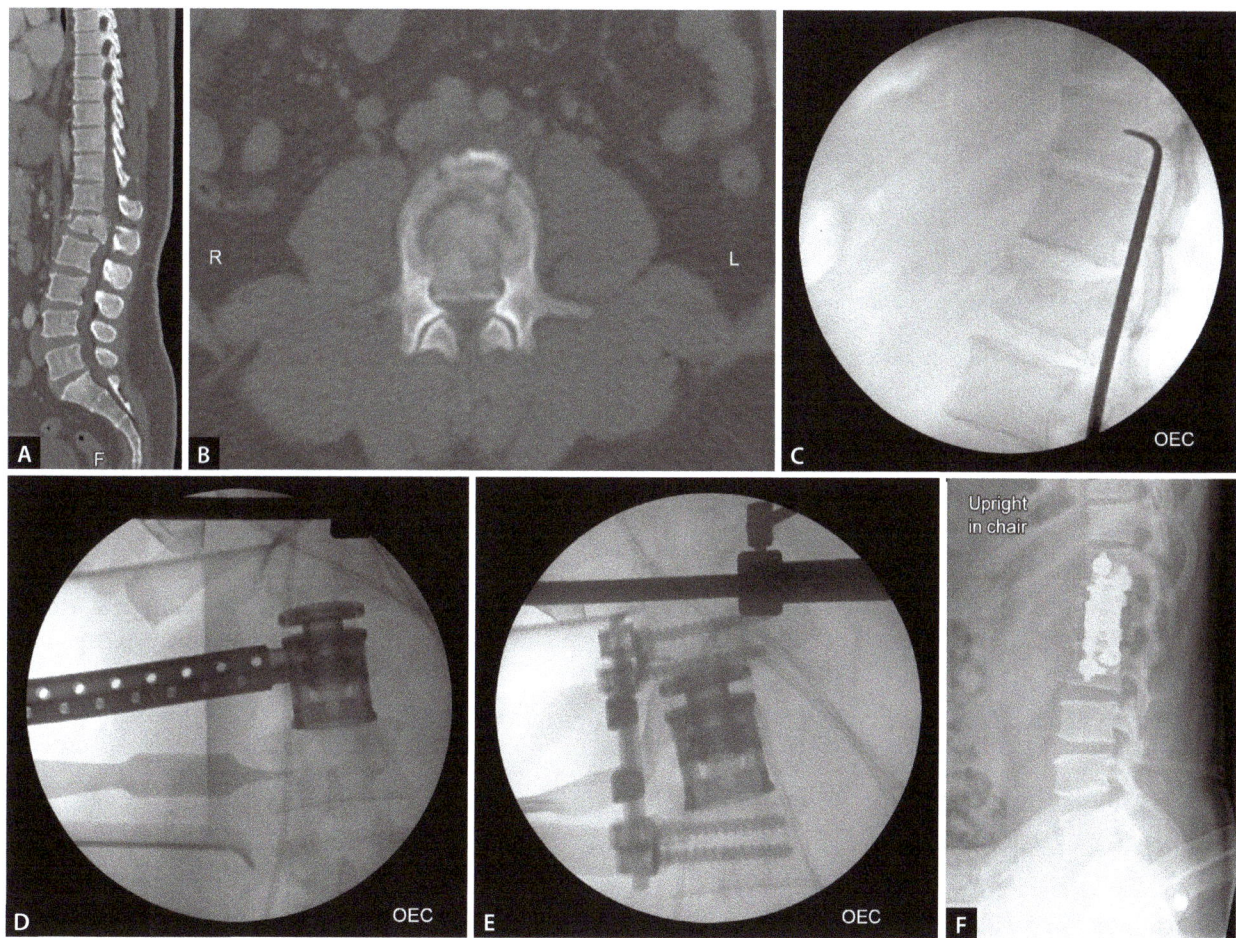

Figs. 2A to F: (A) Sagittal CT-scan view of T12–L1 flexion-distraction and L1 burst fracture; (B) Axial CT view of L1 burst fracture; (C) Intraoperative fluoroscopy is utilized to plan a lateral incision centered over the level of injury; (D) Intraoperative anteroposterior fluoroscopy image showing expandable cage placement into the corpectomy defect; (E) Intraoperative AP fluoroscopy image showing an L1 corpectomy with expandable cage in place. Additionally, a lateral plate and screws instrumentation was placed through the same incision spanning T12–L2; (F) Postoperative lateral X-ray.

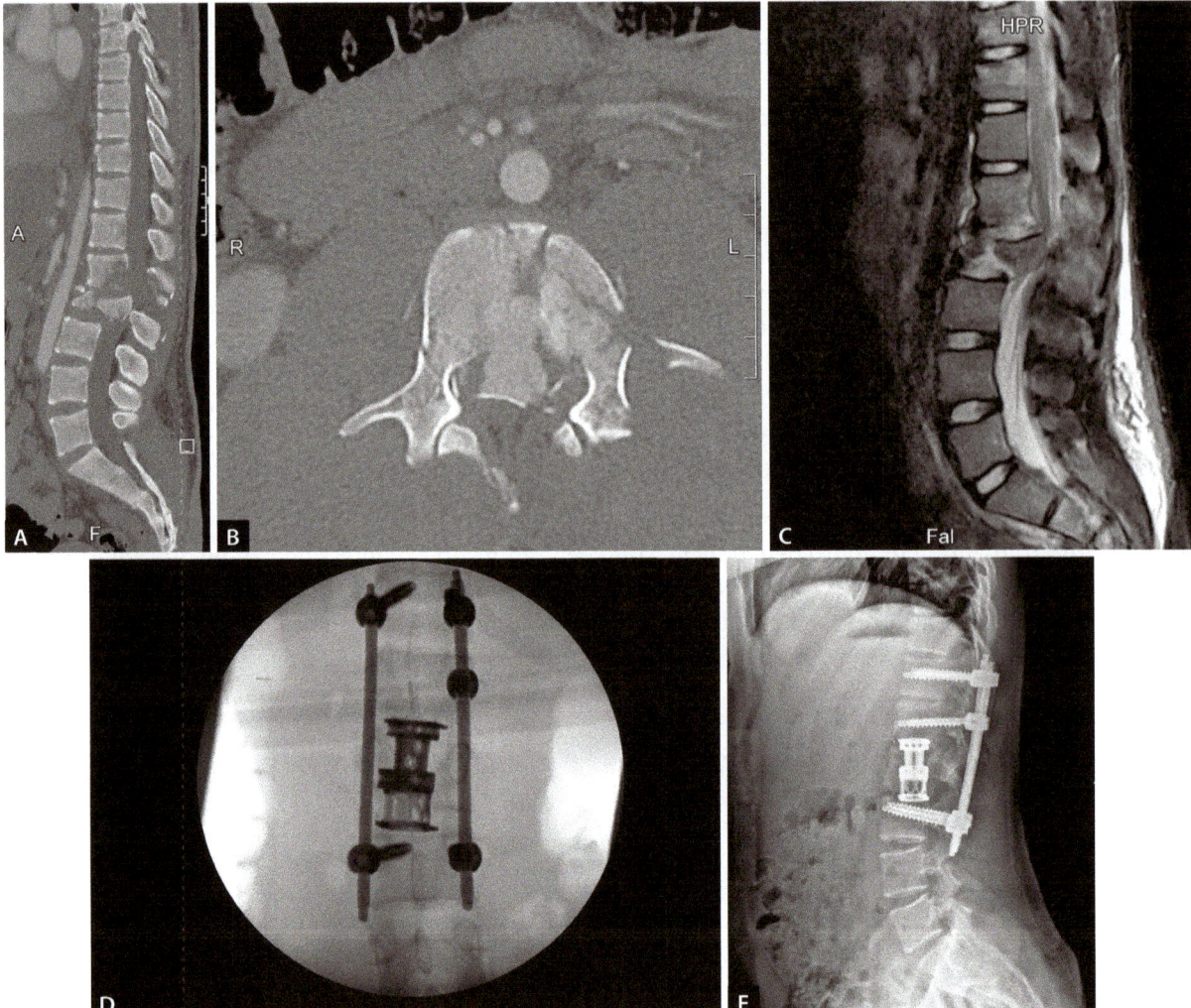

Figs. 3A to E: (A) Sagittal CT view of a L2 burst fracture; (B) Axial view of L2 burst fracture with significant canal compromise; (C) Sagittal T2-weighted MRI scan demonstrates L2 burst fracture with severe canal compromise and impingement of the conus medullaris. Thoracolumbar injury classification and severity classification score of 7 (burst morphology 2 pts, nerve root injury 2 pts, posterior ligamentous injury 3 pts); (D) Intraoperative anteroposterio fluoroscopy image; (E) 1-year postoperative lateral X-ray.

- This technique is best used within the first 48 hours after injury, as the fracture fragments are more mobile.
- Indirect decompression technique requires placement of pedicle screws above and below the injury. Rods are then placed, loose cephalad screws and secured caudally. Distractors are then placed bilaterally to simultaneously distract across the injured segment. Ligamentotaxis then reduces the fragments out of the canal. The cephalad portion of the construct is then tightened to secure the reduction.[9]
  - If unable to achieve adequate reduction of the fragments in the canal, consider a more extensive decompression or an anterior approach decompression.

Caution: Rotation of any of the retropulsed fragments greater than 180° (referred to as the reverse cortical sign) is a contraindication to this technique, as this indicates that the PLL is disrupted.

REDUCTION

Many thoracolumbar fractures are reduced with proper positioning.

- Typical positioning techniques were reviewed previously. There are situations where additional positioning maneuvers can be helpful in achieving reduction.
  - For thoracic extension injuries, typically seen in the ankylosed spine, we position the patient using a Wilson frame on a Jackson table with the legs in a sling to allow for restoration of thoracic kyphosis.
  - For lumbar flexion injuries, using a Jackson frame as outlined in the posterior approach section is the table of choice at our institution. The position of the chest pad should be in the highest safe position (at the level of the axilla) in order to allow the weight of the abdomen to aid in reduction.
  - For thoracic flexion injuries, taking care to elevate the head into a neutral position will aid in improving thoracic alignment.

- For upper thoracic injuries, use Mayfield and/or traction
- For mid thoracic injuries, use a Prone viewer
- For coronal plane deformity, it can be helpful to rest the patient's chest on two hip pad positioners instead of the usual chest pad, as this will aid in guiding the patient into a more neutral position.
- After initial positioning, minor residual deformity can typically be reduced with rod contouring, implementing a cantilever reduction maneuver, followed by compression or distraction maneuvers. Further adjustment may require in-situ bending.

Thoracolumbar spine dislocations pose a unique set of challenges. There are several reduction techniques that can be employed after performing the posterior approach. Reduction maneuvers should be controlled and deliberated. Before reduction techniques outlined below, (1) expose the zone of injury, (2) place pedicle screws above and below the zone of injury, and (3) remove the superior and inferior facets at the site of the dislocation, as these are often blocking the reduction.

Note: Regardless of technique, extreme caution should be used when reducing these unstable injuries in patients who are neurologically intact, or have incomplete neurologic injuries. No further reduction is needed once after sagittal and coronal alignment if achieved with positioning. Neurophysiologic monitoring should always be utilized. If the dislocation if through a disk space, an extracavitary discectomy and grafting should be used for fusion purposes.

- *Distraction across zone of injury* can be accomplished by placing a lamina spreader between the spinous processes at the site of injury. The spine is then gently reduced and stabilized with contoured rods.

  Note: This maneuver can create a flexion moment. In order to reduce, distract between the two pedicles one level above and below of injury.

- *Manual traction and translation* can be accomplished with the use of reduction forceps placed on the spinous processes above and below the zone of injury to allow for control of both segments. If more force, or more controlled force is needed, short temporary rods can be placed into the pedicle screws (horizontal or vertical between two screws) above and below the injury. These rods can then be grasped using rod holders to manually manipulate both cephalad and caudal fragments in order to translate and reduce the spine. Once reduced, the injury is then spanned with bilateral rods.
- *Cantilever reduction* is the preferred reduction technique for patients without complete spinal cord injury. This technique allows for greater control motion in cephalad and caudal segments and minimizes aggressive reduction, thus chance of injury. Pedicle screws are placed at two-levels cephalad and two-levels caudal the zone of injury. Two rods are then contoured in preparation for reduction. The rods are then secured to the proximal segments. A wide laminectomy may be performed if there is concern for postreduction neural compression with ligamentum flavum and/or lamina bone. Rod holders are used to gradually translate the rods to the distal pedicle screws. Rod reduction instruments or screw extenders can be used to aid in gradual controlled reduction. Once the rods are reduced and the rod caps are tightened, crosslinks can be placed for added construct rigidity in rotational injuries with significant instability. The use of crosslinks becomes less critical in longer constructs.

FUSION

Fusion can be achieved with local bone graft, iliac crest autograft, and cancellous allograft.

- Regardless of bone graft used, ensure full decortication of transverse processes and lateral aspects of superior facets to promote fusion.
- A bone mill can be used to morselize local bone graft from the decompression procedure.
- If additional bone graft is needed, cancellous allograft or iliac crest autograft can be used.
- We typically use local bone graft. If local bone graft is scant, we would supplement with allograft. We do not normally use iliac crest graft due to donor site morbidity.

Iliac Crest Bone Graft

- Can extend posterior lumbar midline incision in a subcutaneous fashion lateral to iliac crest
  - If a separate incision is necessary, make an oblique incision in line with iliac crest and over the posterior superior iliac spine (PSIS).
- Subperiosteally dissect caudally along the outer cortex
- Do not extend dissection distally beyond the sciatic notch, sacroiliac joint medially, or 8 cm lateral to the PSIS. This way we reduce risk of iatrogenic injury from exiting NV structures.
- Dissection should be performed cephalad to a line from the longitudinal axis to the PSIS.
- Cancellous or corticocancellous autograft can be harvested with this approach.
- An oscillating saw or osteotomes can be used to make cuts for corticocancellous autograft.
- If no corticocancellous autograft is needed, then a rongeur or osteotome can be used to uncap the PSIS to allow for cancellous bone harvesting with a gouge or curette.
- The iliac tubercle provides the greatest amount of cancellous bone.

CLOSURE

Wound Closure and Dressing

- The wound is copiously irrigated and the fascia is closed with a Vicryl suture in figure-of-8 fashion.
- A second layer of deep closure can be utilized for larger patients in order to close potential dead space.
- Deep dermal Vicryl sutures are placed in a simple buried, interrupted fashion.
- Skin can be closed with a running subcuticular monocryl, running locking nylon suture, or staples depending on the tissue tension and condition.
  - In patients with traumatized tissue, our preference is to use nylon sutures. Staples are usually used when no significant soft tissue injury.
- If closed with monocryl suture, Dermabond® alone or in conjunction with the Prineo® mesh can be used.
- The incision is dressed with folded 4 × 4 gauze and Ioban® is placed over the entire incision. Dressings are usually changed at postoperative day 2, unless there is an incisional vac in place, which in that case would stay longer.

Drains

A small generic hemovac drain is usually placed subfascially and exits at the cephalad end.

Negative Pressure Wound Therapy Systems

- Indicated in patient with significant soft tissue injury or internal degloving injury. Also for patients with history of infection or at high risk of infection (e.g., diabetics). Also, patient who are polytraumatized and are expected a long intensive care unit (ICU) stay.
- Used to remove edema, improve blood flow, and stimulate cellular proliferation
- Continuous suction at −125 mm Hg.
- Negative pressure wound therapy (NPWT) is not regularly applied unless the patient is at risk for wound complications due to comorbidities.
- Use of incisional NPWT has been shown to decrease incidence of wound dehiscence and postoperative surgical site infection.
- Not recommended for patients with CSF leaks, bleeding diathesis, neoplastic or metastatic disease, or allergic reactions to the dressings.

POSTOPERATIVE

Medication

- Low-molecular weight heparin is given up to 24 hours postoperation.
- We avoid the use of nonsteroidal anti-inflammatory drugs (NSAIDs).

Activity and Bracing

- Bracing is not used postoperatively.
- Patients can resume activities as tolerated. There is no activity restrictions, unless concomitant injury preventing weight bearing.

REFERENCES

1. Lee JY, Vaccaro AR, Lim MR, Oner FC, Hulbert RJ, Hedlund R, et al. Thoracolumbar injury classification and severity score: a new paradigm for the treatment of thoracolumbar spine trauma. J Orthop Sci. 2005;10(6):671-5.
2. McCullen G, Vaccaro AR, Garfin SR. Thoracic and lumbar trauma: Rationale for selecting the appropriate fusion technique. Orthopedic Clinics. 1998;29(4):813-28.
3. Fischgrund JS. OKU 9: Orthopaedic Knowledge Update: American Academy of Orthopaedic Surgeons; 2008.
4. Mattei T, Meneses M, Milano J, Ramina R. "Free-hand" technique for thoracolumbar pedicle screw instrumentation: Critical appraisal of current "State-of-Art". Neurology India. 2009;57(6):715-21.
5. Parker SL, Bydon A, Sciubba DM, Wolinsky J-P, Gokaslan ZL, Witham TF, et al. Accuracy of free-hand pedicle screws in the thoracic and lumbar spine: Analysis of 6816 consecutive screws. Neurosurgery. 2011;68(1):170-8.
6. Girardi FP, Cammisa FP Jr, Sandhu HS, Alvarez L. The placement of lumbar pedicle screws using computerised stereotactic guidance. J Bone Joint Surg Br. 1999;81(5): 825-9.
7. Harris EB, Massey P, Lawrence J, Rihn J, Vaccaro A, Anderson DG. Percutaneous techniques for minimally invasive posterior lumbar fusion. Neurosurg Focus. 2008;25(2):E12.
8. Gómez JA, Ludwig SC. Minimally invasive techniques for thoracolumbar spine trauma. Contemp Spine Surg. 2012;13(5): 1-7.
9. Crutcher JJ, Anderson P, King H, Montesano P. Indirect spinal canal decompression in patients with thoracolumbar burst fractures treated by posterior distraction rods. J Spinal Disord. 1991;4(1):39-48.

CHAPTER 22

Open Microdiscectomy and Laminectomy

Tyler Kreitz, Howard An

■ INTRODUCTION

Open microdiscectomy and laminectomy approaches are essential techniques for management of symptomatic disk herniations and spinal stenosis including central, subarticular lateral recess, and foraminal stenosis.

■ INSTRUMENTS SUGGESTED

- Open Jackson frame with leg sling, Wilson frame, or Andrews table. Each allowing for varying degrees of hip flexion thereby opening the interlaminar space facilitating the decompression. The author prefers use of open Jackson frame with leg sling as the open Jackson is used frequently for other spine procedures and allows for operating room consistency. All are good options.
- Intraoperative fluoroscopy
- For open approaches, standard open lumbar decompression sets are utilized including Kerrison and pituitary rongeurs, curettes, Woodson elevator, and a high-speed burr. Additionally, a harmonic bone scalpel may be used to facilitate decompression.
- The author prefers the use of an operative microscope for visualization of neural elements in both microdiscectomy and laminectomy procedures. The microscope is preferred to loupe magnification for excellent visualization, more ergonomic surgeon position, and easier accommodation of instruction with residents and fellows. Alternatively, loupe magnification may be used.

■ SETUP AND APPROACH

- *Table:* Position the patient prone on a radiolucent table. The authors prefer the open Jackson with leg sling to allow for hip flexion and opening of the interlaminar window.
- *Retractor:* For microdiscectomy, a McCullough or Taylor retractor may be used. For laminectomy, a McCullough, Cerebellar, Gelpi, or similar retractors may be used.
- *Localization:* Localize the midline incision using spinal needle localization on lateral fluoroscopy at the levels of interest. The skin incision will likely extend a few centimeters above and below the target disk space depending on the depth of the patient's subcutaneous tissues (i.e., the skin incision should be targeted on the L4–L5 disk space for a L4–L5 microdiscectomy or laminectomy).
- *Incision:*
  - Once the skin is prepped and draped, 0.5% bupivacaine epinephrine may be injected along the length of the incision to reduce postoperative pain and subcutaneous bleeding about the incision. Complete relaxation/paralysis of the patient is preferred to facilitate exposure and promote with hemostasis.
  - For open microdiscectomy or laminectomy, a standard extensile midline approach is used centered about the target levels. The length of the incision typically extends from the pedicle of the cephalad vertebrae to the top of the spinous process of the caudad vertebrae (i.e., for a L4–L5 decompression, the incision extends from the L4 pedicle to the top of the L5 spinous process). Ultimately the length of the incision depends on the size of the patient and deep retractor preference.
  - A scalpel is used to open the skin along the previously marked incision. Bovie electrocautery is used to obtain hemostasis within the subcutaneous tissues. A Weitlaner or Cerebellar retractor may be used to place tension on the tissue and retract facilitating deeper midline Bovie dissection to the level of the lumbodorsal fascia.
- *Fascial incision:* Make a midline fascial incision over the underlying spinous process. Due to the caudal angulation of the lumbar spinous processes, the tip of the cephalad spinous process will likely be in line with the caudal disk

space (i.e., the L4 spinous process is situated dorsal to the L4–L5 disk space).

- *Exposure of posterior elements:*
  - The posterior elements are exposed subperiosteally using Bovie electrocautery. The Bovie is used to elevate the multifidus and short spinal rotator muscles in a subperiosteal fashion from the tip of the spinous process to the lamina, lateral to the facet joint (care used to maintain the facet capsule) and cephalad to the pars interarticularis. Care should be taken to avoid placing the Bovie tip in the interlaminar space to avoid dural injury. Additionally, the preoperative magnetic resonance imaging (MRI) should be evaluated for spinal dysraphism or congenital abnormality potentially exposing dura to injury during exposure. For microdiscectomy, the fascia is split and the posterior elements are exposed on only one side of the spinous process. The upper portion of the caudal lamina is exposed in a similar fashion. A Cobb elevator or rigid suction is used to retract paraspinal musculature facilitating deep exposure. Additionally, a Cobb elevator may be used for blunt dissection of the lamina in index and revision cases. The Cobb is used to sweep soft tissue off of the lamina in a subperiosteal manner using a small packing sponge to facilitate hemostasis and gentle exposure.
  - Dissection is carried out in this fashion unilaterally for microdiscectomy or bilaterally for laminectomy.
  - At this point a deep retractor may be placed. For microdiscectomy, the authors prefer a McCullough retractor. The appropriate depth blade is chosen. The blade end is placed laterally to the level of the facet, and the pick end within the interspinous ligaments at the target level. The retractor is placed and opened. Alternatively, a Taylor retractor may be placed laterally over the facet of the targeted level. The Taylor retractor is malleted into place over the ipsilateral facet and held in place using woven gauze wrapped around the handle and foot of surgeon or assistant on the ipsilateral side. For laminectomy, a McCullough retractor with two blades, two Cerebellar, or Gelpi retractors may be used.
  - Confirmation that the surgeon is at the appropriate level should be done before further work is performed. The author prefers to place a curved micro curette or Woodson elevator underneath the undersurface of the cranial lamina at the target level (i.e., underneath the L4 lamina for a L4–L5 exposure). Double-checking the position of the curved curette on lateral fluoroscopy cannot be over emphasized to prevent wrong level surgery. When placed under the caudad lamina, the curette should be in line or slightly caudal to the target disk level. If necessary, a small amount of bone may be removed from the lower portion of the lamina to facilitate placement of the curette for the marker film.
  - Once the appropriate level is confirmed, complete exposure of necessary landmarks should be performed. For both microdiscectomy and laminectomy, exposure of the lateral border of the cephalad pars interarticularis is necessary for adequate decompression and to avoid over resection of the pars risking iatrogenic fracture. Adequate exposure of the upper border of the caudal lamina should also be performed in order to safely remove the insertion of the ligamentum flavum from its insertion at the top of this lamina.
  - The interlaminar window may be further defined using pituitary rongeurs and curettes to remove soft tissue overlying the ligamentum flavum.
  - In the revision cases, the author prefers the use of large straight and curved curettes to define the bone margins from the adjacent scar and underlying dura. This is performed by carefully scraping the bone edge with a straight curette with sharp side toward the bone, followed by curved curette in a similar fashion facilitating entrance into the canal. This should be done in a controlled fashion, recommending a novice surgeon to use two hands on the surgical instrument to improve control and reduce risk of iatrogenic neural injury.
  - Adequate hemostasis is critical for appropriate visualization. The paraspinal musculature may be infiltrated with 0.5% Marcaine with epinephrine prior to or after deep exposure. After opening the interval with the deep retractors, initial hemostasis can be achieved with Bovie or bipolar electrocautery. Hemostatic agents and gelfoam thrombin may also be used in areas adjacent to neural elements. Adequate hemostasis will improve visualization, reduce blood loss, and reduce the risk of complication throughout the procedure.

MICRODISCECTOMY

- *Laminotomy:*
  - A laminotomy of the cephalad lamina is often necessary for exposure. The extent of laminotomy is determined by the interlaminar window (i.e., less is needed at L5/S1 and more is necessary at more cephalad levels). A high-speed burr (2 mm side-cutting) is preferred for the laminotomy. The burr is used to remove the lower half of the cephalad lamina to facilitate the removal of the underlying ligamentum flavum. The burr is used in a side-cutting fashion to thin or remove the lamina. The

underlying ligamentum flavum is used for depth reference and to protect from iatrogenic dural injury. While progressing cephalad, the surgeon should be mindful of the termination of the ligamentum flavum and increased risk of dural injury using a high-speed burr and similar instruments. Frequently checking the remaining ligamentum and any exposed dura using a Woodson or curved curette is recommended. Additionally, the laminotomy is carried laterally to remove the medial portion of the facet joint facilitating exposure. The laminotomy is limited by the pars interarticularis (at least 9 mm of pars should be maintained to reduce risk of iatrogenic fracture), the insertion of the ligamentum flavum in the cephalad direction (the laminotomy rarely needs to be carried above the insertion of the ligamentum except in cases of cephalad disk extrusion), and laterally by the facet joint. The facet joint may be undercut to facilitate decompression, but at least 50% of the facet joint should be maintained. The author prefers to create a lateral trough for the laminotomy based on maintaining roughly 1 cm of pars interarticularis. The trough may be lateralized at the level of the facet joint as necessary for adequate visualization of the traversing nerve root.
- Next, the ligamentum flavum should be removed. This can be done from the undersurface of the cephalad or caudad lamina. A curved curette is used to loosen the ligamentum attachment from the undersurface of the cephalad lamina. Once loosened, the curette can be flipped caudal underneath the ligamentum creating a plane of dissection over the dura. If the plane between the ligamentum and dura cannot be clearly defined, the surgeon may consider releasing the ligamentum in similar fashion from its insertion on the upper level of the caudad lamina in order to facilitate safe removal and reduced risk iatrogenic dural injury. A series of pituitary and Kerrison rongeurs is then used to remove the ligamentum. Alternatively, the ligamentum can be removed from the insertion on the top undersurface of the caudal lamina in a similar fashion. Once removed, the underlying dura and traversing nerve root will be exposed. If at this point you cannot reliably identify the pedicle and foramen with a Woodson elevator, further lateral resection should be performed. This may be performed using a Kerrison rongeur to undercut the facet.
- *Discectomy:*
  - The disk space is found by identifying the caudal pedicle within the canal using a Woodson elevator or Penfield. Once identified, the traversing nerve root may be gently medialized revealing the underlying disk space just cephalad to the pedicle. A nerve root retractor is used to gently retract the root medially. The disk may be further defined using a Penfield elevator. Once the disk is clearly identified, the bipolar electrocautery may be used to coagulate epidural veins and achieve better hemostasis and visualization.
  - The author prefers to probe the annulus to find the preexisting tear. Once identified, the Penfield is used to widen the annular tear, while simultaneously pushing down on the disk facilitating extrusion of material. Alternatively if no annular tear is identified, a 15 blade is used to create a cruciate annulotomy. A nerve hook or micropituitary may be placed into the disk space to remove any free material.
  - Once satisfied, a ball tip or Murphy probe is passed under the nerve root and thecal sac feeling for additional extruded fragments. Any identified fragments may be removed using pituitary rongeur. Additionally, microirrigation may be used to irrigate the disk space and extrude and remaining free fragments.
  - A sequential and consistent checklist is necessary for evaluation of decompression. The author considers the microdiscectomy and decompression is considered complete when the traversing nerve root is free and mobile at the level of the disk and no ventral compression is found using a Murphy ball tip probe. Additionally, a Woodson elevator may be passed into the lateral recess above the caudad pedicle and foramen below the cephalad pedicle.
  - Depo-medrol (1 mL of 40 mg/mL) may be placed on the decompressed nerve root prior to wound closure.

LAMINECTOMY
- *Exposure:*
  - Similar to the microdiscectomy exposure above, the exposure for laminectomy is carried out to the cephalad and lateral borders of the pars interarticularis of the upper level and carried down to the upper border of the lower lamina (i.e., for a L3–L5 decompression, cephalad to the L3 pars and caudad to the L5 lamina). This is performed bilaterally.
  - A deep retractor is placed (McCullough, Cerebellar, Gelpi, or similar retractor).
  - A Leksell rongeur is used to remove the interspinous ligaments of each level followed by the lower half of the spinous process at the upper level and the complete spinous process at all intervening levels. A pituitary rongeur may be used to remove any remaining soft tissue form the ligamentum flavum. Alternatively, a large straight curette may be used to

further define the lower portion of each lamina to be removed. At this point, the undersurface of each target lamina should be exposed with clear differentiation of the underlying ligamentum.

- *Laminectomy:*
  - The lamina is then thinned using a high-speed burr. The author prefers to create bilateral "troughs" representing the lateral extent of the laminectomy. This is performed widest at the level of the facet joint and narrowest at the level of the pars, with care taken to preserve adequate pars width, creating a diagonal trough on each side. The width of the trough at the pars level maintain at least 9 mm of pars. At the facet level, the trough may be carried to the medial border of the pedicle if adequate facet (50%) is maintained. The medial wall of the pedicle may be estimated by the mid-lateral pars (i.e., the midlateral pars represents the midpoint of the pedicle at L5 and a point more medial as you move cephalad in the lumbar spine). The depth of the trough may be carried to the level of the ligamentum flavum on the lower half of the lamina. Care is taken at the top of the ligamentum attachment, this may be identified by epidural fat overlying the dura. The cephalad insertion of the ligamentum extends further cephalad at its lateral borders than in the midline. Its cephalad lateral termination occurs a few millimeters inferior to the cephalad pedicle.
  - Once bilateral troughs are created, the lamina is thinned in a similar fashion in the midline. Again this may be carried to the depth of the ligamentum on the lower portion of the lamina. Alternatively, the lamina may be thinned to the underlying cortical bone, which will then be removed using Kerrison rongeurs.
  - Once the lamina is thinned, Kerrison rongeurs are used to remove the remainder of the lamina. This may be done more aggressively on the lower portion of the lamina when you are protected by underlying ligamentum flavum.
  - A Woodson elevator, Frazier suction tip, or similar instrument may be used to protect the underlying dura while performing laminectomy above the insertion of the ligamentum.
  - The author prefers to remove the ligamentum flavum en bloc once the boney lamina is completely removed. This is performed with help of Woodson elevator of curved curette to loosen it from its lateral boney attachment and protect the underlying dura, while a Kerrison rongeur is used to remove the ligamentum.
  - The cephalad extent of a laminectomy is performed to the level of the ligamentum attachment on the undersurface of the upper lamina. The caudad extent of the laminectomy is performed to the ligamentum insertion on the upper portion of the lower lamina.

- *Central stenosis:*
  - Central stenosis results from shingling of the lamina due to degenerative disk disease and disk space collapse and resultant in folding and compression by the ligamentum flavum. Additionally, central stenosis may result from underlying congenital stenosis. Decompression of central stenosis is accomplished by a pedicle to pedicle width laminectomy with complete removal of the underlying ligamentum flavum.
  - The cephalad extent of a laminectomy is performed to the level of the ligamentum attachment on the undersurface of the upper lamina. The caudad extent to the ligamentum insertion on the upper portion of the lower lamina.
  - The lateral extent of the laminectomy is performed to the medial border of the pedicle bilaterally. This is performed by undercutting the facet to the medial border of the pedicle, with care to maintain at least 50% of the facet joint.
  - The central decompression is performed once the entire ligamentum is removed, and the Woodson can be freely passed to the medial border of the pedicles bilaterally.

- *Subarticular lateral recess stenosis:*
  - The lateral recess is bordered by the disk ventrally, and superior articular process (SAP) dorsally.
  - Lateral recess stenosis results from compression of the traversing nerve root by superior articular facet arthrosis, and/or ligamentum flavum hypertrophy dorsally, and any disk herniation or bulging at this level ventrally. This is addressed through partial medial facetectomy and removal of any compressive disk material.
  - Decompression of the lateral recess is performed by underbiting hypertrophied SAP and ligamentum at the level of the disk space and by removing any underlying compressive disk material or adhesions.
  - Once complete, a Woodson elevator should be passed freely laterally to the traversing nerve root at the level of the disk. The traversing nerve root should be free and mobile.

- *Foraminal stenosis:*
  - Foraminal stenosis results in compression of the exiting nerve root between the medial and lateral borders of the pedicle. This stenosis results from hypertrophy and subsequent compression from the tip of the SAP and underlying ligamentum flavum as well as foraminal disk herniations.
  - Decompression of the foramen is performed by first identifying the foramen. This is done by palpating the medial border of the cephalad pedicle using a Woodson elevator. The Woodson is then passed

inferior to the pedicle into the foramen in the direction of the exiting nerve root (i.e., caudal and lateral).
- An isolated foraminotomy may be performed with unilateral exposure and laminotomy as in the case of microdiscectomy.
- Once identified, the foramen is decompressed by passing a series of Kerrisons into the foramen to undercut and remove the overlying facet and ligamentum hypertrophy. Care is taken to protect the underlying exiting nerve root and avoid directing a Kerrison cephalad or across the path of the nerve root. Sequential use of small to larger Kerrisons, 2 mm progressing to 3 mm, may be used to create working space within the foramen. Special curved foraminotomy Kerrisons or foraminotomy rasps may also be used to facilitate the foraminotomy. Foraminotomy Kerrisons curve upward in order to protect the underlying nerve root, while the foraminotomy rasps may be used to remove overlying bone increasing the working space within the foramen. Foraminal decompression is deemed adequate when the Woodson elevator may be freely passed into the foramen over the underlying exiting nerve root.
- *Extraforaminal stenosis:*—results in compression of the exiting nerve root lateral to the lateral border of the cephalad pedicle, typically by overgrowth of the lateral portion of the facet or lateral disk herniation. Extraforaminal stenosis is best addressed with a lateral facetectomy and discectomy via a far lateral or Wiltse type approach as discussed in a separate chapter.

CLOSURE

- The wound is thoroughly irrigated. Hemostasis is achieved with hemostatic agents, bone wax, bipolar, and Bovie electrocautery. The author does not routinely use vancomycin powder in laminectomy or microdiscectomy cases unless the patient is at significant risk of postoperative infection due to medical comorbidities.
- Remove the deep retractors slowly, maintaining meticulous hemostasis. Ensure no active bleeding is identified prior to closure. We perform fascial closure with #1 Vicryl in a figure-of-8 fashion, followed by 2-0 Vicryl deep dermal interrupted stitches, and a running 3-0 monocryl with for epidermal closure. The use of a deep fascial drain is recommended in multilevel cases using appropriate surgical discretion.
- *Pearls:*
  - For microdiscectomy, the extent of cephalad and caudad exposure of the nerve root depends on the size of herniated nucleus pulposus (HNP) and the location of HNP.
  - For a large central HNP, a normal annulotomy and posterolateral discectomy should be done first, followed by use of Woodson elevator to move and push down the HNP and avoid undue retraction of the traversing nerve.
  - Likewise, for foraminal HNP, use Woodson to push the HNP medially to preserve the facet joint resection.
  - For laminectomy for multiple level central stenosis, the lateral trough and extend of the decompression becomes narrower as you move to cephalad levels to prevent iatrogenic pars fracture as the pars is more medial at those levels. Therefore, laminectomy and undercutting the facets make the decompression more lateral at the level of the facet and more medial at the pars, creating an hourglass appearance of the final laminectomy.
  - The foot plate of the Kerrison rongeur should be used in a direction and angle that is parallel to that of the dura to avoid "side-biting" the dura. The thecal sac is ovoid, as such the foot plate should up angles up or down with the upslope or downslope of the thecal sac when moving laterally away from midline.
  - Maintaining a working plane is between dura and overlying ligamentum or scar is important to reduce the risk of dural tear. This may be done with consistent use of a Woodson elevator to palpate and create a free working plane.
  - Adherent ligamentum or scar may be left on the thecal sac to reduce the risk of dural tear, as long as it is free laterally and does not compress a nerve root.

SECTION 3

Miscellaneous

- **Minimally Invasive Surgical Discectomy and Laminectomy**
  Sheeraz Qureshi

- **Extraforaminal Approaches for Microdiscectomy and Foraminal Decompression in the Lumbar Spine**
  Barrett S Boody, Glenn S Russo, Rick C Sasso

- **The Fellows Manual: Techniques of Spine Surgery Minimally Invasive Transforaminal Lumbar Interbody Fusion**
  Peter B Derman, Sravisht Iyer, Dil V Patel, Joon S Yoo, Kern Singh

- **Lateral Lumbar Interbody Fusion**
  Corey T Walker, David S Xu, Juan S Uribe

- **Ante-Psoas Interbody Fusion**
  Neel Anand, Sheila Kahwaty

- **Navigation Techniques**
  Peter R Swiatek, Wellington K Hsu

- **Technical Pearls in the Management of Spinal Cord Injury**
  Daniel Franco, Aria Mahtabfar, Glenn Gonzalez, James Harrop

- **Dural Repair Strategies**
  Fadi Al-Saiegh, Anthony Stefanelli, Srinivas Prasad

- **Minimally Invasive Sacroiliac Joint Fusion**
  Matthew J Sabatino, Glenn S Russo, Peter G Whang

CHAPTER 23

Minimally Invasive Surgical Discectomy and Laminectomy

Sheeraz Quereshi

INTRODUCTION

The use of minimally invasive surgical (MIS) techniques in spinal surgery has shown tremendous increase in recent years[1-4] due to a growing body of literature demonstrating the efficacy and advantages of these techniques and due to technological advances and innovations in imaging modalities, instrumentation, and surgical techniques that are making MIS increasingly feasible, efficient, and safe.[5-11] MIS lumbar microdiscectomy and laminectomy are commonly performed procedures for surgical decompression (Figs. 1A to D).

INSTRUMENTS SUGGESTED

- Jackson table with a Wilson frame
- Intraoperative fluoroscopy or navigation system
- Operating microscope
- Table-mounted tubular retractor system—consisting of multiple dilators of increasing diameter, a table clamp, and a rigid holding arm. Typically a 15- or 16-mm tube is used for discectomies and 18- or 19-mm for laminotomies/laminectomies.[4]
- Intraoperative neurophysiologic monitoring
- Bayoneted instruments such as various Kerrison rongeurs, conventional and ball-tip nerve hooks, and pituitaries are helpful to maximize visualization around the working instruments.
- Surgical power drill, with a 15-cm curved drill shaft and a 3-mm fluted matchstick drill bit.

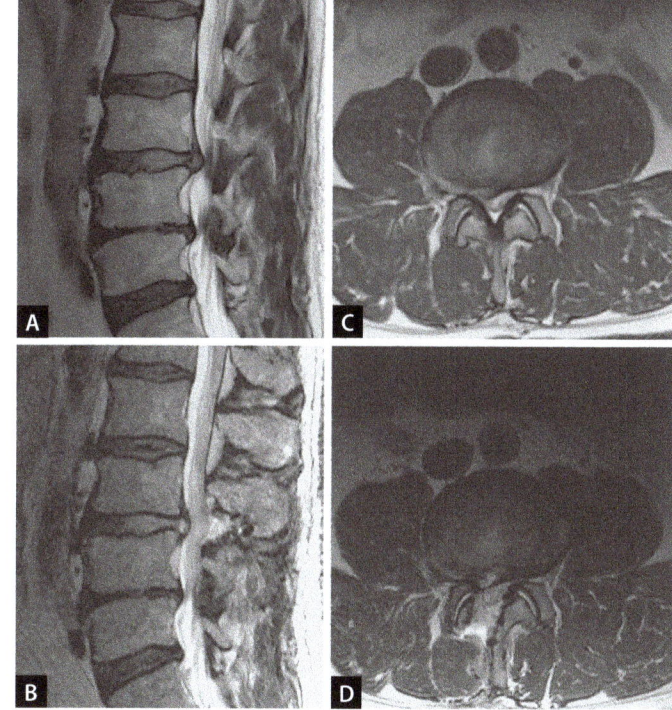

Figs. 1A to D: T2-weighted magnetic resonance imaging images of 60-year-old male with 3 months of debilitating bilateral lower extremity pain in buttocks and posterior thigh, without numbness and tingling. Patient is unable to sit or stand for lower than 5 minutes. Preoperative sagittal (A) and axial (B) images show right-sided L3–L4 paracentral-subarticular disk herniation causing central stenosis. Patient underwent L3–L4 right-sided laminotomy, microdiscectomy, and bilateral decompression. 6-week postoperative sagittal (C) and axial (D) images show decompression of central stenosis. Postoperatively the patient had 80% relief of preoperative symptoms by 2 weeks postoperatively.

OPERATING ROOM SET-UP

- Surgeon and operating microscope should be positioned on the same side as targeted disk herniation or more severe stenosis. Assistant may stand on the opposite side.
- Fluoroscopy or navigation may be used. If fluoroscopy is utilized, it should be positioned on the opposite side of the bed as the surgeon and the microscope. When not in use, it should be slid parallel to the operating table.
- Neuromonitoring should be placed at the cranial end of the patient.

- Microscope and fluoroscope should be positioned on opposite sides of the table, so as to allow for the fluoroscope to be brought into the operative field while the surgeon is under the microscope.

APPROACH

- *Patient-positioning:*
  - General endotracheal anesthesia is induced on a regular operating room bed in supine position.
  - After induction of anesthesia, the patient is flipped to the prone position on a radiolucent Jackson table with a Wilson frame.
  - Arms are held in at 90° of shoulder abduction and 90° of elbow flexion.
  - All bony prominences are padded and eyes are free of any type of compression.
  - Skin is prepped and draped in usual fashion with a water-tight seal around surgical field.
- *Retractor placement:*
  - Under fluoroscopic or navigation guidance, the target level is identified **(Fig. 2)**.
  - A small incision is made approximately 1–1.5 cm lateral to the midline on the side of predominant symptoms and a blunt dilator is passed through the incision under navigation or fluoroscopic guidance until it reaches the inferior edge of the lamina **(Fig. 3)**. This is confirmed on lateral imaging or using computed tomography (CT)-guided navigation.
  - Once it is satisfactorily positioned, dilators of increasing diameter are inserted using twisting motion to enlarge the approach in order to accommodate the tubular retractor.
  - Using navigation or fluoroscopic guidance, an appropriately-sized tubular retractor is docked over the intervertebral space of interest and a working channel is established. The inferior edge of the lamina, and the inferior edge and base of the spinous process should be visible.
  - Fluoroscopy is then used to confirm dilator placement directly at the inferior edge of the lamina, with minimal soft-tissue interposition.
- *Visualization:*
  - The remaining surgical procedure is performed under microscopic visualization.
  - Intervening soft-tissue is cleared from the view through the tubular retractor.

DECOMPRESSION

Microdiscectomy

- For microdiscectomy, a unilateral approach was utilized using a 15 or 16 mm working tube docked at the inferior edge of the ipsilateral superior lamina **(Fig. 4)**.

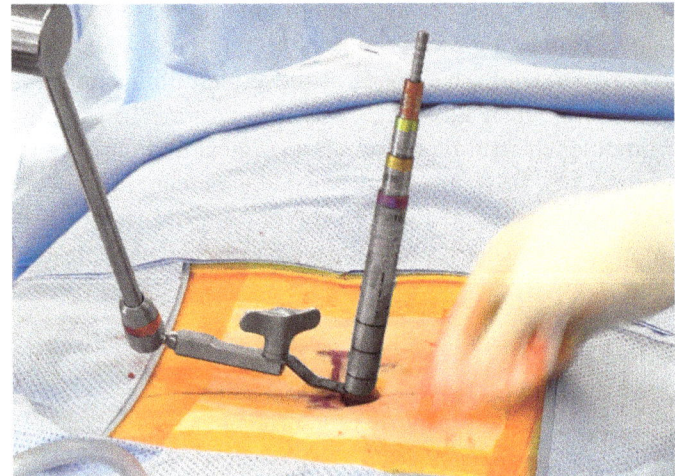

Fig. 3: Intraoperative imaging showing 18 mm incision with sequencing dilators of initial guidewire localized to inferior L4 lamina.

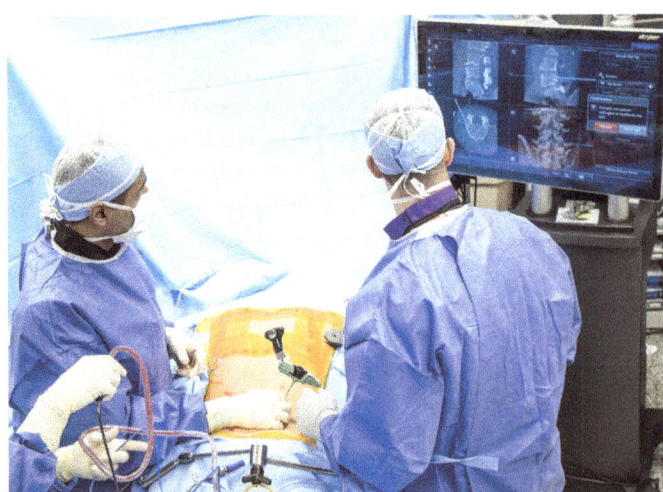

Fig. 2: Intraoperative imaging with patient positioned prone. Intraoperative imaging-guided navigation being utilized for guide wire localization.

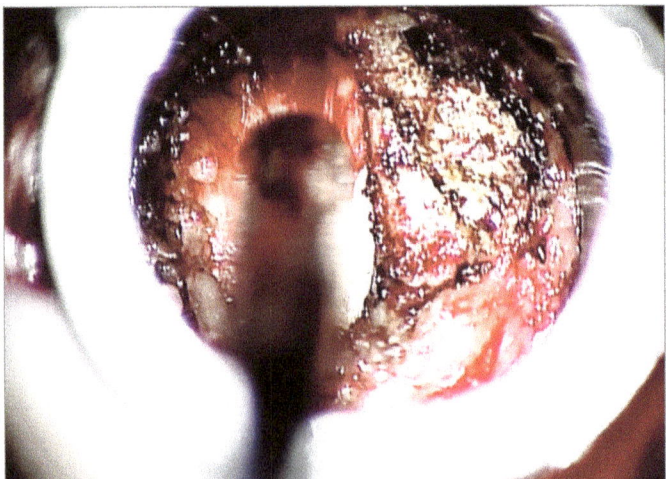

Fig. 4: Intraoperative image of initial anatomic landmarks during microscopic visualization with inferior edge of superior lamina (right) and underlying ligamentum flavum (left).

- Under microscopic visualization, intervening soft tissues are removed. Underlying ligamentum flavum (LF) is visualized caudally and maintained to protect underlying neural structures.
- A unilateral laminotomy is performed using a high-speed side-cutting burr and/or 2- and 3-mm 45° Kerrison rongeurs starting at the interior edge and working superiorly to the cranial insertion of the LF.
  - Care is taken with burring technique to avoid vertical drilling through bone. The blunt tip may be placed on the LF and used to remove away the inferior edge of the lamina.
  - Laminotomy should be carried medially until the midline raphe of the LF is visible. This may be identified due to exposed intervening epidural fat.
  - Partial medial facetectomy may also be performed to increase exposure laterally. Care should be taken not to violate the pars interarticularis laterally.
- The ipsilateral LF is the removed either from the detached cranial insertion on the superior lamina or from the midline raphe between the leaves of the LF.
- The dural sac and nerve roots are then visualized. Traversing nerve root may be gently mobilized medially and axillary region of the exiting nerve root may be explored.
  - Coagulation of epidural bleeding should be performed using bipolar electrocautery and hemostatic agents.
- Herniated disk material may now be visualized and removed. Multiple attempts are made to remove all loose disk fragments. An annulotomy may be performed to remove a symptomatic disk protrusion.
  - Pulsatile movement of the dural sac and freely mobile nerve roots must be visualized to confirm adequate decompression **(Fig. 5)**
- The wound is then copiously irrigated once again, to ensure that all disk fragments are removed.

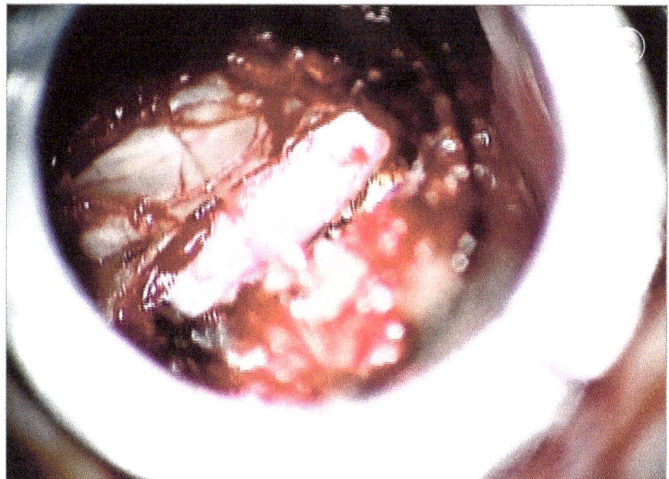

Fig. 5: Intraoperative imaging showing fully decompressed thecal sac (upper left) and traversing nerve root (center).

Laminectomy

- For laminectomy, a unilateral approach is also utilized with 18- or 19-mm working tube docked at the inferior edge of the medial ipsilateral superior lamina. Intervening soft tissues are removed.
- Under microscopic visualization, a combination of high-speed side-cutting burr and/or 2- and 3-mm 45° Kerrison rongeur is used to perform laminectomy.
  - Resection begins at inferior edge of lamina and extends cranially to insertion of LF.
  - Partial medial facetectomy may be performed for additional lateral decompression.
  - Medially, resection is extended to midline exposing midline raphe of LF with intervening epidural fat.
  - Underlying ipsilateral LF may be removed from the midline from medial to lateral.
- Operating table may then be tilted away from the surgeon and the tubular retractor may be angled further medially to perform contralateral laminectomy.
  - Spinous process may be left intact and undercut using side-cutting drill and 2-mm rongeurs to remove ventral bone from lamina completely exposing contralateral LF up to cranial insertion.
  - LF is left in place contralaterally to protect underlying dura. A number 9 suction tip may be used to gently retract the LF ventrally during bony resection.
- Contralateral LF may then be carefully removed using a 90° Kerrison rongeur.
- Contralateral exiting nerve root should then be followed out to the contralateral foramen. Additional bony resection may be required to fully decompress the contralateral foramen laterally including partial ventral facetectomy.
  - This may require additional tilting of the operating table and angling of the working tube.
- Bilateral lateral recess stenosis may also be addressed with a 2 mm Kerrison rongeur.
- Confirmation of adequate decompression is determined by palpation of the contralateral inferior pedicle and visualization of bilateral exiting nerve roots with at least 10 mm of free excursion.
  - The preoperative sagittal magnetic resonance imaging (MRI) should be studied to identify additional areas of LF hypertrophy that may often be missed more caudally.
- The wound is then copiously irrigated.

CLOSURE

- Once meticulous hemostasis is achieved, the tubular retractor is removed.
  - Bipolar cautery as well as thrombin-soaked hemostatic matrix or temporary packing can be helpful in achieving hemostasis.

- The tubular retractor is removed slowly, ensuring that no active bleeding is seen. Hemostasis is essential to prevent the occurrence of a postoperative hematoma, which can cause severe pain and muscle spasms.
- Muscle is infiltrated with local anesthetic.
- Layered would closure is performed with 2-0 absorbable braided suture in the fascia followed by buried 3-0 absorbable monofilament suture in the skin.

REFERENCES

1. Al-Khouja L, Shweikeh F, Pashman R, Johnson JP, Kim T, Drazin D. Economics of image guidance and navigation in spine surgery. Surg Neurol Int. 2015;6(11):323.
2. Kobayashi K, Ando K, Nishida Y, Ishiguro N, Imagama S. Epidemiological trends in spine surgery over 10 years in a multicenter database. Eur Spine J. 2018;27(8):1698-703.
3. Martin B, Brodke DS, Mirza SK, Spina N, Lawrence B, Spiker WR. Trends in lumbar fusion procedure rates and associated hospital costs for degenerative spinal diseases in the United States, 2004-2015. Spine (Phila Pa 1976). 2018;44(5):1.
4. Boukebir MA, Berlin CD, Navarro-Ramirez R, Heiland T, Schöller K, Rawanduzy C, et al. Ten-step minimally invasive spine lumbar decompression and dural repair through tubular retractors. Oper Neurosurg. 2017;13(2):232-44.
5. Kraus MD, Krischak G, Keppler P, Gebhard FT, Schuetz UHW. Can computer-assisted surgery reduce the effective dose for spinal fusion and sacroiliac screw insertion? Clin Orthop Relat Res. 2010;468(9):2419-29.
6. Overley SC, Cho SK, Mehta AI, Arnold PM. Navigation and robotics in spinal surgery: Where are we now? Clin Neurosurg. 2017;80(3):S86-99.
7. Amiot LP, Lang K, Putzier M, Zippel H, Labelle H. Comparative results between conventional and computer-assisted pedicle screw installation in the thoracic, lumbar, and sacral spine. Spine (Phila Pa 1976). 2000;25(5):606-14.
8. Yu X, Xu L, Bi L. Spinal navigation with intra-operative 3D-imaging modality in lumbar pedicle screw fixation. Zhonghua Yi Xue Za Zhi. 2008;88(27):1905-8.
9. Roser F, Tatagiba M, Maier G. Spinal robotics: current applications and future perspectives. Neurosurgery. 2013;72 Suppl 1:12-18.
10. Schizas C, Thein E, Kwiatkowski B, Kulik G. Pedicle screw insertion: robotic assistance versus conventional C-arm fluoroscopy. Acta Orthop Belg. 2012;78(2):240-5.
11. Kumar A, Merrill RK, Overley SC, Leven DM, Meaike JJ, Vaishnav A, et al. Radiation exposure in minimally invasive transforaminal lumbar interbody fusion: The effect of the learning curve. 2019;13(1):39-45.

CHAPTER 24

Extraforaminal Approaches for Microdiscectomy and Foraminal Decompression in the Lumbar Spine

Barrett S Boody, Glenn S Russo, Rick C Sasso

■ INTRODUCTION

Foraminal and extraforaminal pathology, such as bony stenosis and disk herniations, are sources of pathology resulting in lumbosacral radiculopathy that can be difficult to diagnose. A lumbar magnetic resonance imaging (MRI) is a highly reliable imaging study to diagnose foraminal and extraforaminal disk herniations.[1] Findings of focal eccentricity of the disk contour, obliteration of perineural fat within the foramen, changes in thickness of the nerve root, and displacement of the nerve root are all suggestive of foraminal or extraforaminal disk herniations.[2]

Far lateral or extraforaminal approaches are powerful techniques for extraforaminal or foraminal pathology resulting in lumbar radiculopathy. These approaches are commonly performed from L2 to L5, but the L5–S1 extraforaminal approach has also been described with successful results. Lee et al. reported a retrospective series of 52 L5–S1 extraforaminal decompressions with 96% of patients reporting good to excellent outcomes.[3] However, access medial to the pedicle into the spinal canal is limited with far lateral approaches and concomitant pathology within the spinal canal may require both a combined hemilaminotomy and extraforaminal approach using a midline-based incision.[4]

While open approaches have historically been the gold standard, minimally invasive approaches have been well described for the treatment of extraforaminal disk herniations and foraminal stenosis.[5,6] Akinduro et al. performed a systematic review of open versus minimally invasive extraforaminal approaches for disk herniations. While they found similar rates of complications and reoperations between groups, minimally invasive approaches resulted in lower estimated blood loss, shorter operative time, shorter hospitalizations, and shorter return to work. However, since there were no head-to-head trials comparing open to minimally invasive approaches, they cautioned reporting the superiority of one technique to the other.[7]

■ INSTRUMENTS SUGGESTED

- Open Jackson, Allen table, or Wilson frame
- Intraoperative fluoroscopy or digital flat plate intraoperative imaging
- *Microscope (optional):*
  - Helpful for assistants to visualize the surgical field through limited exposures
  - We prefer loupe magnification due to ease of workflow.
- Intraoperative neuromonitoring [considered, but not required. The use of triggered and/or spontaneous electromyography (EMG) for nerve identification can be helpful if unfamiliar with the approach and dissection.]
  - Use of triggered EMG cannot be reliably performed with neuromuscular blockade
  - We do not routinely use neuromonitoring for these cases.
- *For minimally invasive surgical (MIS) approaches:*
  - Table-mounted tubular retractor system with lighting options
  - *Expandable or static tubes:*
    - Expandable tubes may improve working room for instruments through the opening of the retractor, but may result in more "shallow" docking and require more soft tissue dissection.
    - Adjustable depth custom retractors
  - Bayoneted instruments such as Kerrisons, nerve retractors, Woodson elevators, and pituitaries are helpful to maximize visualization by removing the surgeon's hand from the surgical field.
- *For open approaches:*
  - Standard open lumbar decompression sets are utilized.
  - Deep Gelpi, Cerebellar, or McCullough retractors can be used for exposure.

APPROACH

- This can be performed using an MIS or open parasagittal Wiltse approach.
  - Additionally, this can be done in an open fashion through an extensile midline longitudinal skin incision with a parasagittal fascial incision. This is our preferred technique if a combined procedure is planned.
- A lighted retractor can be helpful for relatively deep dissections. Alternatively, we prefer the use of a headlight for adequate visualization.

Minimally Invasive Surgical Approach (Figs. 1A to E)

- *Table:* Position the patient prone on a radiolucent table. The authors prefer the open Jackson or Allen tables for unencumbered anteroposterior (AP) and lateral fluoroscopy.
- *Retractor:* Attach the post for the tubular retractor to the side-rail contralateral to the side of approach, opposite of the surgeon.
- *Draping:*
  - Drape widely. Larger patients will require a more lateral incision to allow for a straight "line-of-sight" approach through the Wiltse interval between the multifidus and erector spinae.
  - The distance from the incision to midline can be estimated preoperatively using the axial images on the MRI.
- *Fluoroscopy:*
  - Using lateral fluoroscopy and a spinal needle, identify the pedicle above and below the extraforaminal pathology (i.e., for L4–L5 extraforaminal disk, identify where the L4 and L5 pedicle would be) and/or the transverse processes at each pedicle level.
  - The trajectory of the spinal needle and eventually the retractor should be in-line with the disk space, accounting for the lordosis of the lumbar spine.
  - Your skin incision should extend from the pedicle above to the pedicle below the surgical level and lateral to the midline at the appropriate distance. On average this will be approximately 2.5–3 fingerbreadths from the midline as determined by either palpation of spinous processes or AP fluoroscopy.
- *Dissection:*
  - Hemostasis is critical to this approach. Muscular arterial bleeders and facet branches of the segmental

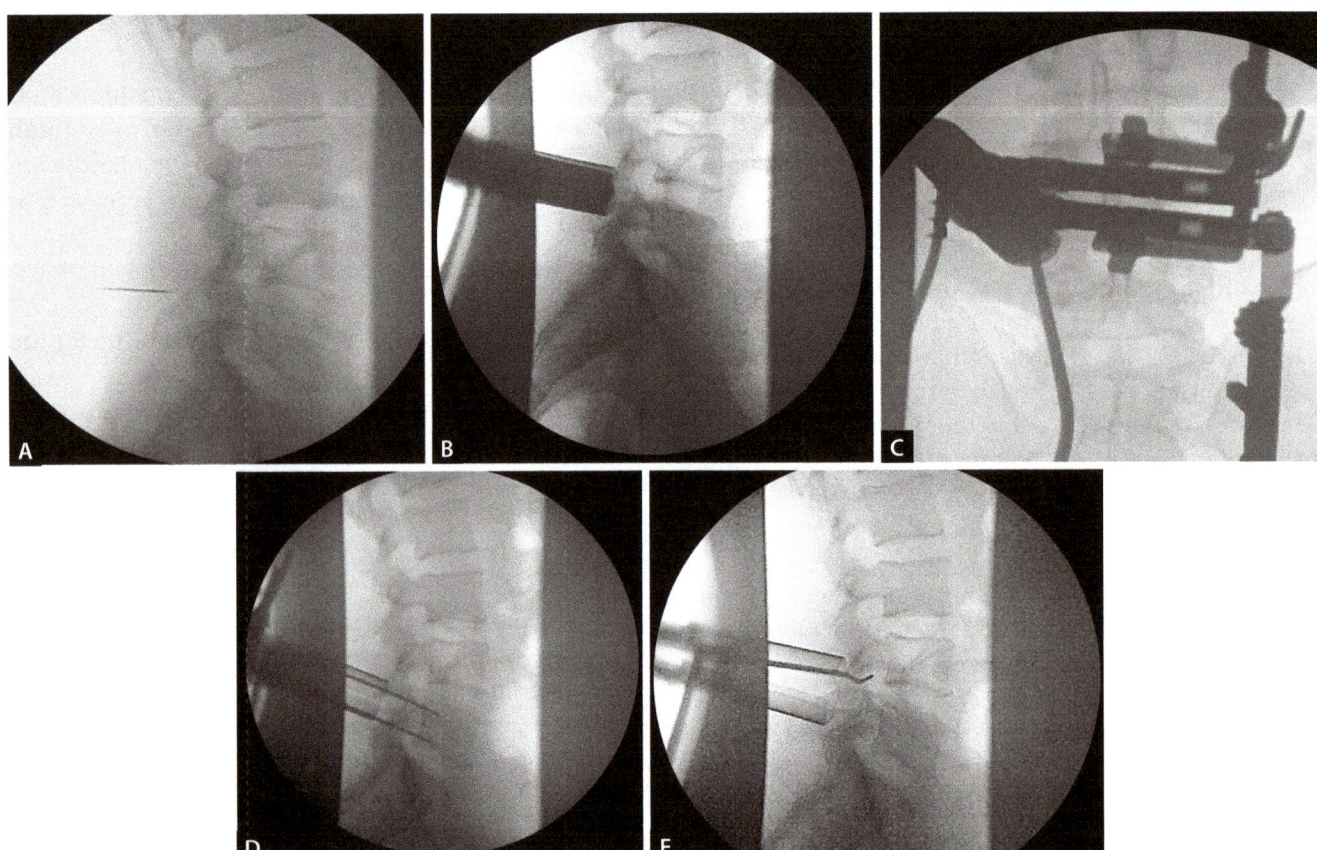

Figs. 1A to E: Minimally invasive right L4–L5 far lateral microdiscectomy. After needle localization (A), an expandable tubular retractor was placed through the Wiltse interval onto the right L5 pedicle and confirmed with lateral and anteroposterior fluoroscopy (B and C, respectively). After removal of dilators, the L5 transverse process was identified with bayoneted forceps (D). The tube was expanded under lateral fluoroscopic images to reach the L4 pedicle and a Woodson elevator was used to identify the L4 pedicle (E) prior to beginning exiting nerve decompression.

artery can cause significant bleeding and will significantly compromise visualization through tubular access.

- Following skin incision, dissect down to the fascia and obtain strict hemostasis of the approach prior to fascial incision.
- Palpate the interval between the multifidus and erector spinae. Next, infiltrate the muscular plane and adjacent muscles with 20-30 cc of 0.25% Marcaine with epinephrine and wait 60-120 seconds for the epinephrine to create regional vasoconstriction.
- Incise the fascia with electrocautery, bluntly dissecting using your finger within the interval and palpate the transverse process and upslope to the superior articular facet (similar to the percutaneous approach for lumbar pedicle screws) for the pedicles above and below the surgical level.
- Sweep your finger between the two transverse processes so there are no fascial or muscular bands that could restrict tube movement or adjustments.
- Consider placing Floseal or gelfoam-thrombin in this space and pack with a Raytec for 1-2 minutes to reduce muscular bleeding.

- *Visualization:* Place the initial dilator at the start point for a percutaneous pedicle screw (on the transverse process toward the upslope of the superior articular facet). If you use a static tube, start at the cephalad pedicle since exiting nerve exposure is the first step of the decompression. If you use an expandable, you can start at either the cephalad or caudad pedicle and expand toward the other.

- *Confirm retractor position:*
  - Confirm on lateral fluoroscopy that your tubular retractor is seated to the depth of the transverse process. The tip of the initial dilator should be at the dorsal aspect of the pedicle on lateral fluoroscopy.
  - A common mistake here is to dock on a large, overgrown facet or dock excessively lateral due to the size of the lateral facet osteophytes. If the facet overgrowth causes the tube to be docked significantly laterally to where you cannot identify the pars safely, you can consider a "shallow dock" at the level of the facet and remove lateral osteophytes with a burr or rongeur prior to "final docking" at the level of the transverse process. Additionally, you may consider switching to an open technique for improved anatomy identification.
  - Continue to dilate and measure the depth of the retractor blades. Place your retractor and secure it to the table. Before removing your dilators, confirm your position with AP and lateral fluoroscopy. Reconfirm you are at the correct level, your retractor is angled toward the extraforaminal space, in line with the surgical level disk space, that the deepest aspect of the tube is below the facet joint on the lateral view. Also use AP fluoroscopy to confirm that your retractor is angled slightly medially and also is lateral to the facet on the AP view.
    - A common mistake is to dock on the facet and have your retractor be too shallow, increasing the soft tissue dissection and bleeding.
  - Once you have confirmed your retractor location, you can expand the blades. After expansion, confirm on lateral fluoroscopy that the expandable tube has not migrated.

Open Approach (Figs. 2A to C)

- *Localization:*
  - Localize the incision using needle localization on lateral fluoroscopy at the foramen of interest.
    - The authors prefer a midline incision with a parasagittal fascial incision to decrease the risk of skin necrosis should a midline revision procedure be required in the future.

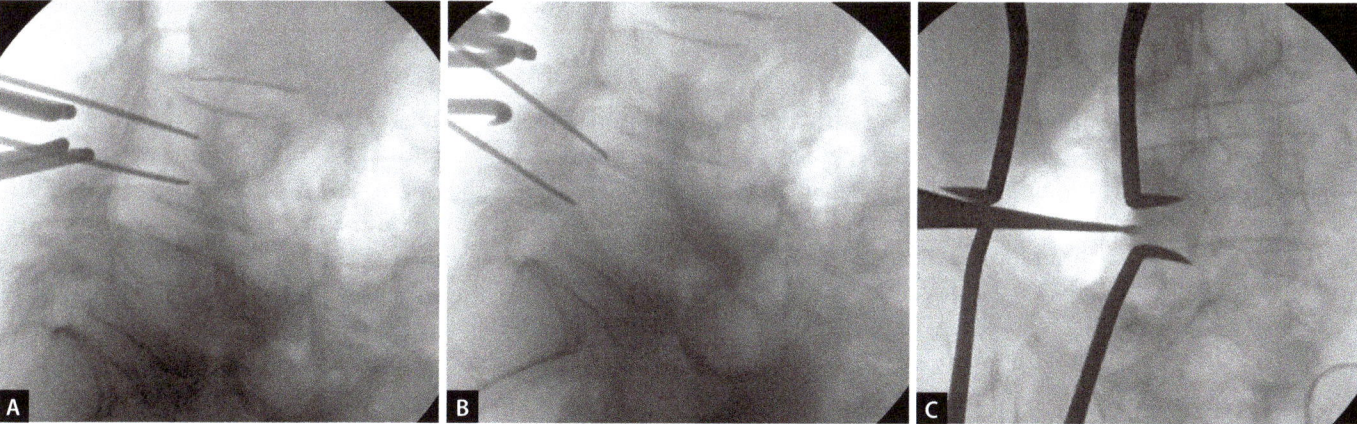

Figs. 2A to C: Open approach right L4–L5 far lateral microdiscectomy. After placement of deep Gelpi retractors, bayoneted forceps were placed over the transverse process of L4 and L5 (A and B, respectively) and lateral fluoroscopic views were obtained to confirm the correct surgical level. Next, the right lateral pars of L4 was identified with a curette on anteroposterior fluoroscopic image (C) prior to beginning exiting nerve decompression.

- For a midline incision, the skin incision will likely extend from the spinous process above and below (i.e., for a L4–L5 extraforaminal approach, the skin incision will likely extend from the spinous process of L3 to L5). Continue the dissection down to the fascia with meticulous hemostasis. Mobilize the skin incision and expose the fascia by clearing the attachments to the subcutaneous tissues on the side of interest. If the skin is not properly mobilized, this will prohibit use of the deep Gelpi retractors.
- For a parasagittal incision, localize and use fluoroscopy similar to the skin incision used for the MIS approach. The length of incision will be dependent on the size of the patient.

- *Fascial incision:*
  - Make a parasagittal fascial incision between the multifidus and the erector spinae. You can identify this with palpation, finding a small valley between the two muscle groups. Additionally, it will confirm you are in correct interval/plane if you are able to bluntly dissect down to the transverse processes.
    - The length of the fascial incision/dissection should extend beyond the transverse process above and below the surgical level.
  - Place two deep Gelpi retractors (or other preferred retractors) within the Wiltse interval, roughly at the level of the pedicle above and below the surgical level.
    - An assistant positioned across the table retracting the soft tissues and multifidus medially with an army-navy or Hibbs retractor at the level of the pars can assist with the exposure.
  - Additionally, confirm with lateral fluoroscopy you are at the appropriate level using bayoneted forceps placed over an exposed transverse process before beginning the decompression.
- *Hemostasis:* Although the field of direct visualization is larger than the MIS approach, hemostasis is still critical for the open approach. Similarly, you can infiltrate the paraspinal musculature with 20–30 cc of 0.25% Marcaine with epinephrine prior to entering the Wiltse interval. After opening the interval with the Gelpi retractors, initial hemostasis can be achieved with Floseal or gelfoam-thrombin in this space and packing with a Raytec for 1–2 minutes followed by bipolar cautery. Using electrocautery prior to identification of landmarks can potentially result in nerve injury.

EXPOSURE

- Begin exposure with known landmarks. The authors prefer to expose both the caudal and cephalad transverse processes in order to expose the entire extraforaminal space, providing visualization of both the exiting nerve and disk space.
  - A common error is losing perspective of depth and position in space with the Wiltse approach. To avoid this, make sure you can identify sequentially the cephalad transverse process, facet joint, and then pars at the surgical level (if not occluded by significant degenerative overgrowth).
  - Blunt or manual palpation of landmarks is a safe way to orient yourself before using sharp dissection or electrocautery.
  - Beginning dissection too lateral without orienting using bony landmarks can result in inadvertent entry below the intertransverse membrane without recognizing the depth of dissection, with potential nerve injury or segmental artery injury.
- First, identify the transverse process of the cephalad pedicle and use electrocautery to expose the upslope to the facet and lateral aspect of the facet. Make sure the dissection does not go deeper than the transverse process with electrocautery, as this can cause nerve injury.
- Continue dissecting caudad and identify the pars interarticularis and continue down to the caudad lateral facet joint transverse process.
  - Overgrown degenerative facets can obstruct visualization of the pars.
  - If necessary, resect a small amount of the lateral facet using burr or Kerrisons to visualize the pars. Visualizing the pars is key to safely performing this procedure.
- Ensure that the landmarks are cleared of soft tissue and achieve meticulous hemostasis. Commonly, a large facet bleeder will be encountered during dissection. Use bipolar cautery and Floseal/gelfoam-thrombin for hemostasis.
- Alternatively, you may begin with exposure of the caudad transverse process and proceed proximally. The key here is sufficient exposure of anatomy and hemostasis that you can safely find the exiting nerve and extraforaminal pathology.

DECOMPRESSION

- First identify the nerve root.
  - Extraforaminal disk herniations are most likely to displace the nerve dorsally and cephalad, resulting in a nerve location that is commonly directly ventral to the pars and just caudad to the cephalad pedicle.
  - Identify the junction between the intertransverse membrane and pars and use a burr to thin the lateral aspect of the pars/facet, usually about 2–3 mm of lateral resection at this level. Next, use a Woodson elevator or forward angle curette medially beneath the pars to enter the foramen and identify the ventral pars.
    - Identifying the nerve in relation to its position adjacent to the pars is a safe and reliable way to

identify the nerve. Identifying the nerve within the soft tissues of the extraforaminal window can be difficult due to bleeding and distorted anatomy from disk herniations. Additionally, identifying the nerve in the extraforaminal space can be difficult, as disk herniations and intertransverse membrane can be mistaken for nerve, or vice-versa.
- Next, a plane between the intertransverse membrane and the nerve can be developed using a Woodson elevator. Only after a plane is identified should the membrane be resected with a Kerrison rongeur. This will expose the nerve and enable the nerve to be safely distinguished from the disk herniation.
    - The intertransverse membrane is a thick, fibrous membrane, similar to the posterior longitudinal ligament (PLL) in an anterior cervical discectomy and fusion (ACDF) approach. Multiple perforating bleeders will be encountered and hemostasis should be achieved with bipolar cautery.

- *Neuromonitoring:*
    - Avoiding the use of neuromuscular blockade can assist with nerve identification during decompression. An irritable nerve will commonly create spontaneous depolarizations with contact from instruments and create spontaneous EMG (if using neuromonitoring) or leg twitches and can be clinically appreciated.
    - Additionally, if using neuromonitoring, a nerve stimulator can be helpful for identifying a displaced nerve.

- *Discectomy:*
    - Only after you have identified the nerve root can you begin to remove extraforaminal disk herniations. Make sure you identify the plane between the nerve and disk herniation prior to disk removal.
    - Use a Woodson elevator, D'Errico, or Frazier suction tip to protect the nerve as you remove the disk herniation with a micropituitary.
        - Minimize manipulation of the nerve within the extraforaminal window as the dorsal root ganglion is exceptionally sensitive to traction and compression and even minimal manipulation can result in difficult to control neuropathic pain postoperatively.
    - Removal of disk fragments and dissection in this area can create significant venous and arterial bleeding. Although it can be tedious, deal with the bleeders using bipolar and Floseal or gelfoam-thrombin as they arise, do not wait until after finishing the discectomy. Bleeding will obscure landmarks and increase the risk of inadvertent nerve injury due to poor visualization.

- *Evaluate decompression:*
    - Following removal of visualized extraforaminal disk, trace the nerve on all sides (ventral, dorsal, cephalad, and caudad) from the inferomedial cephalad pedicle out into the extraforaminal space to confirm your decompression.
    - After confirming the decompression, irrigate to remove small disk fragments and inflammatory mediators from the surrounding areas.
    - Identify the disk space next and look for annular defects.
    - Identify any loose pieces of disk within annular defects and remove these with a micropituitary or nerve hook.

- *Foraminal stenosis:*
    - Foraminal stenosis can be addressed as well from the extraforaminal approach after removing extraforaminal disk herniations (if present).
    - Using a burr, thin the lateral aspects of the facet joint from the pars to the cephalad aspect of the caudad pedicle. The superficial aspects of the facet (dorsal to the pars) can be left alone to maintain as much facet as possible. Bony overgrowth from degenerative disease extending laterally can be resected as needed to improve visualization.
    - Next, use a Kerrison rongeur to further resect superior articular facet overgrowth within the foramen. Always know where the exiting nerve root is prior to making passes or taking bites with the Kerrison rongeur.
        - Avoid aggressive bites in the cephalad area which can injure the exiting nerve root.
        - Bites with the Kerrison medial to the medial aspect of the caudad pedicle risk injury to the traversing nerve root at this level.
    - Continue foraminal decompression until the nerve can be easily traced from the inferomedial cephalad pedicle to the extraforaminal window without compression.
        - Keep in mind that although the nerve may be decompressed in this current, static state, that the patient may experience dynamic foraminal decompression. Ensure that an adequate margin of decompression is achieved around the exiting nerve root.

CLOSURE

As you remove the retractor, obtain meticulous hemostasis. Bipolar cautery as well as Floseal or gelfoam-thrombin and temporary packing can be helpful. Ensure no active bleeding is identified prior to closure. We perform fascial closure with #1 Vicryl in a figure-of-8 fashion for open cases and #0 Vicryl for MIS cases, followed by 2-0 Vicryl deep dermal interrupted stitches, and a running 3-0 monocryl for epidermal closure.

POSTOPERATIVE MANAGEMENT

- We commonly recommend no formal postoperative restrictions and can be safely discharged home the same day as the procedure.
- Occasionally, patients may report neuropathic pain in the distribution of the decompressed nerve. Oral or intravenous (IV) steroids and gabapentin can be helpful adjuncts for these patients.
- Standing X-rays are obtained at the first postoperative visit to evaluate for fracture or new postoperative listhesis at the surgical levels. Subsequent X-rays are ordered on an as-needed basis.

REFERENCES

1. Moon KP, Suh KT, Lee JS. Reliability of MRI findings for symptomatic extraforaminal disc herniation in lumbar spine. Asian Spine J. 2009;3(1):16-20.
2. Lee IS, Kim HJ, Lee JS, Moon TY, Jeon UB. Extraforaminal with or without foraminal disk herniation: Reliable MRI findings. Am J Roentgenol. 2009;192(5):1392-6.
3. Lee S, Kang JH, Srikantha U, Jang IT, Oh SH. Extraforaminal compression of the L-5 nerve root at the lumbosacral junction: clinical analysis, decompression technique, and outcome. J Neurosurg Spine. 2014;20(4):371-9.
4. Bae JS, Kang KH, Park JH, Lim JH, Jang IT. Postoperative clinical outcome and risk factors for poor outcome of foraminal and extraforaminal lumbar disc herniation. J Korean Neurosurg Soc. 2016;59(2):143-8.
5. Siu TL, Lin K. Microscopic tubular discectomy for far lateral lumbar disc herniation. J Clin Neurosci. 2016;33:129-33.
6. Phan K, Dunn AE, Rao PJ, Mobbs RJ. Far lateral microdiscectomy: a minimally-invasive surgical technique for the treatment of far lateral lumbar disc herniation. J Spine Surg Hong Kong. 2016;2(1):59-63.
7. Akinduro OO, Kerezoudis P, Alvi MA, Yoon JW, Eluchie J, Murad MH, et al. Open versus minimally invasive surgery for extraforaminal lumbar disk herniation: A systematic review and meta-analysis. World Neurosurg. 2017;108:924-38.e923.

CHAPTER 25

The Fellows Manual: Techniques of Spine Surgery Minimally Invasive Transforaminal Lumbar Interbody Fusion

Peter B Derman, Sravisht Iyer, Dil V Patel, Joon S Yoo, Kern Singh

DISCLOSURE

No funds were received in support of this work. No benefits in any form have been or will be received from any commercial party related directly or indirectly to the subject of this manuscript.

INTRODUCTION

Decompression, disk space preparation, and interbody cage placement through the transforaminal space are accomplished via a muscle-preserving paraspinal (Wiltse) approach using tubular retractors. Percutaneous pedicle screw and rod instrumentation are placed. This method allows for a direct decompression of the neural elements in addition to access to the interbody space for fusion. Indications are identical to those of traditional open transforaminal lumbar interbody fusion (TLIF). In overweight and obese individuals, minimally invasive techniques are especially beneficial as the increased technical and physical demands of performing operations on such patients are less marked with tubular retractors than with traditional open techniques.

INSTRUMENTS SUGGESTED

Four-post Jackson frame:
- Intraoperative fluoroscopy
- Local anesthetic
- Jamshidi needles
- Kirschner wires
- Tubular dilators
- Nonexpandable tubular retractors
- Kerrison and pituitary rongeurs (combination of straight and bayoneted)
- Straight and curved bayoneted curettes
- High-speed burr with 3 mm side-cutting tip
- Paddle distractors
- Interbody trial spacers
- Interbody cage
- Pedicle taps
- Percutaneous pedicle screws
- Contoured rods
- Set screws.

APPROACH

- *Patient positioning:*
  - Following intubation, neuromonitoring leads are placed, and the patient is positioned prone on a standard four-post Jackson frame.
  - The arms are abducted and flexed to 90°, allowing space for the fluoroscopy arm. The lower extremities are positioned on a flat board with hips in extension to promote lumbar lordosis. Knees are flexed to take tension of the sciatic nerve **(Fig. 1)**.
  - Padding is placed under pressure points. Pelvic pads should be placed approximately 1 inch below the anterior superior iliac spines to maximize lumbar lordosis.
- *Draping:*
  - Widely drape the entire lumbar spine to allow for identification of surface anatomy such as the iliac crest, posterior superior iliac spine, and spinous processes for improved orientation.
  - If a unilateral approach is planned, the hemilaminotomy is typically performed on the side of greatest symptoms or pathology. The surgeon will stand on that side, and the tubular retractor arm is affixed to the operating table on the contralateral side so that it is out of the surgeon's way. For bilateral approaches, retractor arms are placed on both sides of the table. Bilateral approaches for bilateral complete facetectomies are most often used in the setting of severely collapsed disk spaces in need of additional mobilization.

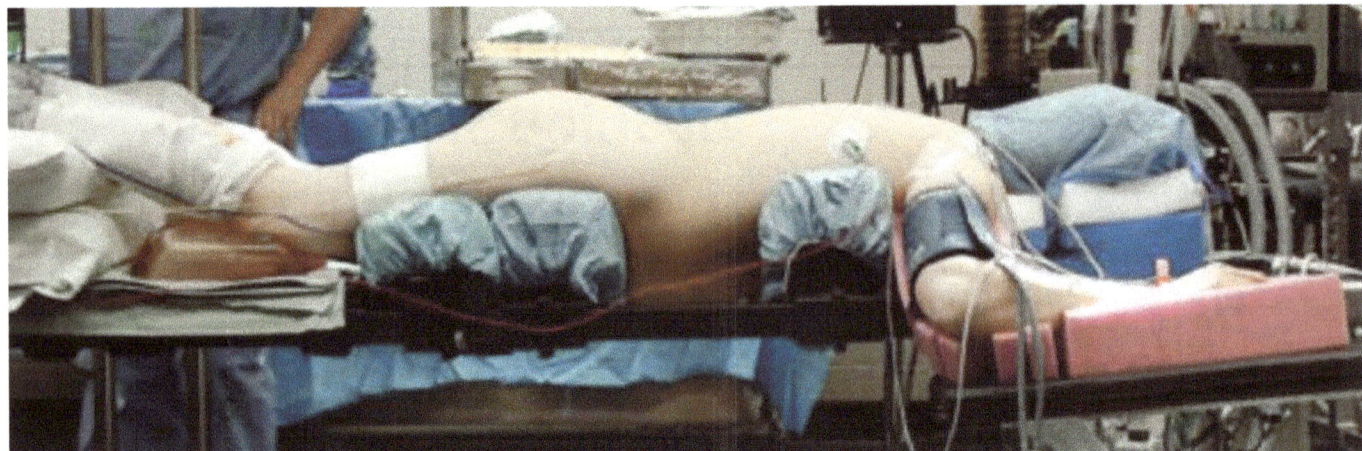

Fig. 1: Patient in prone positioning on a Jackson table with adequate padding, with shoulders abducted and arms flexed.

- *Fluoroscopy:*
  - The fluoroscopy unit should be located on the side opposite from the surgeon.
  - Using fluoroscopic imaging, the appropriate lumbar level is identified. At the superior endplate of the cephalad vertebral body, the C-arm is positioned for an anteroposterior (AP) view.
  - AP fluoroscopic alignment is correct when the pedicles are equidistant from the spinous process and the endplates are clearly visualized.
- *Incision:*
  - A 2–3 cm incision extending from approximately 5 mm lateral to the cranial pedicle to 5 mm lateral to the caudal pedicle is marked on the side of the greatest pathology. Incisions are placed slightly more laterally in obese patients to allow for a sufficiently medialized pedicle screw trajectory.
  - Bilateral instrumentation is performed so a similar incision can be marked on the contralateral side. Depending on patient anatomy, two small percutaneous incisions can be used on the contralateral side rather than a single incision connecting the two percutaneous pedicle screw insertion sites.
  - Local anesthetic is infiltrated into the deep and superficial soft tissues overlying the projected pedicle screw and retractor trajectories using a spinal needle. Be careful not to puncture the dura and perform a spinal anesthetic. While the effect of local anesthetic is greatest before incision is made, the deep soft tissues can be infiltrated after the fascia has been incised if there is any concern regarding the appropriate depth (e.g., obese patients).
  - The skin overlying the marked incisions is incised with a scalpel. Unipolar electrocautery is then used to dissect through the subcutaneous tissue and to incise the fascia in line with the intended pedicle screw trajectory.
- *Guidewire placement:*
  - The pedicle screw start point is located at the intersection of the transverse process and the pars interarticularis at the lateral aspect of the facet. Under fluoroscopic guidance, the Jamshidi needle is carefully advanced toward this point. The ideal starting position is at 2 o'clock on the right pedicle and 10 o'clock on the left pedicle.
  - Once the Jamshidi tip is resting on the optimal start point, use a mallet to tap the handle to create an entry point. It may be beneficial to exaggerate the lateral-to-medial trajectory during this step to prevent the tip from slipping. Once the entry point has been established, the Jamshidi is redirected into the trajectory of the pedicle and advanced using manual pressure or careful taps with a mallet.
  - The Jamshidi needle is advanced into the pedicle in 5 mm increments. At 20 mm, the Jamshidi needle is presumed to have traversed the entire length of the pedicle and is now entering the posterior aspect of the vertebral body. Contact with the medial border of the pedicle prior to 20 mm is suggestive of a medial pedicle wall breach. This can be avoided by careful attention to tactile cues and through the use of fluoroscopy.
  - A Kirschner guidewire is placed into the needle shaft. The tip of the guidewire should be advanced until it lies within the mid-vertebral body. This increases purchase and reduces the chance of inadvertent guidewire dislodgement. However, advancing the guidewire past the mid-vertebral body increases the risk of anterior cortical perforation and visceral injury. The Jamshidi is removed, and the free end of the guidewire is temporarily snapped to the drapes.
  - A Kirschner guidewire is placed through the contralateral pedicle with a Jamshidi needle following a similar technique.

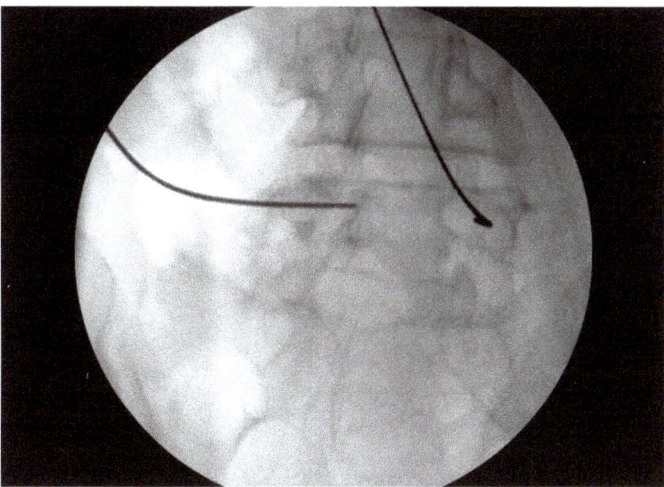

Fig. 2: Fluoroscopic image taken intraoperatively shows the center placement of the guidewires within the pedicle.

- Oblique or "owl-eye" fluoroscopic images may be taken at this point to ensure the guidewires traverse within the confines of the pedicles **(Fig. 2)**.
- Next, the fluoroscopy unit is directed at the superior end plate of the caudal vertebral body. Identical steps are performed to place guidewires bilaterally at this level.
- If a unilateral approach is planned (as is typically the case), the pedicle screws and rod can be placed on the contralateral side utilizing the steps described in the "Percutaneous Pedicle Screw Placement" section below. The cranial set screw is tightened down, while the caudal set screw is applied loosely to allow the rod to slide during paddle distraction later in the case.

■ *Tubular retractor placement:*
- Nonexpandable tubular retractors are used. Expandable retractors require additional muscle resection, and the visualization provided by a nonexpandable retractor is sufficient to safely and effectively perform the procedure.
- A dilator is inserted between the guidewires on the side of the approach.
- If a unilateral decompression is planned, the tubular retractor can be placed in the same trajectory as the pedicle screws. However, a more vertical trajectory is necessary to undercut the contralateral lamina for a bilateral decompression via a unilateral hemilaminotomy. In this case, the initial dilator can be placed through the fascial incision made for the percutaneous screws, but the tip is then medialized before progressing through the paraspinal musculature to create a less medial-to-lateral angle. A "T-cut" can also be made in the fascia if it is impeding appropriate dilator placement.
- The initial dilator is directed toward the inferior border of the cranial lamina at the spinolaminar junction. Starting with the tip of the first dilator on the lateral border of the spinous process and then sliding down on bone to the spinolaminar junction can help prevent plunging into the interlaminar space, which may be especially large at more caudal levels. Tactile feedback is used to confirm the location of the dilators on bone, but fluoroscopy images can provide confirmation if there is any question.
- Sequential dilation is performed at the level of the disk space.
- Maintain constant gentle downward pressure onto the lamina during dilation to prevent surrounding soft tissues from entering the field. However, be careful not to plunge into the interlaminar window.
- A tubular retractor is inserted, secured to the operating room (OR) table, and position confirmed on fluoroscopy to ensure proper retractor depth and position.
- The upslope of the lamina toward the midline should be visualized at the spinolaminar junction once the tube is in place.
- If a microscope is used, the bed can be rotated to allow for a more favorable viewing angle. However, this is typically not necessary if the procedure is performed using loupes.

DECOMPRESSION

■ *Laminectomy:*
- Excision of remaining soft tissue and musculature with electrocautery and a pituitary rongeur improves visualization of the lamina, pars interarticularis, and facet joint.
- Using a microscope or loupes for optimal visualization, a hemilaminotomy is performed using a high-speed burr.
- The laminectomy is extended cephalad to the origin of the ligamentum flavum. The laminectomy provides local bone autograft, which should be collected using a suction trap and saved in a cannister as a bulking agent for interbody fusion.
- If bilateral decompression is to be performed via a unilateral approach, the tubular retractor is then angled medially. The spinous process and contralateral lamina are undercut with the ligamentum flavum providing a safety barrier between the dura and the burr.
- A raphe in the ligamentum flavum marks the midline. Bony decompression should be extended across the raphe and into the contralateral lateral recess to ensure complete decompression. The majority of the boney decompression is performed with the burr, but a Kerrison rongeur can be used to clean up the edges.

- *Resection of ligamentum flavum:*
  - The ligamentum is then reflected from the midline to either side of the spinal canal using a curved microcurette.
  - Using a Kerrison punch, the ligamentum flavum is removed.
  - The underlying thecal sac and traversing nerve roots should now be exposed and decompressed.
- *Facetectomy:*
  - The tubular retractor should be redirected over the ipsilateral facet joint. Using the burr, the laminectomy is extended laterally, transecting the pars interarticularis at the level of the superior aspect of the underlying disk space. An osteotome can also be used to complete this cut. Lateral fluoroscopic guidance can be used to confirm the site of the osteotomy to prevent excessive pars resection. The remaining pars is left intact to protect the exiting nerve root and to direct the cage during insertion.
  - The amputated inferior articular process is removed in a single piece. It is then debrided of soft tissue and cartilage, morselized, and saved as autograft for interbody fusion.
  - The superior articular process of the inferior level is then resected using a burr, followed by a Kerrison. The superior articular process should be completely removed flush to the superior wall of the pedicle to maximize the working window to the disk space; but be careful not to violate the pedicle, which is easy to do if not cognizant when using the burr.
  - If bilateral facetectomies are to be performed, the identical process is performed via a second tubular retractor on the contralateral side.
- *Discectomy:*
  - Bipolar electrocautery is then used to coagulate epidural veins overlying the disk space. The transforaminal space should now be completely visualized **(Fig. 3)**.
  - The bounds of the working window are the traversing nerve root located medially, exiting nerve root located superolaterally under the pars (often not directly visualized), and the pedicle of the caudal vertebra located inferiorly.
  - A #15 blade scalpel is utilized to create a wide rectangular annulotomy, which is placed sufficiently lateral that no retraction of the neural elements is necessary during disk space preparation or cage insertion.
  - The intervertebral disk is excised using pituitary rongeurs, straight and curved curettes, and rasps. A narrow osteotome and lateral fluoroscopy can be helpful to gain access to a difficult-to-access disk space. Offset instruments facilitate contralateral discectomy. The use of shavers is avoided to prevent endplate violations and subsequent subsidence and pseudoarthrosis. However, paddles are utilized to help distract the disk space.

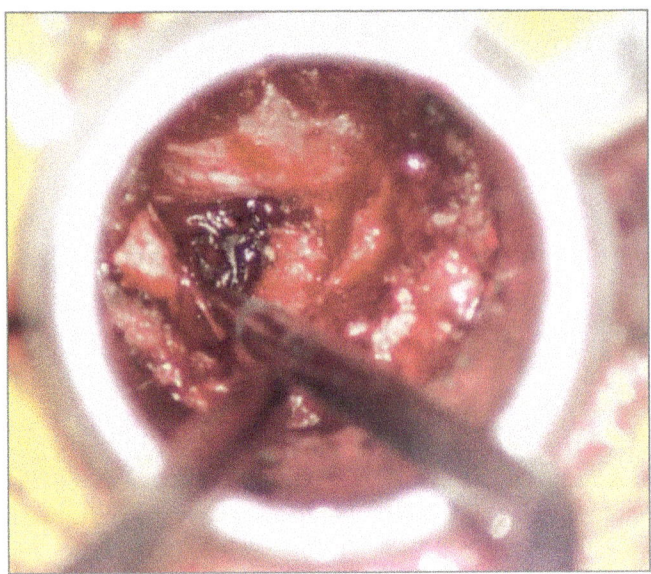

Fig. 3: The intervertebral disk space is visualized through a tubular retractor following coagulation of the overlying epidural veins.

  - In a unilateral approach, the previously placed rod on the contralateral side can be locked down while a paddle is in place to hold the disk space distracted and facilitate disk preparation. If performing bilateral approaches, a paddle can be left on one side while the surgeon performs disk preparation on the other, moving back and forth to sequentially mobilize the space.
  - Lateral fluoroscopy should be periodically used to assess working depth to ensure the anterior longitudinal ligament remains undisturbed.
  - Work from posterior to anterior in the disk space with your preparation to maximize direct visualization.
  - Thorough endplate preparation is imperative. The greatest portion of the procedure should be spent on this step. However, great care should be taken to avoid endplate violations.

INTERBODY CAGE PLACEMENT

- A trial interbody spacer or paddle is fitted into the disk space to assess sizing.
- The disk space is filled with local bone with or without iliac crest autograft. A bone graft substitute can be added as an extender. Autograft is applied first to the anterior portions of the disk space. Bone morphogenetic protein use is avoided out of concern for ectopic bone growth in the foramen and the development of associated postoperative radiculopathy.

- Under lateral fluoroscopic guidance, the interbody cage is partially inserted into the disk space. The retractor arm is then loosened to allow more a more medial insertion trajectory, and the cage is inserted the rest of the way. It should be placed into the anterior third of the disk space to maximize lordosis. Anterior placement on the apophyseal ring also reduces the chance of subsidence.
- A wide variety of cage designs are available, but expandable cages are easier to insert and center; and articulating banana-shaped implants may allow for greatest restoration of lordosis.
- Additional bone graft is placed posterior to the intervertebral cage, optimizing fusion potential.
- Endplate violations are associated with cage malpositioning, subsidence, and pseudoarthrosis. Inadequate discectomy is another common cause of pseudoarthrosis.

PERCUTANEOUS PEDICLE SCREW PLACEMENT

- The Kirschner wires are released from the drapes. Undersized pedicle taps are placed over the guidewires and advanced through the pedicles.
- Cannulated pedicle screws are inserted over the Kirschner wires and into the pedicles. Guidewires are removed when the screws reach the posterior aspect of the vertebral bodies.
- Lateral fluoroscopic imaging is used to confirm that the taps and pedicle screws are collinear with the Kirschner wires as they are advanced through the pedicles. Not doing so can result in kinking and breaking of the guidewires within the bone—broken fragments can be exceptionally difficult to access and remove.
- Following insertion of the screws, an electromyography (EMG) probe is used to stimulate each. The pedicle screw extensions are aligned, and a contoured rod is then passed under the fascia.
- The pedicle screws are secured to the rods with set screws. AP and lateral fluoroscopy are used to confirm appropriate positioning of instrumentation. The set screws are final tightened, and the associated extensions are removed. Final AP and lateral fluoroscopy images are taken.

CLOSURE

- The wounds are copiously irrigated, and meticulous hemostasis is obtained. Electrocautery, topical hemostatic agents, packing, and bone wax may be utilized as needed. Attention to hemostasis is imperative prior to closure to avoid epidural hematoma and cauda equina syndrome.
- The incisions are closed in a layered fashion using absorbable suture followed by a commercial skin sealant and a sterile dressing.

CHAPTER 26

Lateral Lumbar Interbody Fusion

Corey T Walker, David S Xu, Juan S Uribe

INTRODUCTION

Lumbar lateral interbody fusion is a minimally invasive retroperitoneal transpsoas approach to the lumbar disks for arthrodesis. The technique allows for access down to the L4/L5 disk level, providing an opportunity for robust disk space disk preparation, large-footprint interbody placement, and disk height restoration that creates indirect neural decompression and correction of sagittal and coronal malalignment.

INSTRUMENTS SUGGESTED

- Amsco bed or other bed that allows for bed "breaking"
- Intraoperative fluoroscopy
- Intraoperative neuromonitoring [the use of triggered and/or spontaneous electromyography (EMG) for nerve identification is essential during the approach and dissection]. We prefer to use directional stimulation with the dilator probes to help identify the location of the lumbosacral plexus, particularly at the lower levels (L3/L4 and L4/L5) prior to and during tubular retractor placement through the psoas muscle.
- A table-mounted tubular retractor system dedicated for lateral approaches should be used.
  - Lighted retractor options are helpful.
  - Long, minimally invasive surgical (MIS) instruments such as scalpels, Kerrisons, pituitaries, curettes, Cobbs, and box cutters are required for discectomy and disk space preparation.

APPROACH

- The approach is performed by performing a lateral incision orthogonal to the disk space as determined with preprocedural fluoroscopy.
- Progressive dilation in the retroperitoneal space through the psoas muscle creates the corridor of approach.
- Once the retractor is in place, the discectomy is performed and the lateral interbody is placed; a staged circumferential fusion can be performed by placing posterior pedicle screws at the fusion level(s).
- Multiple levels can be approached through a single incision (particularly in cases of degenerative scoliosis that are approached on the concavity) or multiple incisions.
- The side of approach is determined based on provider preference and careful analysis of the psoas, vascular and urological anatomy, and the direction of the scoliosis.

Minimally Invasive Surgical Lateral Approach

- *Table:* Position the patient in the lateral decubitus position on the radiolucent table.
- *Positioning:*
  - A quick anteroposterior (AP) and lateral X-ray shot can help get the patient in a lateral position where the targeted vertebral levels are orthogonal to the table surface.
  - A bump can be placed under the top of the iliac crest and axilla to help prop up the down side of the body and obtain a more neutral spine.
  - The patient's thorax and lower body are taped in the lateral position to prevent body shifting **(Fig. 1)**.
  - The knees need to be padded in a flexed position with pillows between the knees and ankles to allow for maximal psoas relaxation.
  - The bed can be bent or broken at the level of the patient's iliac crest. While some surgeons prefer not to brake the bed due to concern for neural traction, breaking the bed helps to create space between the iliac crest and ribs. This can be particularly helpful for approaching the L4–L5 level which comes close to the iliac crest.

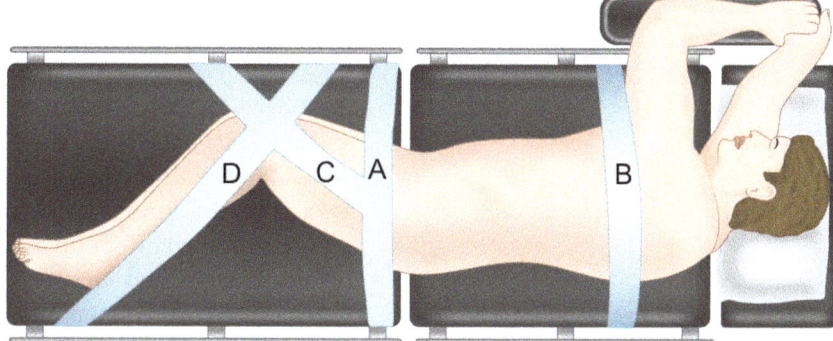

Fig. 1: Picture of patient positioning and strategic taping to keep patient in correct position and pull down on the iliac crest.

- *Retractor:* Attach the post for the tubular retractor to the contralateral side-rail (the abdominal side).
- *Draping:*
  - The level and location of the incision is generally determined prior to draping using fluoroscopy by finding "true" AP and lateral images and marking the disk space location trajectory on the skin.
  - If single-position percutaneous pedicle screw fixation is intended, the posterior lumbar spine should be draped into the field as well to expose the skin entry points.
- *Fluoroscopic localization:*
  - Fluoroscopy imaging is the most important tool for determining true AP and lateral images and guiding the surgeon to the disk space. Inappropriate preoperative fluoroscopy may cause the surgeon to enter a disk space obliquely.
  - Your skin incision should be approximately 4 cm in length centered over the disk space entry point. We target the posterior one-third mark of the disk space for our entry point. A radio-opaque target can be used to identify the skin entry point.
- *Accessing the retroperitoneal corridor:*
  - The incision is made parallel to the external oblique fibers and dissection is made down to the fascia. Blunt dissection through the abdominal musculature is performed using tonsillar hemostats down through each layer (external oblique, internal oblique, and transversus abdominis) to the transversalis fascia, which is carefully opened to expose the underlying retroperitoneal fat. This fat needs to be visualized to confirm access into the retroperitoneal space.
  - Blunt finger dissection is performed to gain access to the psoas. Posterior palpation of the retroperitoneal wall is used to feel the quadratus lumborum. Deep to this, the transversus process can be felt posteriorly and then finger dissection is used to sweep the bowel and peritoneum anteriorly up and over the psoas muscle. The psoas muscle fibers can be palpated to ensure there is no bowel or fat on top of the psoas prior to placing the dilator.

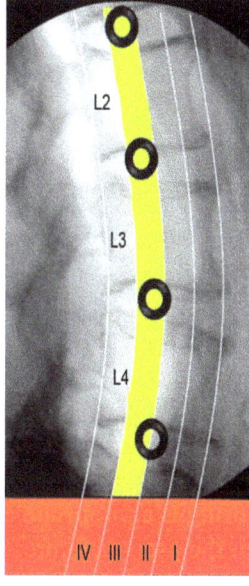

Fig. 2: Lateral radiograph of the lumbar spine showing the relative safe zone (Zone III) with the recommended optimal dilator placement locations at each intervertebral disk space that will prevent nerve injury.

- *Retractor placement:*
  - Fluoroscopic placement of the dilator is performed. Directional EMG from the dilators can be performed to ensure the lumbosacral plexus is posterior to the entry point, particularly at the L4/L5 disk space, where the plexus courses most anteriorly **(Figs. 2 and 3)**.[1] Low stimulation of the plexus or anterior localization of the plexus warrants immediate repositioning of the dilator more anterior. If continued stimulations that are outside of what is expected to occur, the surgeon should abort treating the level at that time to prevent plexus injury.
  - Stimulation during progressive dilator and retractor placement can ensure that the plexus is not too close to the retractor.
  - Lateral boney osteophytes may make retractor placement difficult. An AP fluoroscopy image can help to ensure that the retractor blades are centered over the disk space if they are being diverted rostrally or caudally by a lateral boney osteophyte.

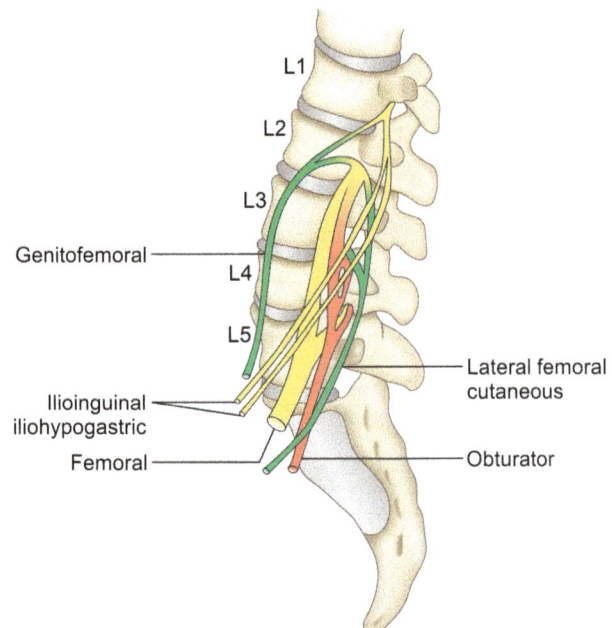

Fig. 3: Schematic drawing of the lumbar plexus from a lateral view. The locations of the major motor and sensory nerves are illustrated in relation to the disk spaces.

- The retractor is then attached to the bed-rail mount to hold it in place. Placement of a leveling device on the retractor may be helpful to ensure that the retractor is perfectly upright and not angled.
- *Confirm retractor position:*
  - If the monitoring is appropriate and the retractor is placed within the psoas, a fluoroscopic image can be used to confirm placement of the retractor.
  - A single click dilation of the retractor can then be used to perform direct visualization of the retractor. Any nerves or blood vessels in the field need to be dissected away, or the retractor needs to be replaced. Direct EMG stimulation of the field can be confirmed to ensure that no nerves are coursing through the field if desired.
  - A posterior intradiscal shim can then be placed into the disk space to dock the retractor. AP fluoroscopy can be used to confirm placement of the shim in the disk space. The retractor then is dilated to expose the remainder of the disk space anterior to the shim. The retractor should only be opened as wide as needed to pass instruments and the interbody to avoid overdistraction of the psoas muscle.
  - An anterior shim should be used to protect the anterior structures during instrument placement and discectomy maneuvers.
  - Care should be performed to identify the anterior longitudinal ligament (ALL) and avoid violation. ALL violation warrants placement of a lateral vertebral screw to prevent graft migration, and also likely necessitates pedicle screw fixation. Maintenance of the ALL helps to keep an anatomical border between the disk space and the great vessels.
- *Discectomy:*
  - A box-shaped disk annulotomy is performed with a scalpel blade to expose the disk space.
  - A Cobb can be used to the strip the disk off the superior and inferior endplates. AP fluoroscopy can be used to maintain depth of instruments. The contralateral annulus is opened carefully with the Cobb during this maneuver to help open up the disk space and release the downside of the disk for disk height restoration. A pituitary is then used to remove loose disk fragments.
  - A box cutter can then be used to remove large amounts of disk down through the contralateral annulus. Care should be performed during this maneuver not to damage the endplates. AP fluoroscopy can be used to ensure an appropriate angle of the instrument parallel to the endplates. Anterior angling of the box cutter can result in ALL damage and vascular injury, so care should be made to ensure that the instrument enters the disk space in an orthogonal manner.
  - It may be helpful to have an assistant at either end of the bed helping to ensure that your instruments are straight upright and entering the disk space in an orthogonal manner.
  - End plate preparation can then be finalized while the interbody is being prepared by the scrub technician. A uterine curette, side-angle rasp or other form of curette can be used to gently scrape the disk off the endplates and prepare the bone for fusion. Care should be made to not disrupt the endplate integrity, particularly in patients with weaker bone quality.
- *Interbody placement:*
  - An interbody device is placed after the disk is prepared for fusion. The interbody should be sized for the patient's anatomy. The goal is to span the epiphysial ring of the vertebral bodies without oversizing the body so it extends into the psoas.
  - An oversized graft with too much height may allow for increased disk height but raises the risk for graft subsidence. Surgeons should take into account the patient's bone quality, preoperative disk height, and sagittal alignment goals. A hyperlordotic implant can be used to help improve lordosis. However, subsidence can result in pseudoarthrosis and segmental kyphosis, so a balance of disk height restoration should be weighed with subsidence risk. A young healthy individual typically does not have a disk height over 10 mm, therefore, for most patients, a 8-mm or 10-mm sized interbody is sufficient.
  - Shimmed slides can be placed on the outside of the interbody during placement to help "shoe-horn" the implant into the disk space and prevent endplate damage.

- Recombinant human bone morphogenetic protein-2 (rh-BMP2) can be considered for lateral interbody fusion, but typically is not necessary unless there is a strong concern for poor fusion potential.
- AP and lateral fluoroscopy area used during and after interbody placement to make sure the graft is not too far anterior or posterior. Posterior grafts place the contralateral nerve root at risk, while anterior grafts may raise the risk for vessel injury.

■ *Retractor removal:*
- Prior to retractor removal, hemostasis must be performed. Floseal is used to stop any oozing prior to removing the retractor, as psoas hematoma can result in undesired postoperative neural complications and a retroperitoneal hemorrhage can be life-threatening.
- Slow removal under direct visualization allows for hemostasis during retractor removal. Any small bleeders can be bipolared carefully before visualization is lost with retractor removal.
- The fascia is then closed carefully to prevent hernias. If the bed was broken at the beginning of the case, it should be unbroken prior to fascial closure to help make sure there are not any areas of fascial dehiscence. The subcutaneous and dermal layers can be closed in a standard fashion using Vicryl sutures and dermabond on the skin.

PITFALLS

- Maintenance of positioning with taping helps to prevent patient movement throughout the case. Patient movement may disrupt the true AP and lateral fluoroscopy images that guide the surgeon throughout the case. Small disruptions in alignment result in higher risk of neurovascular structures throughout the procedure.
- Avoid electrocautery of the abdominal musculature below the level of the fascia. Subcostal, ilioinguinal, and iliohypogastric nerve fibers run within the muscle fibers. Injury to these nerves can result in abdominal "pseudohernia" postoperatively.
- During retroperitoneal exposure, access should be performed with care to anteriorly retract all peritoneal and retroperitoneal structures. Peritoneal, bowel, and ureteral/kidney injury can occur during dilator placement. During passage of progressive dilators, placing a finger anterior to the dilator can help protect these structures.
- Overdissection rostrally and caudally of the retroperitoneal space beyond what is needed for dilator placement is unnecessary and can cause tearing of small retroperitoneal vessels that raise the risk for retroperitoneal bleeding postoperatively.
- Posterior dilator placement at the L4/L5 disk space places the lumbosacral plexus at risk of injury. Use of directional EMG monitoring is imperative to maintain a posterior position of the plexus relative to the dilators prior to retractor placement and dilation.
- Take care to protect the vertebral endplates during each of the discectomy maneuvers. Disruption of the endplates and oversizing the height of grafts can result in subsidence, which may compromise the goals of surgery, including indirect decompression and sagittal alignment correction.
- Entry and removal of all tools and implants during surgery must be performed in an orthogonal manner. Slight changes in alignment or trajectory at the patient's skin incision can result in significant malposition at the level of the disk.

REFERENCE

1. Uribe JS, Arredondo N, Dakwar E, Vale FL. Defining the safe working zones using the minimally invasive lateral retroperitoneal transpsoas approach: an anatomical study. J Neurosurg Spine. 2010;13(2):260-6.

CHAPTER 27

Ante-Psoas Interbody Fusion

Neel Anand, Sheila Kahwaty

INTRODUCTION

Ante-psoas interbody fusion is a modification of the lateral transpsoas approach for minimally invasive lumbar interbody fusion. The ante-psoas technique relocates the access to the disk space from a transpsoas approach to a pre-psoas approach. The ante-psoas approach is a useful technique for performing, in a single position, discectomy, restoration of disk height and lumbar lordosis, and obtaining interbody fusion with indirect decompression, particularly in multilevel adult deformity corrections. The approach allows access to multiple lumbar levels without repositioning of the patient. It is recommended to pair the ante-psoas interbody fusion with percutaneous posterior instrumentation and fusion, either performed on the same day or staged to several days later.

INDICATIONS/CONTRAINDICATIONS

- Indications for the ante-psoas approach include idiopathic scoliosis, degenerative scoliosis, iatrogenic scoliosis, kyphosis, flat-back syndrome, low-grade spondylolisthesis, and single-level or multi-level degenerative disk disease/stenosis/facet arthropathy.
- Contraindications include high-risk medical comorbidities, osteoporosis (bone density scan T score of −3.0 or worse), history of complex intra-abdominal surgery or trauma, presence of vascular structures obstructing access to the disk space.
- Relative contraindication includes osteopenia (T score of −1.0 to −2.5) or osteoporosis (T score of −2.5 to −3.0). Patients in this category are still eligible for surgery if they undergo treatment of the osteoporosis with parathyroid hormone agents, such as teriparatide or abaloparatide.

PREOPERATIVE PLANNING

- History and physical evaluation
- Standing 36-inch scoliosis X-rays to assess global alignment, deformity parameters (including Cobb angle), and spinopelvic parameters.
- Magnetic resonance imaging (MRI) lumbar spine without contrast to assess stenosis, disk herniations, spinal anomalies, and soft tissue anatomy. MRI is the preferred image to assure unobstructed access to the disk through the ante-psoas approach and evaluate the vascular anatomy.
- Computed tomography (CT) lumbar spine without contrast to assess bony anatomy and rule out spondylolysis or bony fusion of interbody segments or facet joints.
- Bone density scan of the hips and spine to assess bone quality.

INSTRUMENTS SUGGESTED

- Flat top Jackson table with rolled blanket for kidney bump or Sliding 3100 Skytron table with kidney rest
- Intraoperative fluoroscopy
- Table-mounted tubular retractor system (e.g., Medtronic Thompson retractor system)
- Long-handled discectomy instruments
- Interbody trials and spacers (e.g., Medtronic Divergence system, Medtronic Clydesdale system)
- Fusion augmentation materials [e.g., recombinant human bone morphogenetic protein 2 (rhBMP-2) and demineralized bone matrix]
- Intraoperative neuromonitoring/somatosensory evoked potentials (SSEPs)—not required for ante-psoas approach.

POSITIONING

- Patient is positioned in a right lateral decubitus position (left side up) on a flat top Jackson table or Sliding table, regardless of deformity alignment. A right side approach

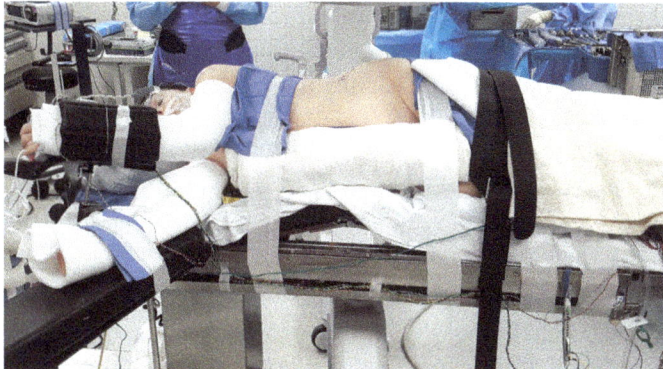

Fig. 1: *Patient secured in a right lateral decubitus position for multilevel lumbar access via ante-psoas interbody fusion approach.* Correct positioning for the ante-psoas interbody fusion approach includes appropriate padding of the axilla, arms and legs, deployment of the kidney rest, adequate exposure for all lumbar levels, and securing the patient to the table.

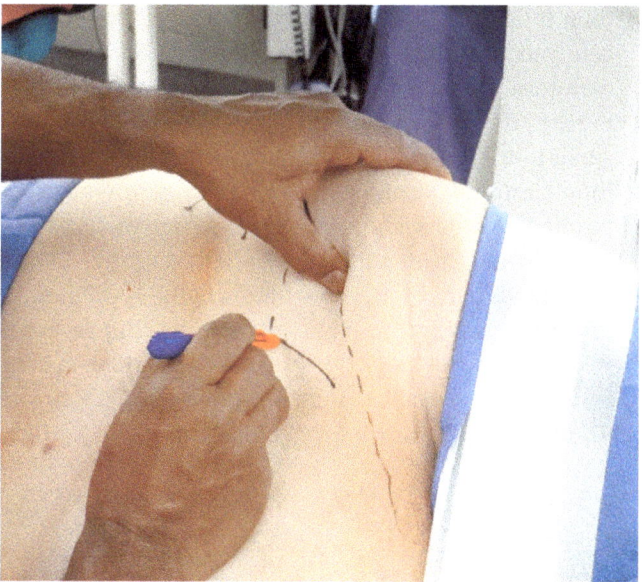

Fig. 2: *Marking of the L5–S1 ante-psoas interbody fusion incision.* An oblique incision is made approximately two finger breadths anterior to the anterior superior iliac spine in between the angle of the L5–S1 disk space.

may be considered if the left side is inaccessible, if vascular anatomy prevents access, or in the case of revision approaches, but caution should be taken given the proximity to the inferior vena cava on the right side. An axillary roll is placed under the right axilla. The left arm is secured. A pillow is placed under the right knee to pad the peroneal nerve. The kidney rest is deployed or a rolled blanket kidney bump is placed under the right side to open the left flank. Rolled blankets (~0.5 m long) are placed lengthwise against the patient's abdomen and back and the patient is secured in place with tape across the iliac crest, chest, greater trochanter, and legs **(Fig. 1)**.

- The surgeon stands at the patient's abdomen.
- C-arm is positioned at the patient's back.
- The tubular retractor system is mounted along the table rail at the patient's back, at the level of the shoulder.
- Patient is wired for SSEPs as an option. This is not mandatory as the access is pre-psoas.

APPROACH TO L5–S1

- Prior to draping, a straight, anatomic lateral view X-ray of the spine is used to identify and mark the anterior and posterior margins of the disk space at L5–S1 (no tilting of the C-arm is used during marking of the disk). A diagonal line is extended toward the pubis in line with the angle of the L5–S1 disk space. Another line is drawn straight from the posterior margin of the L5–S1 disk space to the abdomen. An oblique incision is made between these lines, approximately two finger breadths anterior to the anterior superior iliac spine **(Fig. 2)**.
- SSEP neuromonitoring is run throughout the case (not required).
- A vascular surgeon makes the incision in the left lower abdominal quadrant. The fascia is incised lateral to the rectus sheath. The transversalis fascia is then divided lateral to the rectus abdominis, allowing access to the retroperitoneal space. Careful attention is paid in identifying the peritoneum and ureter and mobilizing these structures as needed. The left iliac vessels and middle sacral vessels are visualized and mobilized as needed to gain access to the L5–S1 disk space.
- A table-mounted tubular retractor system, such as the Medtronic Thompson retractor system, is used to maintain the access. A post is attached to the contralateral side rail by the patient's shoulder. Three blades are positioned: One superiorly retracting the left common iliac vein and artery (dark blue blade, approximately 14 cm in length), one blade retracting the bifurcation cephalically (light blue blade, approximately 14 cm in length), and one inferiorly by the right common iliac vein and artery (green blade, approximately 17 cm in length) **(Fig. 3)**.
- A needle is positioned in the center of the L5–S1 disk space and the level is confirmed under lateral view fluoroscopy. It is essential to obtain a clear view of the L5 and S1 endplates and posterior margins, thus some Ferguson angle (tilt of the C-arm in line with the lumbosacral angle) may be required.
- A slit incision is made in the anterior annulus with a long knife in line with the disk space. A straight, large, long-handled Cobb elevator [from the Medtronic direct lateral interbody fusion (DLIF) set] is used to enter the disk space and is deepened to the posterior margin of the disk space under fluoroscopy.
- In severely collapsed disk spaces, an osteotome may be introduced in line with the disk space to create a path for discectomy. The osteotome depth and angle are monitored with fluoroscopy. The initial osteotome is

then followed by a bullet-nosed dilating osteotome to gently distract the disk space in preparation for the Cobb elevators.

- Further discectomy ensues with large Cobb elevators, small long-handled straight and angled curettes, large long-handled straight and angled curettes, rasps, pituitary rongeurs, and Kerrisons. Instrumentation depth is confirmed under lateral view fluoroscopy. Careful attention is paid to avoid disruption of the endplates.
- The posterior longitudinal ligament (PLL) is gently released with a small long-handled straight curette, followed by a small long-handled angled curette under lateral fluoroscopy. Release of the PLL allows for greater disk height restoration, direct and indirect decompression, and angular correction of the disk space.
- If epidural bleeding is encountered, achieve hemostasis with thrombotic agents, such as Floseal or Gelfoam with thrombin.
- Disk space trials are then used to gently dilate the disk space. Sequential smooth trials with rounded ends, such as the Medtronic DLIF Clydesdale trials, are initially used to open up the disk space under lateral fluoroscopy. An 8 mm height × 45 mm length is used first, followed by a 10 mm height × 45 mm length trial, followed by a 12 mm height × 45 mm length trial. Fluoroscopy is used to ensure that the trial is following the correct angle of the disk and to ensure that the posterior height is increasing appropriately, without subsidence into the endplates. Paddle distractors may also be used if preferred **(Figs. 4A and B)**.
- Following dilation with the Clydesdale trials, the Medtronic Divergence trials are used, beginning with a medium-sized footprint trial with 10 mm of height and 12° of lordosis. Adjust the size of the trial footprint as necessary to fit the anterior-posterior and left to right dimensions of the disk space. Progressively increase the height and lordosis of the trials to achieve adequate coverage of the disk space, as well as desired height and lordosis. For example, when using the Medtronic Divergence system, the first trial used is a 10 mm height × 12° of lordosis, followed by a 12 mm height × 12° of lordosis, followed by a 14 mm height × 12° of lordosis trial. If a greater lordotic angle is required, a 16 mm height × 18° of lordosis trial is then used. A key requirement is to choose a trial, and ultimately a spacer, that provides at least 4–6 mm of posterior height **(Figs. 5A and B)**.

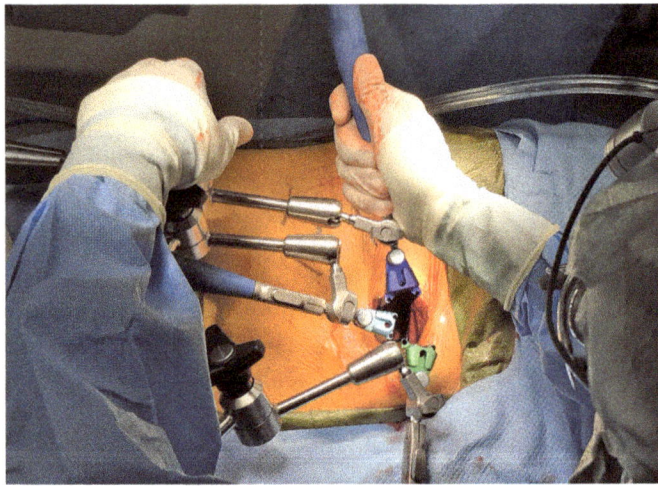

Fig. 3: *Placement of the table-mounted retractor system.* Retractor blades are positioned by the vascular surgeon. The dark blue retractor is placed superiorly retracting the left common iliac vein and artery. The light blue retractor is placed cephalically retracting the bifurcation. The green retractor is placed inferiorly retracting the right common iliac vein and artery.

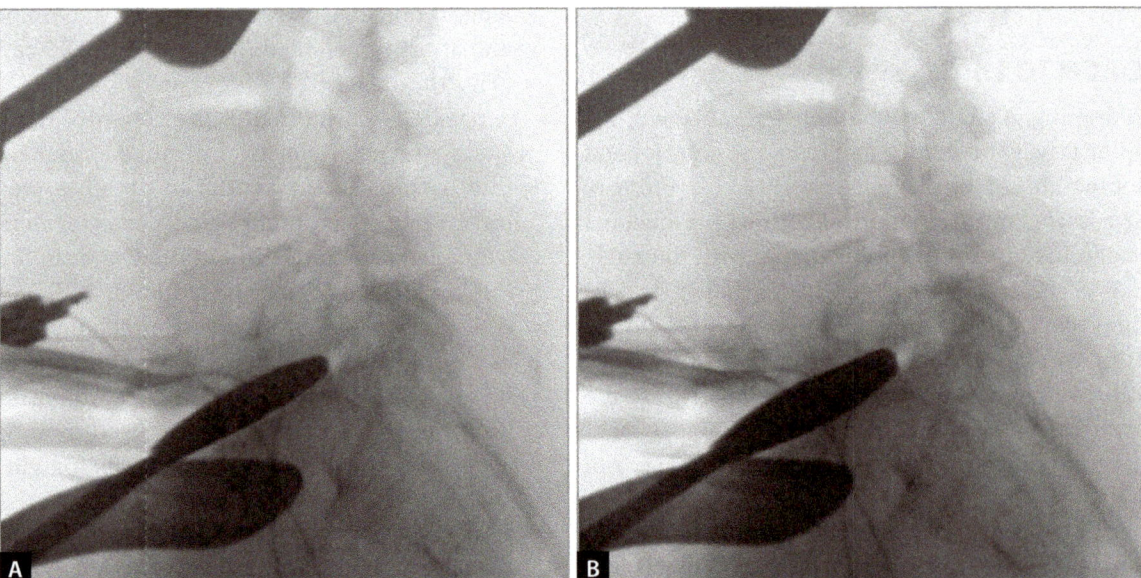

Figs. 4A and B: *Use of smooth biconvex trials allows for gradual dilation of the L5–S1 disk.* Medtronic Clydesdale trials are used sequentially to open the disk at L5–S1. Note the increase in posterior height achieved without endplate subsidence.

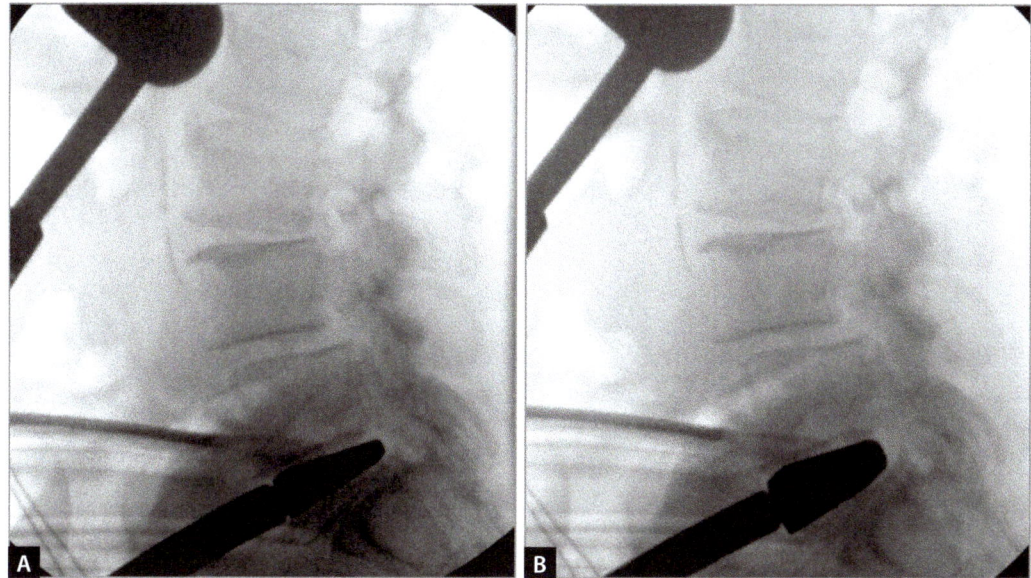

Figs. 5A and B: Trialing of the L5–S1 disk space is seen. (A) The trial does not adequately increase the posterior disk height; (B) A larger trial is seen with satisfactory posterior disk height.

- An anteroposterior (AP) X-ray is taken with the trial in place to confirm that it is well centered between the pedicles of L5 and S1. To obtain a clear view of the L5–S1 disk space and pedicles, the C-arm machine will need to be positioned in the same angle as the disk space **(Fig. 6)**.
- A corresponding polyetheretherketone (PEEK) spacer is then chosen along with an anterior plate, which is sized according to the anterior height (14 mm anterior height will have a 14 mm plate).
- A long-handled screwdriver, with a guide for the screws, is mounted obliquely to the plate and spacer. The handle should be mounted on the left side of the spacer, which will correspond to the right side of the patient **(Fig. 7)**.
- The spacer is packed with fusion augmentation materials, such as rhBMP-2 (approximately 4 mg) and Grafton putty.
- The disk space is thoroughly irrigated.
- The PEEK spacer is then impacted into the disk space under lateral fluoroscopy with a mallet **(Fig. 8)**. Great attention is paid to assure protection of the soft tissues during the implantation of the spacer and placement of the screws.
- An awl is passed through the guide and impacted into the sacrum, approximately 20 mm. This is confirmed on lateral fluoroscopy. A 30 mm screw is then passed through the guide and implanted into the sacrum. This process is repeated for a second sacral screw.
- The awl is then passed through the guide and impacted into L5, approximately 20 mm. This is confirmed on lateral fluoroscopy **(Fig. 9)**. A 25 mm screw is then passed through the guide and implanted into L5. This process is repeated for a second L5 screw.
- The screwdriver and guide are then removed. All screws are then tightened.

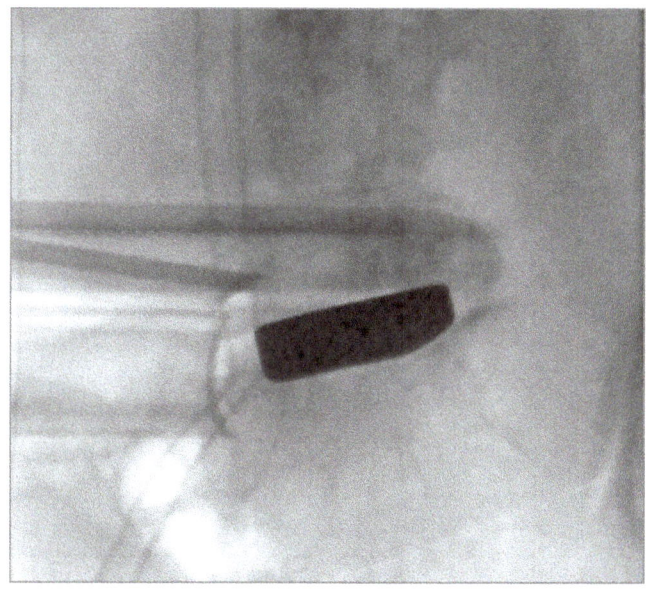

Fig. 6: *Anteroposterior X-ray of L5–S1 trial implant.* The implant should be centered and aligned within the pedicles of L5 and S1.

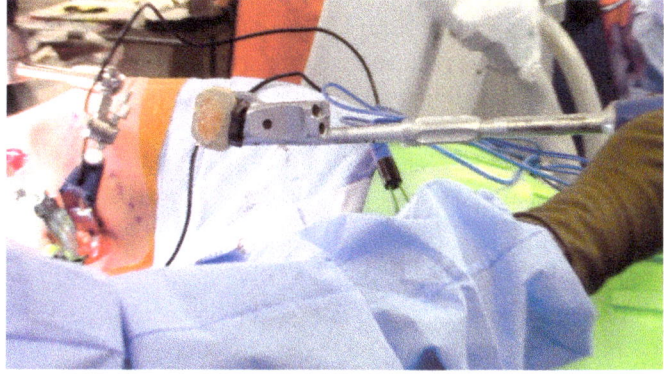

Fig. 7: *Implant handle.* The handle is attached to the spacer and plate at an oblique angle. Note that the screw guide is also mounted on the handle.

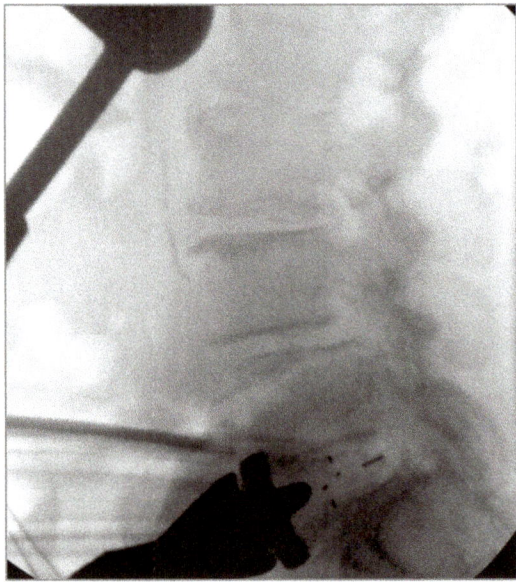

Fig. 8: *Implantation of the L5–S1 interbody spacer with plate.* The implant is impacted into the L5–S1 disk space. The plate rests on the anterior borders of the L5 and S1 vertebrae.

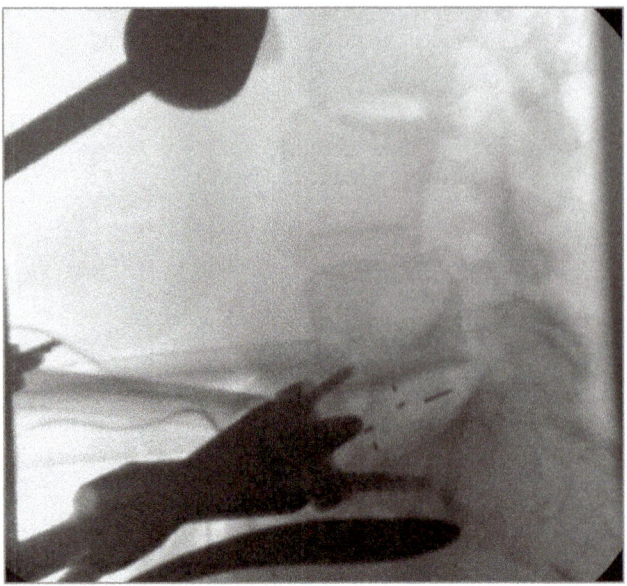

Fig. 9: *Securing the spacer with an anterior plate and screws.* With the guide still in place, an awl is passed through the guide and impacted into the sacrum and L5 bilaterally. Screws are then placed, 30 mm in the sacrum and 25 mm in L5, to secure the spacer and plate.

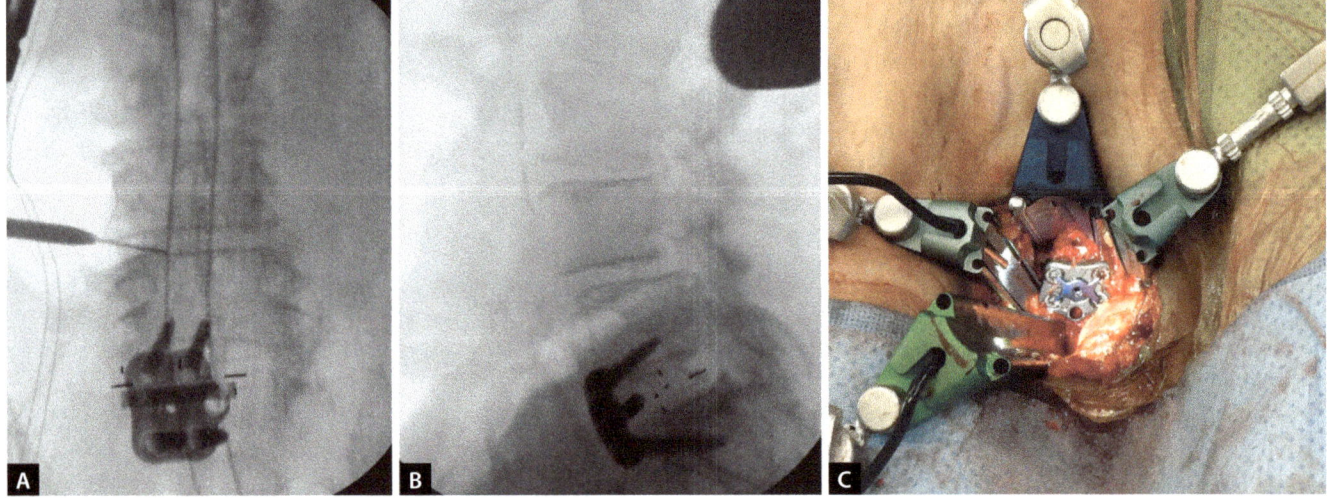

Figs. 10A to C: *Final anteroposterior and lateral X-rays and visualization of the L5–S1 implant.* The spacer and plate are firmly secured at L5–S1.

- Final position of the graft is then confirmed visually and with lateral and AP X-rays **(Figs. 10A to C)**.
- Grafton putty is packed on either side of the spacer.
- If only L5–S1 is being addressed, please skip ahead to the "Closure" section.
- If additional lumbar levels are being addressed, please see the sections below.

■ APPROACH TO L4–L5

- Prior to draping, lateral fluoroscopy is used to identify and mark the anterior and posterior margins of the disk space at L4–L5. If the procedure includes other proximal levels, it is recommended to mark the borders of those disk spaces as well.
- SSEP neuromonitoring is run throughout the entirety of the case (again not a requirement).
- An oblique 2.5 cm incision is made in line with the external obliques, approximately 2.5 cm in front of the anterior margin of the L4–L5 disk space, keeping in mind that L3–L4 will likely be accessed through this same incision **(Fig. 11)**.
- The external oblique muscle and the internal oblique muscle are split in line with their fibers **(Fig. 12)**. The transversalis fascia is entered with finger dissection, reaching back toward the iliac crest, to access the retroperitoneal space. If the L5–S1 disk space was addressed as above, the right hand can be used to help create access to the retroperitoneal space at L4–L5. If

the L5–S1 disk space was not approached previously, then finger dissection is used to sweep under the iliac crest and under the 12th rib to enter the retroperitoneal space. Finger dissection is used to sweep the peritoneum anteriorly, while palpating for the psoas tendon and carefully identifying the aorta.

- Similar to the access for an anterior cervical procedure, the access for the L4–L5 ante-psoas interbody fusion lies in a plane between vascular structures (aorta) and muscles (psoas). The psoas tendon serves as an excellent landmark for the anterior margin of the disk space and mobilizes easily. Gentle, shallow, retraction above the psoas muscle with handheld retractors, such as the Medtronic Thompson retractors, allows for visualization of the psoas tendon **(Fig. 13)**.

- Take care to assure that the ureter and sympathetic chain are not in the field.
- Under direct visualization, a probe is docked onto the anterior one-third of the disk space at L4–L5 and held in place with a Kocher. A lateral view X-ray is taken to confirm the position and the picture is saved and used as a reference **(Fig. 14)**. The probe is then advanced into the disk space, approximately half the length of the disk space. This is confirmed on AP view X-ray. Make note to position the C-arm in line with the lordotic angle of the

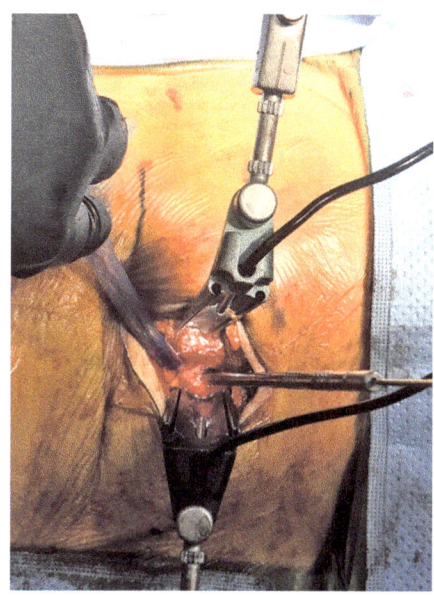

Fig. 13: *Psoas tendon.* Shallow docking of handheld retractors reveals the psoas muscle. The psoas tendon serves as the primary landmark for the anterior margin of the disk space and mobilizes easily. The ante-psoas approach accesses the disk space just anterior to the psoas tendon.

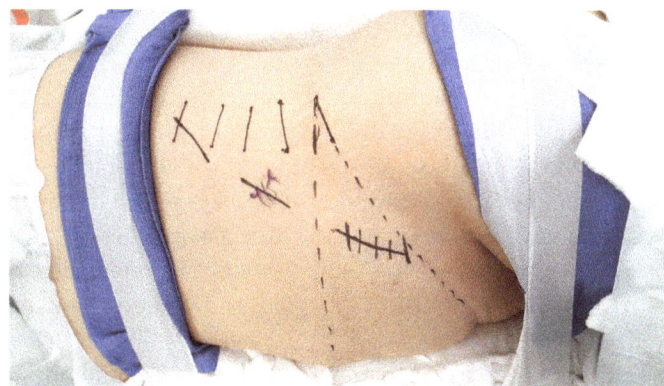

Fig. 11: *Localizing of the lumbar disks and corresponding incisions.* The anterior and posterior borders of the disk spaces at L4–L5, L3–L4, L2–L3, and L1–L2 are marked under fluoroscopy. Incisions for access to the disks are marked just anterior to the disk spaces, one for L4–L5 and L3–L4 and one for L2–L3 and L1–L2.

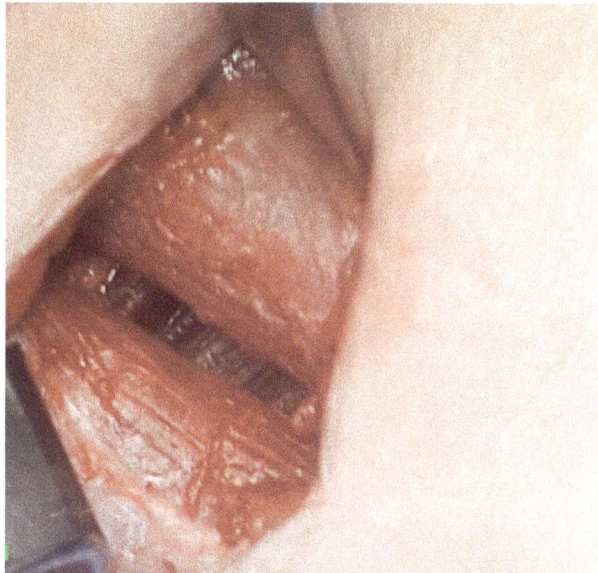

Fig. 12: *Visualization of the external and internal oblique muscles.* The external and internal oblique muscles are split in line with their fibers. The transversalis fascia is then entered with finger dissection to access the retroperitoneal space.

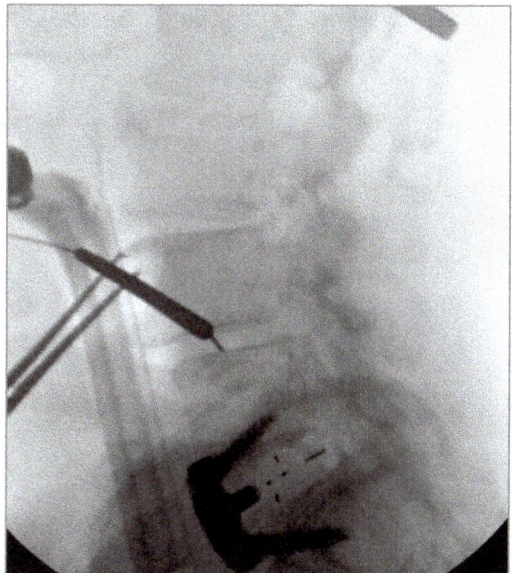

Fig. 14: *Probe docked in the anterior third of the L4–L5 disk space.* Optimal placement of the initial probe is within the anterior one-third of the disk space. This position allows for the greatest restoration of lordosis.

disk for good visualization of the L5 superior endplate and both L5 pedicles.

- Sequential dilators are carefully passed over the initial probe all the way down to the disk. Great attention is paid to assure protection of the soft tissues during the passage of the dilators. An AP X-ray is taken to confirm position of the dilators. Appropriately-sized round retractor blades (usually 15 mm in length) are passed over the dilators and secured in place by attaching the retractor to a table-mounted post. All other handheld retractors used for visualization of the pre-psoas space are removed **(Fig. 15)**.
- Once secured, the retractor is gently expanded in the cephalad-caudal plane. No direct retraction of the psoas is performed. All dilators, except the initial probe, are then removed. A tubular light is used with the retractor to increase visualization down the tube. The retractor blades may be angled outward to also increase visualization as needed.
- A long Penfield #4 and a long, flat suction cannula (such as a Thompson cannula) are used to further expose the disk and visualize the anterior longitudinal ligament (ALL). The retained initial probe is used as a reference for the anterior-posterior entry point into the disk.
- A long 15 blade scalpel is used to create a linear incision of the disk (not a box cut incision) at the insertion site of the initial probe. The initial probe is then removed.
- Under direct visualization, a straight, small, long-handled Cobb elevator (from the Medtronic DLIF set) is used to enter the disk space and is deepened to the contralateral margin of the disk space with a mallet under AP view fluoroscopy. The Cobb enters the disk space at an angle, underneath the psoas muscle body, and is gradually straightened perpendicular to the patient's body while being impacted. This allows for the psoas muscle to be gently rolled away from the disk as it is not attached to the anterior part of the spine but rather just lies on it. A lateral view X-ray may be taken at this time to confirm the anterior-posterior position of the Cobb elevator to ensure the correct trajectory and avoid entering the canal inadvertently. Visualizing the ALL also serves as a landmark of the anterior border of the disk space. The Cobb elevator is rotated slightly to gently open up the disk space and is then removed.
- In severely collapsed disk spaces or in the case of ipsilateral intervertebral segment autofusion, an osteotome may be introduced in line with the disk space to create a path for discectomy. The osteotome depth and angle is monitored with AP view fluoroscopy. The initial osteotome is then followed by a bullet-nosed dilating osteotome to gently distract the disk space in preparation for the Cobb elevators.
- Under direct visualization, a straight, large, long-handled Cobb elevator (from the Medtronic DLIF set) is then passed down the same opening, perpendicular to the patient's body, and across the disk space with a mallet to the contralateral margin of the disk space under AP view fluoroscopy. Again, the Cobb elevator is rotated slightly to gently open up the disk space and is then removed **(Fig. 16)**.
- Further discectomy ensues with a long-handled uterine curette and straight double-sided rasp. Special attention is paid to not violate the endplates, the ALL, or the contralateral annulus during the discectomy. Disk material and redundant ipsilateral annulus are removed

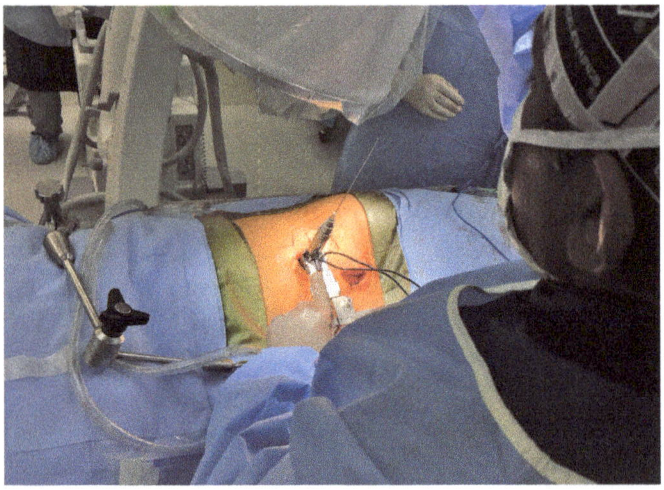

Fig. 15: *Placement of a table-mounted retractor.* A table-mounted arm secures the round retractors in place over the initial probe. Note the oblique angle of the retractor, consistent with the pre-psoas approach.

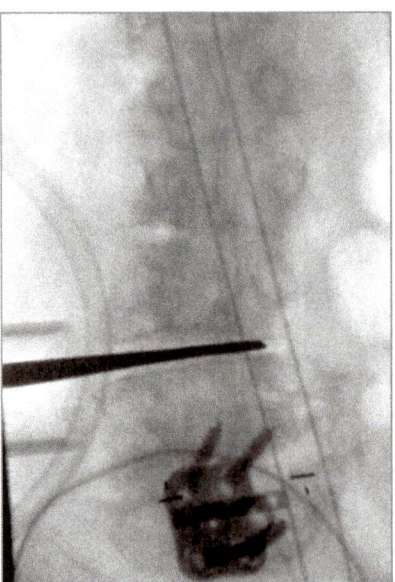

Fig. 16: *Cobb elevator opens the L4–L5 disk space.* A Cobb elevator is passed down the disk space opening and across the disk space to the contralateral border of the disk space. Fluoroscopy is used to ensure that the instruments are in line with the disk space and do not violate the endplates.

with a long pituitary rongeur and Kerrison. Instrumentation depth is confirmed under AP fluoroscopy.
- Disk space trials are then used to gently dilate the disk space under direct visualization and AP view fluoroscopy. Sequential smooth 18 mm wide trials with rounded ends and 6° of lordosis (Medtronic Clydesdale trials) are implanted into the disk space, perpendicular to the patient's body. An 8 mm height × 50 mm length is used first, followed by a 10 mm height × 50 mm length trial. The length of the trial is adjusted as necessary to cover the disk space from lateral border of ipsilateral L5 pedicle to lateral border of contralateral L5 pedicle (available lengths include 45, 50, 55, 60 mm). AP view fluoroscopy is used to ensure that the trial is following the correct angle of the disk, appropriately dilating the disk space, and avoiding subsidence into the endplates **(Figs. 17A to C)**.
- Further discectomy and endplate preparation is achieved with passage of a Medtronic combo tool and a pituitary rongeur. A 12 mm height × 50 mm length trial is then impacted into the disk space. A lateral view X-ray can be taken at this time to confirm the anterior-posterior position of the trial in the disk space. The trial is removed and the disk space is irrigated.
- A 12 mm height × 50 mm length × 12° lordosis spacer is then chosen and attached to the Medtronic inserter. The spacer is packed with fusion augmentation materials, such as rhBMP-2 (approximately 3–4 mg) and Grafton putty. Under direct visualization, the spacer is then implanted with a mallet into the L4–L5 disk space under AP view fluoroscopy **(Figs. 18A to D)**.
- With the inserter still attached, a lateral view X-ray is taken to confirm the final position. The ideal position for

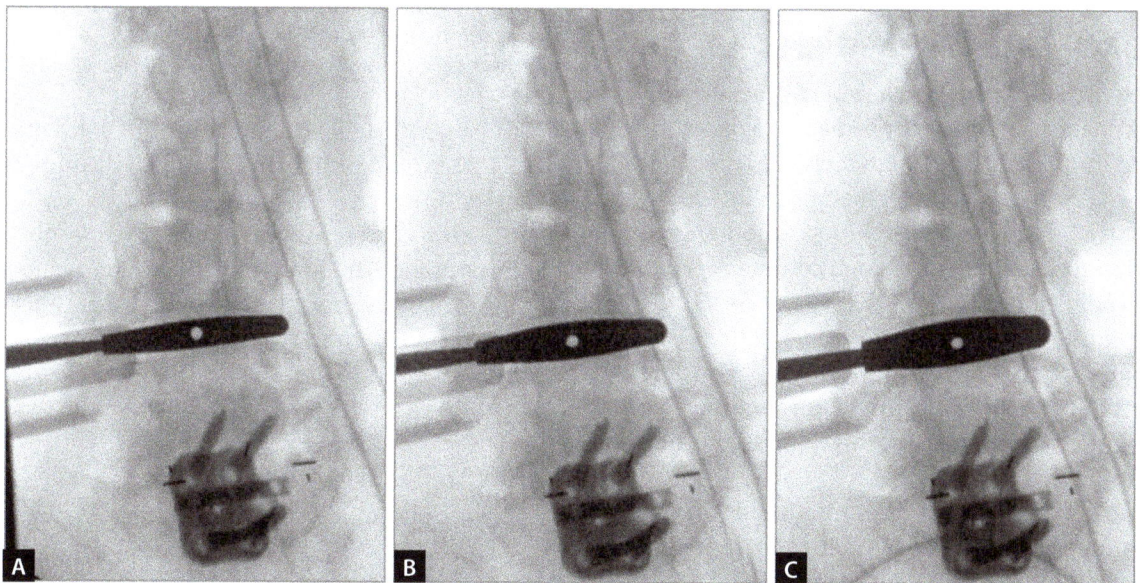

Figs. 17A to C: *Sequential trials placed at L4–L5.* Sequential Medtronic Clydesdale trials are impacted into the L4–L5 disk space following the discectomy. An 8 mm height trial is placed (A), followed by a 10 mm trial (B), followed by a 12 mm trial (C).

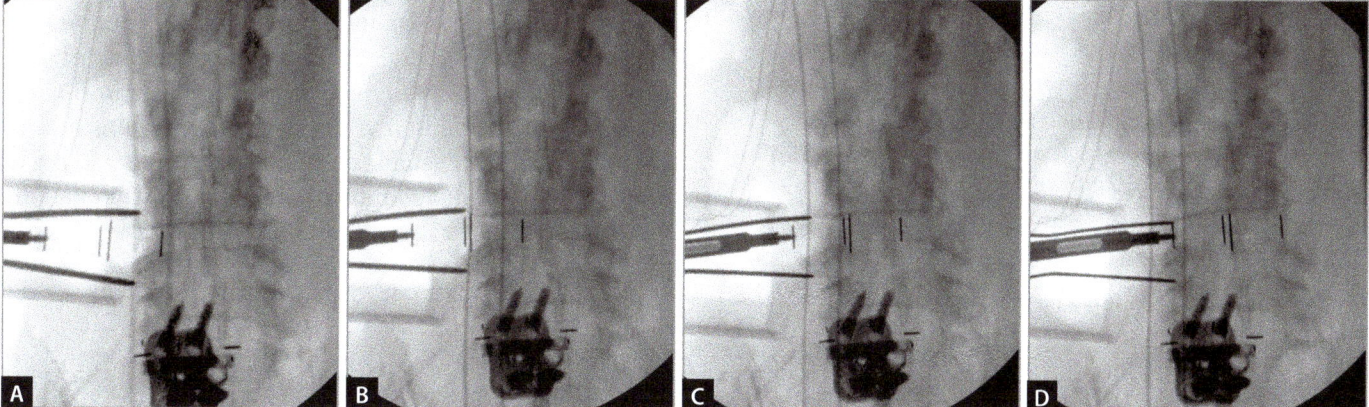

Figs. 18A to D: *Final placement of the L4–L5 implant.* A Medtronic Clydesdale spacer is implanted across the L4–L5 disk space. Note the restoration of the disk height and coronal realignment of the L4–L5 disk during the implantation of the spacer.

the implant is within the anterior third of the disk space, just behind the ALL. This ensures optimal lordosis.
- Lateral plating is not routinely used so as to not restrict further deformity reduction and correction during the posterior instrumentation stage. Percutaneous pedicle screw and rod instrumentation accompanies lateral interbody fusion, usually staged by several days. In the event that the ALL is released or resected, a lateral plate and screws may be considered to provide additional stability at that segment.
- The inserter is then removed and the area is irrigated again. Grafton putty is packed over the spacer.
- If only L4–L5 is being addressed, the retractor is then loosened and removed slowly while looking down the tube to confirm adequate hemostasis and ensure that the peritoneum was not violated. Closure then proceeds. If additional levels are planned, please see the section below.

APPROACH TO LEVELS ABOVE L4–L5

- For additional lumbar levels, a similar process to the L4–L5 level ensues. Often two or three disk spaces may be accessed through the same skin incision. Usually, L4–L5 and L3–L4 are accessed through one skin incision, while L2–L3 and L1–L2 are accessed through another incision.
- The technique is replicated at each additional level, with minimal adjustments:
  - The surgeon's right hand is used to clear the retroperitoneal space as the surgery progresses proximally. A leading finger under the fascia is present during the passage of the initial probe and dilators through the fascia.
  - At L1–L2 and L2–L3, attempt to stay below the diaphragm. This may be achieved by using the right hand to keep the diaphragm out of the way or by holding the patient's breath in expiration while passing the initial probe and retractors.
  - L1–L2 and L2–L3 often are accessed on opposite sides of the rib (one above and one below). A rib resection is not required; simply drop the initial probe between the ribs and proceed as described above.
  - A 6° lordotic cage is typically implanted at the L1–L2 disk space, rather than a 12° lordotic cage.
- Final AP and lateral X-rays are taken and attention is directed to closure **(Fig. 19)**.

CLOSURE

- Closure is obtained in a layered method.

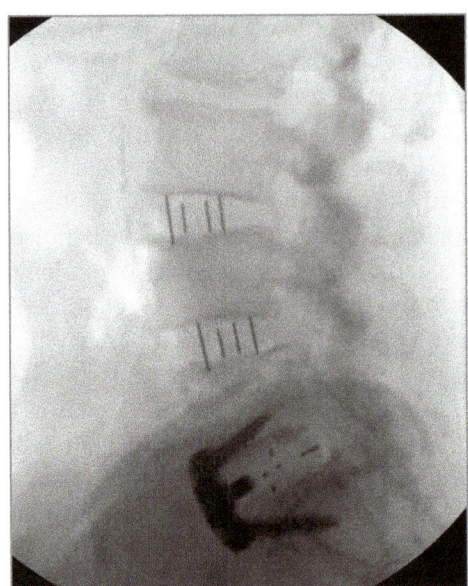

Fig. 19: *Final lateral X-ray of multilevel interbody spacer placement in a single patient position.* Final X-ray reveals adequate placement of the interbody spacers at L3–L4, L4–L5, and L5–S1 via the ante-psoas approach.

- Closure of the fascial layer is obtained with a running 1-PDS suture or interrupted 0-Vicryl suture with a CT-1 or CT-X needle.
- Closure of the subcutaneous layer is obtained with interrupted 2-0 Vicryl suture with a CT-2 needle.
- Closure of the dermis is obtained with interrupted 3-0 Vicryl suture with a SH (small half circle) needle.
- The incision is dressed with Steri strips and a gauze dressing.

FINAL RECOMMENDATIONS

If used for adult deformity correction, it is recommended to stage the posterior instrumentation to a later day (usually 2–3 days later). Patients are encouraged to ambulate between stages and no brace is required, unless the patient has significant osteoporosis or an endplate/vertebral body fracture was identified during the first stage interbody fusion procedure. Endplate subsidence or graft migration has not been observed between stages. It is recommended for the patient to undergo an intervening standing AP and lateral scoliosis X-ray between the two stages to finalize the upper instrumented vertebra (UIV) for the posterior instrumentation and confirm restoration of lumbar lordosis. The UIV is determined as the first parallel, nonrotated, healthy disk space. Additionally, staging allows for reassessment of preoperative leg symptoms to determine if adequate indirect decompression was achieved with the interbody spacers.

CHAPTER 28

Navigation Techniques

Peter R Swiatek, Wellington K Hsu

■ INTRODUCTION

Spine surgeons rely on the safety and efficacy of their operative techniques to appropriately treat patients with debilitating spinal disorders. With the ubiquitous acceptance of pedicle screw-based fixation and complication rates ranging from 14 to 54% using standard insertion methods, the need to improve accuracy of screw placement has led to the evolution of imaging-based navigation in spine surgery.[1-3] Over the last several decades, spine surgery has experienced the emergence of various navigation technologies. In 1995, the first navigated pedicle screw was placed in a patient using preoperative computed tomography (CT) and intraoperative fluoroscopic imaging.[4,5] Since then, navigation technology has evolved to include advanced intraoperative fluoroscopic, CT-based, and robotic navigation. Recent reports show that these technologies have improved accuracy of pedicle screw placement and decreased complications related to errant pedicle screws, including decreased return to the operating room (OR) for revision of misplaced screws.[6,7] This chapter will serve as a technique guide for utilizing advanced image-guided navigation.

■ STEREOTACTIC NAVIGATION

Traditionally, surgeons have relied upon two-dimensional (2D) fluoroscopic imaging in multiple planes to triangulate their instruments to complex three-dimensional (3D) spinal anatomy. This process has become even more complicated with the rise in minimally invasive exposures that hide important landmarks during instrumentation.[8] Computer-based stereotactic navigation is an attempt to shift the 2D view of surgical anatomy into a 3D view of the surgical landscape through which surgical instruments can be tracked. A number of commercially available systems are available for intraoperative spinal navigation **(Table 1)**.

All systems require a registration process to establish the spatial relationship between the surgical anatomy and the imaging data.[9] Methods include paired-point, surface matching, and automated registration. Paired-point registration requires the surgeon to select three discrete landmarks on preoperative or intraoperative imaging. The surgeon then touches the corresponding landmarks, or fiducials, with the navigation probe.[10] The chief disadvantage of paired-point matching is that accuracy of navigation is dependent on the surgeon's ability to exactly match the preselected landmark with the surgical anatomy.[9] Surface-based point matching is an adjunctive method of registering through which the surgeons maps multiple random points on the surgical anatomy to the imaging data.[10] Automated registration, regarded as the most accurate and user-friendly form of registration, requires no surgeon input and thus results in less registration error. A reference frame with reflective optical spheres is fixed to a specific point on the surgical anatomy. A second frame is included in the CT scanner or fluoroscope.[9] Advantages of automated registration include the ability to image multiple levels in a single sequence and the increased image accuracy.[10] Examples of intraoperative CT scanners include O-arm™ (Medtronic, Minneapolis, MN) and Brainlab Airo® Mobile intraoperative CT (Brainlab AG, Feldkirchen, Germany).

Type of intraoperative imaging modality, such as fluoroscopy versus CT, and timing of imaging (pre- or intraoperative) are also significantly different among today's available navigation technologies.[11-13] Many systems promote preoperative CT-based navigation that is registered through the aforementioned matching processes.[8] Fluoroscopic navigation involves preoperative anteroposterior (AP) and lateral imaging of the target surgical anatomy and interpolation of the data to create a 3D rendition. Unlike the preoperative CT imaging, however, fluoroscopic navigation does not provide axial views of the spine.[9]

TABLE 1: Catalog of common spine navigation systems.					
Navigation system	Imaging system	Company	Date introduced	Type of registration	Type of preoperative imaging
StealthStation™ S8	O-arm™, iMRI, iCT, and C-arms	Medtronic, Minneapolis, MN	Spring 2017	Automatic (O-arm™)	CT
Brainlab® Spinal Navigation	Airo® Mobile Intra-operative CT, MRI, and C-arms	Brainlab AG, Feldkirchen, Germany	Fall 2013	Automatic (Airo®), surface matching, or paired point	CT
NAV3i™ Platform, Spine Map® 3D	MRI, CT, and C-arms	Stryker, Kalamazoo, MI	Fall 2015	Automatic	CT
7D Surgical System Machine-vision Image Guided Surgery (MvIGS)	IGS	7D Surgical, Toronto, ON	Spring 2017	Paired Point (Flash Registration™)	CT
Pulse™	CT, C-arms (Cios Spin®, Siemens, Malvern, PA), Less Ray	NuVasive, San Diego, CA	Summer 2019	Automatic (Cios)	CT

Source: Medtronic, Brainlab, Stryker, 7D Surgical, and NuVasive product brochures published online.
(CT: computed tomography; iCT: intraoperative computed tomography; IGS: image-guided surgery; iMRI: intraoperative magnetic resonance imaging; MRI: magnetic resonance imaging)

Compared to standard fluoroscopy, isocentric fluoroscopy involves C-arm imaging through a 180° arc in the OR at the start of the case. Its advantages include the increased resolution of the virtual landscape and inclusion of axial spine views compared to standard fluoroscopy.[9] Intraoperative cone-beam CT scans utilize a 360° arc of motion around the patient. These methods increase resolution associated with automated registration compared to other preoperative imaging techniques.[9]

Recent advances in spine navigation are focused on increasing cost-effectiveness and accuracy and reducing radiation exposure. For example, the 7D Surgical System (7D Surgical, Toronto, ON) offers a novel registration method, which eliminates intraoperative CT or fluoroscopy, decreasing processing times to <20 seconds. Using a machine vision image-guided surgery (MvIGS) technology, which is a light source and camera embedded in the overhead surgical light, reflection of light off the surgical anatomy is digitized and mapped to a preoperative CT, creating a 3D landscape for navigation.[14]

RADIATION EXPOSURE

Radiation exposure to patient and surgeon is a significant concern in spine surgery given reliance on preoperative or intraoperative imaging. For example, 1 minute of fluoroscopy is equivalent to 30 mSev (milli-Sievert) or 150 chest X-rays[15] and one abdominal CT scan may expose the patient to radiation ranging anywhere from 1 to 31 mSev.[16-20] Given the reliance on imaging in spine surgery, surgeons and patients are exposed to 10- to 12-times the amount of radiation compared to nonspine cases.[21]

For the surgeon, non-navigated posterior lumbar spine instrumentation using 2D fluoroscopic imaging has been associated with a nearly 10- to 13-fold increase in radiation exposure compared to the same procedure using 3D image-guided fluoroscopic navigation.[22,23]

The impact of image-guided navigation on the patient, however, is less certain. Radiation exposure during non-navigated procedures is highly variable and dependent upon some patient-specific factors, such as body habitus and operative levels, and surgeon-specific factors, such as number of images needed to perform a given procedure and settings used for intraoperative imaging.[24] For example, several recent studies utilizing cadavers and patients demonstrate increased radiation exposure to the cadavers/patients when CT navigation is used compared to 2D fluoroscopy.[25,26] On the contrary, Villard et al. showed a decreased radiation exposure to patients with CT navigation, although their results failed to reach statistical significance.[22] Notably, Kelft et al. showed that use of intraoperative CT, specifically O-arm™, exposed the patient to a mean radiation dose comparable to one-half to that of a standard 64 multislice CT scan.[27]

INTRAOPERATIVE COMPUTED TOMOGRAPHY NAVIGATION GUIDE

At our home institution, we utilize an intraoperative cone-based CT with the Medtronic StealthStation™ Surgical Navigation System and O-arm™ system (Medtronic, Minneapolis, MN). Over the past decade, the evolution of technique and experience has led to a significant decrease in OR time and increase in efficiency when image navigation is used. The most common surgical cases that we use intraoperative CT for are those involving percutaneous screws and greater than three-level open lumbar fusions. Cases are carefully selected based upon its efficiency and risk–benefit ratio compared to open or fluoroscopic techniques.

Setup and Preparation

- A large OR is essential, as navigation equipment can be cumbersome.
- The patient is initially positioned prone on a radiolucent Jackson table, allowing for the intraoperative CT to circumferentially image the patient without interference.
    - The patient's arms may be placed in the 90-90 position for lumbar procedures or at the patient's side for thoracic/cervical procedures.
- For the thoracic and cervical spine, care must be taken to ensure that the gantry angle is appropriate to visualize the lateral mass/pedicle.
- The navigation system, including infrared optical detector and navigation screens, is generally placed at the foot of the bed to accommodate for anesthesia needs **(Fig. 1)**.[28]
    - During the navigation process, we recommend that surgeons primarily view the axial and sagittal CT images and then utilize the fluoroscopic AP and lateral views to double-check general position.
- The passive reference frame is then affixed to the spinal anatomy.
    - The surgeon should ensure that no soft tissue is pushing on the array.
    - For open cases, we recommend attaching the reference frame to the spinous process of the spinal segment caudal to the lowest instrumented level. This provides the shortest distance between the array and infrared camera, enhancing the accuracy of the imaging.
    - For cervical cases in which the camera and navigation system are placed by the patient's head, the reference frame can be affixed to the most cephalad exposed spinous process.[29] For upper cervical cases, we recommend utilizing an intact subaxial cervical spinous process for the attachment of the reference arc and placement of the stealth camera lateral to the patient to ensure the optical visualization of the instruments and anatomy.
    - For minimally invasive lumbar cases, the frame can be attached to an iliac post that is fixed to the posterior superior iliac spine. It is important to angle the array perpendicular to the floor or in a slight caudal position. An array placed with a cephalic tilt may obstruct L4, L5, or S1 screw placement **(Fig. 2)**.
- The reference frame should be placed as close as possible to the levels of instrumentation.
    - One disadvantage of navigation when using an iliac post in minimally invasive spine (MIS) cases is that this distance between reference frame and site of instrumentation is typically increased which may compromise accuracy.[28]

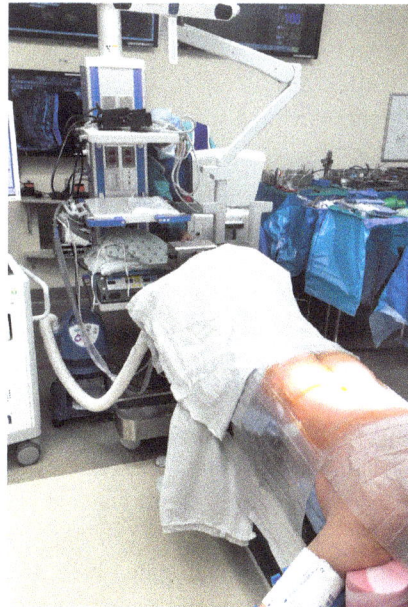

Fig. 1: *Preoperative setup for patient and navigation system.* Patient is positioned with arms abducted and externally rotated. Infrared camera station is positioned at foot of patient with cameras directed at the operative site. Navigation screen is also positioned at the foot of the bed, in a position that is easily visible to surgeons during pedicle screw preparation and placement.

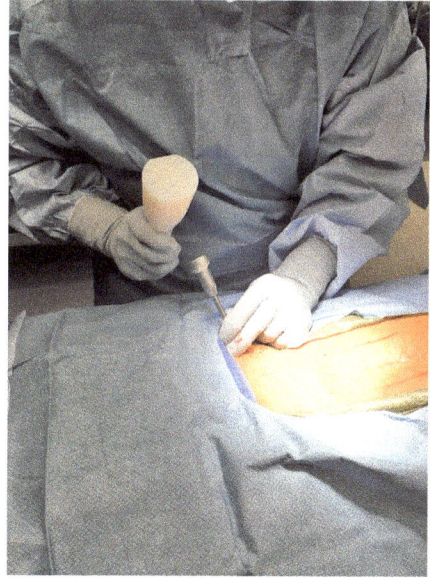

Fig. 2: *Reference frame insertion.* For minimally invasive surgery, the surgeon uses a plastic mallet to insert the reference frame into the posterior superior iliac spine through a percutaneous incision.

- In lumbar surgery, instrumenting three levels from the reference arc has been associated with an inaccuracy of up to 3 mm in 7% of patients when using 3D fluoroscopy,[30] which may also be applicable to CT imaging.
- Registration of the instruments prior to placement of the reference arc reduces variability in the movement of the arc after placement.[28]

■ Once the reference array is placed, the surgeon can prepare for the O-arm™ spin.
- When the O-arm™ is centered over the levels of interested, the position of the array is checked. Additionally, during the imaging process, the array is checked to ensure adequate registration.
- After removal of the O-arm™, the infrared camera is positioned either at the foot of the table (i.e., for lumbar procedures) or at the head of the table (i.e., for thoracic/cervical procedures) to ensure a direct line-of-sight between reference frame and camera **(Fig. 3)**.
- At this time, the surgeon should remind the surgical team that the reference array should not be touched or otherwise altered.
- The navigation system utilizes passive arrays, reflecting light off the spheres to the infrared camera. Any distortion in either reflecting light toward the camera or sensing the light that is reflected may reduce accuracy.
- Although the spherical attachments on the navigated instruments should kept clean of blood and tissue with the generous use of wet and dry laparotomy sponges, the surgeon should refrain from touching the reference array.

■ Additional steps may be taken to ensure accuracy in the registration process.
- Freedman et al. describes placing small screws in the lamina at the planned levels of instrumentation to serve as fiducial markers, particular in large, open deformity cases requiring instrumentation of multiple levels.[28]
- The levels are recorded after insertion of the markers to ensure that all markers are removed prior to the end of the case.
- These screws are then mapped during the registration process, along with other key bony landmarks.
- During the case, the surgeon can test the accuracy of the navigation by placing a ball tip probe on the head of the screw and checking that the navigation appropriately represents the ball-tip probe's position.
- If the navigation is found to be inaccurate at any point, the surgeon can attempt to make adjustments.
- The risk–benefit ratio of these additional steps on the increased OR time must be weighed by the surgeon and institution.

Intraoperative Imaging

■ Preparation for intraoperative CT imaging starts with preparing the wound.
- We use sterile saline solution to fill the wound and place sterile towels over the wound. Because the saline solution has a similar density to blood and surrounding tissues, imaging is more accurate than if left open to air.
- Two drapes are used to circumferentially wrap the patient, leaving a small opening for the reference arc.

■ Next, the O-arm™ is then centered over the surgical site with both AP and lateral spot images taken for localization.
- Adjustments are made to ensure a perpendicular orientation of the beam to the surgical anatomy and that the surgical anatomy is centered within the field of planned CT imaging.[28]
- The upper body warmer should be turned off to decrease imaging artifacts.[31]
- At this time, personnel should vacate the OR during the spin to minimize radiation.

■ O-arm™ image captures is initiated **(Fig. 4)**.
- During the 30 seconds of image capture, the patient should be held apneic to limit motion artifact during creation of the 3D image.[28]
- During the O-arm™ spin, multiple 2D images are captured and digitized into a 3D landscape of surgical anatomy.[28]

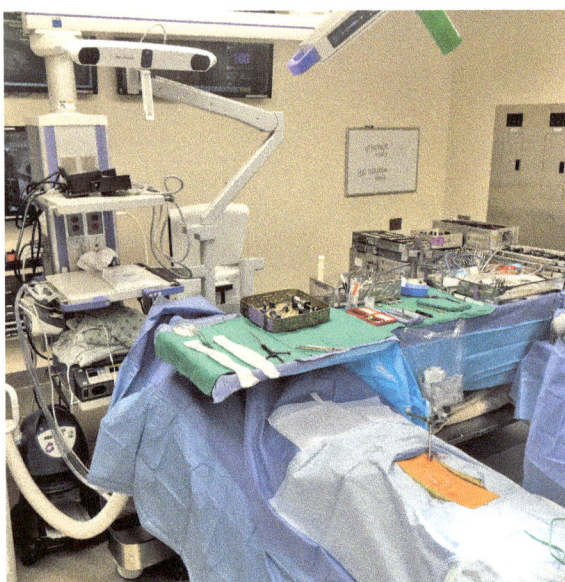

Fig. 3: *Reference frame position relative to infrared camera. The reference frame is positioned with spheres directed at the infrared camera. Care is taken to avoid altering the position of the reference frame or obstructing the line of sight between the infrared camera and reference frame.*

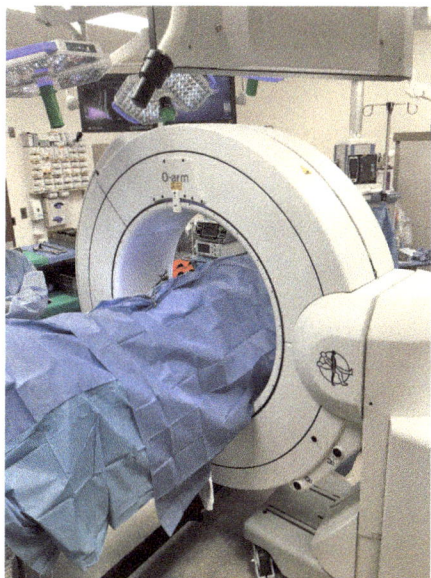

Fig. 4: *Intraoperative computed tomography scan.* Patient is covered with sterile drapes and two allis clamps. The reference frame is left exposed above the drapes. The O-arm™ is positioned at the operative spinal levels.

- Multiple "spins" of the O-arm™ may be required depending on the number of levels to be instrumented.[28]
  - If the levels of interest cannot all be captured in a single O-arm™ spin, then the visible levels after one spin should to be instrumented.
  - Then, additional rounds of imaging with the O-arm™ and instrumenting should be performed until all levels of interest are instrumented.
- Most machines have two settings for image quality: Standard and high definition.
  - We recommend high definition for obese patients, those with metallic implants, or levels involving the cervical or cervicothoracic region.[28]

Pedicle Screw Placement

- An intraoperative probe can be used to localize the level of interest and mark the incision.
- Dissection should be carried out in the typical fashion, with an understanding that the intraoperative anatomy has been statically mapped to the 3D navigation.
  - Any additional manipulation on the intraoperative anatomy or any blocks to a direct line-of-sight between the infrared camera and the reference probes will alter the accuracy of the instrumentation. Therefore, we recommend making more a generous fascial dissection and skin release.
- For open spine cases, we recommend identifying pedicle screw trajectories immediately after imaging and before any decompression. This ensures that the navigation is as accurate as possible, as duration between imaging and instrumentation may decrease accuracy.[28,30]

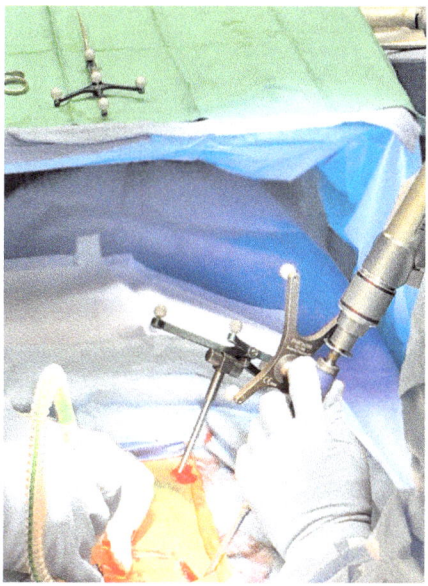

Fig. 5: *Navigating the awl-tip tap for pedicle screw placement.* The surgeon uses the tap on a power driver to prepare the pedicle for screw placement. The "x-shaped" attachment to the driver is positioned with spheres facing the infrared camera. The surgeon triangulates axial and sagittal trajectory during tapping using the navigation interface at the foot of the bed.

- Start point is determined and pedicle screw prepared for insertion.
  - Start point is determined using the navigated awl-tip tap **(Fig. 5)**.
  - The surgeon then advances the 5.5-mm awl-tip tap with a power drill in the optimal trajectory utilizing the axial and sagittal CT images typically displayed on the left side of the screen.
    - Once the outer cortex of the pedicle is breached, the drill is stopped to double-check position. Minor changes in the direction of the instrument in this position to optimize trajectory are possible at this point because the awl-tap is at the surface of the bone.
  - Once the awl-tap has been advanced into the vertebral body, the optimal screw size is measured on the CT imaging.
- The pedicle screw may be advanced by hand or by using a separate power drill to increase the efficiency of workflow.
  - The tip of the pedicle screw can be used to locate the hole from the awl-tap utilizing the sagittal and axial CT images **(Figs. 6A and B)**.
  - In addition to improving workflow and speed, power drivers offer the benefit of decreased toggle, creating a tighter path and improving pullout strength.
- After all pedicle screws are inserted, we obtain 2D fluoroscopic imaging to confirm screw placement.
- Any additional spins of the O-arm™ would be reserved for cases in which screw placement is concerning for proximity to critical structures.[28]

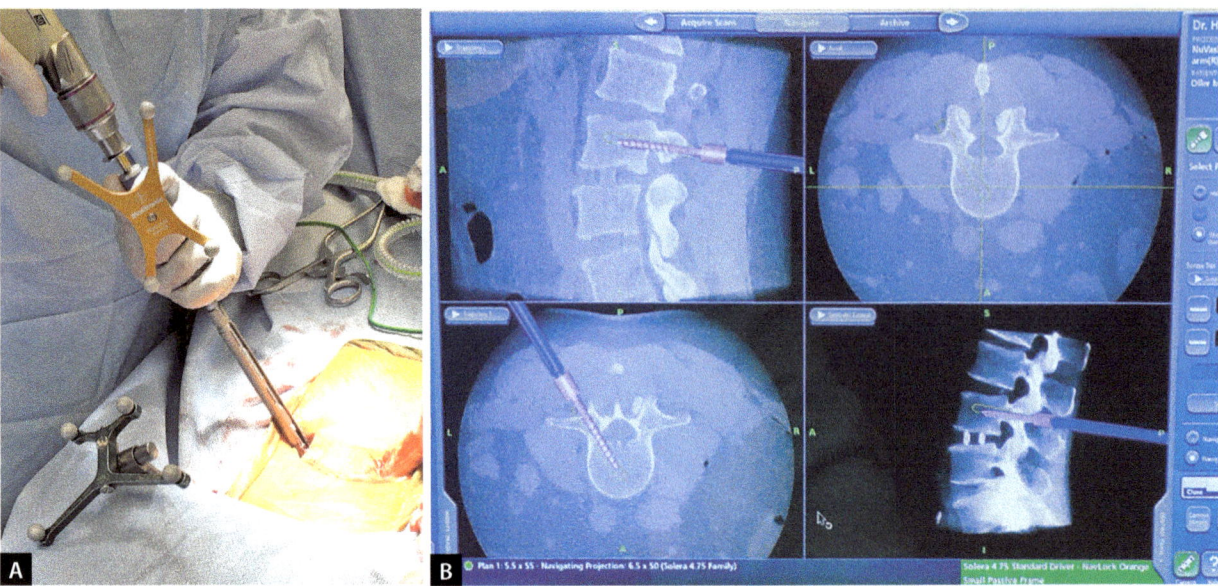

Figs. 6A and B: *Navigating pedicle screw placement.* (A) The surgeon uses a power driver to insert the pedicle screw. The "X-shaped" attachment must be facing the infrared camera; (B) The surgeon triangulates axial and sagittal trajectory of the screw using the navigation interface at the foot of the bed. The previous trajectory of the tap appears as a green outline. The screw appears in pink.

BOX 1: Key considerations for spinal navigation.

- Book a large OR with a flat Jackson and room for the CT
- Position navigation equipment by patient's head
- Can place screws in lamina of instrumented levels for use as fiducial markers
- Attach reference frame to bony prominence, usually spinous process
- Accuracy decreases with distance from reference frame and increased duration
- Keep reference frame between camera and area of instrumentation
- Register surgical instruments prior to imaging to save time
- Drape patient circumferentially prior to CT imaging
- Ask anesthesia to hold patient apneic for 30 seconds during 3D imaging
- Protect reference from any inadvertent adjustment
- Check accuracy of instruments after imaging by touching down on landmarks
- After drilling holes, manually check five walls with ball-tip probe
- Routinely check accuracy of navigated instruments

(CT: computed tomography; OR: operating room; 3D: three-dimensional)

- If at any time during the navigation process there is a question of accuracy using visual landmarks, all instrumentation should be stopped.
- The surgeon would check the accuracy of instruments, make adjustments, consider a respin of the O-arm™, or abandon CT-based navigation and proceed with 2D fluoroscopic navigation.[28]

CONCLUSION

Spinal navigation has evolved significantly over the last two decades. Benefits to surgeons and patients include increased accuracy of instrumentation, improved OR efficiency, and decreased radiation exposure. For spine fellows and new adopters of spinal navigation, we are hopeful that key points discussed in this chapter will serve to enhance surgeons' comfort and familiarity with spinal navigation **(Box 1)**. Looking forward, new advances in robotic technology, higher resolution imaging with less radiation, and quicker registration will continue to shape the future of spinal navigation. Further studies will be needed to elucidate the impact and benefit of new technologies on patient care.

REFERENCES

1. Amiot LP, Lang K, Putzier M, Zippel H, Labelle H. Comparative results between conventional and computer-assisted pedicle screw installation in the thoracic, lumbar, and sacral spine. Spine (Phila Pa 1976). 2000;25(5):606-14.
2. Laine T, Lund T, Ylikoski M, Lohikoski J, Schlenzka D. Accuracy of pedicle screw insertion with and without computer assistance: a randomised controlled clinical study in 100 consecutive patients. Eur Spine J. 2000;9(3):235-40.
3. Vaccaro AR, Rizzolo SJ, Allardyce TJ, Ramsey M, Salvo J, Balderston RA, et al. Placement of pedicle screws in the thoracic spine. Part I: Morphometric analysis of the thoracic vertebrae. J Bone Joint Surg Am. 1995;77(8):1193-9.
4. Nolte LP, Visarius H, Arm E, Langlotz F, Schwarzenbach O, Zamorano L. Computer-aided fixation of spinal implants. J Image Guid Surg. 1995;1(2):88-93.
5. Nolte LP, Zamorano L, Visarius H, Berlemann U, Langlotz F, Arm E, et al. Clinical evaluation of a system for precision enhancement in spine surgery. Clin Biomech (Bristol, Avon). 1995;10(6):293-303.
6. Noriega DC, Hernandez-Ramajo R, Rodriguez-Monsalve Milano F, Sanchez-Lite I, Toribio B, Ardura F, et al. Risk-benefit analysis of navigation techniques for vertebral transpedicular instrumentation: a prospective study. Spine J. 2017;17(1):70-5.

7. Sembrano JN, Santos ER, Polly DW Jr. New generation intraoperative three-dimensional imaging (O-arm) in 100 spine surgeries: does it change the surgical procedure? J Clin Neurosci. 2014;21(2):225-31.
8. Ringel F, Villard J, Ryang YM, Meyer B. Navigation, robotics, and intraoperative imaging in spinal surgery. Adv Tech Stand Neurosurg. 2014;41:3-22.
9. Kalfas I. Image-guided spinal navigation: principles and clinical applications. In: Youmans and Winn Neurological Surgery, volume 331. Netherlands: Elsevier; 2017. pp. 2702-6.
10. Holly LT, Bloch O, Johnson JP. Evaluation of registration techniques for spinal image guidance. J Neurosurg Spine. 2006;4(4):323-8.
11. Austin MS, Vaccaro AR, Brislin B, Nachwalter R, Hilibrand AS, Albert TJ. Image-guided spine surgery: a cadaver study comparing conventional open laminoforaminotomy and two image-guided techniques for pedicle screw placement in posterolateral fusion and nonfusion models. Spine (Phila Pa 1976). 2002;27(22):2503-8.
12. Lavallee S, Sautot P, Troccaz J, Cinquin P, Merloz P. Computer-assisted spine surgery: a technique for accurate transpedicular screw fixation using CT data and a 3-D optical localizer. J Image Guid Surg. 1995;1(1):65-73.
13. Merloz P, Tonetti J, Eid A, Faure C, Lavallee S, Troccaz J, et al. Computer assisted spine surgery. Clin Orthop Relat Res. 1997;(337):86-96.
14. 7D Surgical System. 7D Surgical. [online] Available from: https://7dsurgical.com/7d-surgical-system/. [Last accessed March, 2022].
15. DOD U. The Effects of Nuclear Weapons, Revised ed. 1962. [online] Available from: https://www.deepspace.ucsb.edu/wp-content/uploads/2013/01/Effects-of-Nuclear-Weapons-1977-3rd-edition-complete.pdf. [Last accessed March, 2022].
16. Fujii K, Aoyama T, Yamauchi-Kawaura C, Koyama S, Yamauchi M, Ko S, et al. Radiation dose evaluation in 64-slice CT examinations with adult and paediatric anthropomorphic phantoms. Br J Radiol. 2009;82(984):1010-8.
17. Smith-Bindman R, Lipson J, Marcus R, Kim KP, Mahesh M, Gould R, et al. Radiation dose associated with common computed tomography examinations and the associated lifetime attributable risk of cancer. Arch Intern Med. 2009;169(22):2078-86.
18. Pantos I, Thalassinou S, Argentos S, Kelekis NL, Panayiotakis G, Efstathopoulos EP. Adult patient radiation doses from non-cardiac CT examinations: a review of published results. Br J Radiol. 2011;84(1000):293-303.
19. Tsapaki V, Rehani M, Saini S. Radiation safety in abdominal computed tomography. Semin Ultrasound CT MR. 2010;31(1):29-38.
20. Huda W, Nickoloff EL, Boone JM. Overview of patient doradiation exposure duringsimetry in diagnostic radiology in the USA for the past 50 years. Med Phys. 2008;35(12):5713-28.
21. Jones DP, Robertson PA, Lunt B, Jackson SA. Radiation exposure during fluoroscopically assisted pedicle screw insertion in the lumbar spine. Spine (Phila Pa 1976). 2000;25(12):1538-41.
22. Villard J, Ryang YM, Demetriades AK, Reinke A, Behr M, Preuss A, et al. Radiation exposure to the surgeon and the patient during posterior lumbar spinal instrumentation: a prospective randomized comparison of navigated versus non-navigated freehand techniques. Spine (Phila Pa 1976). 2014;39(13):1004-9.
23. Smith HE, Welsch MD, Sasso RC, Vaccaro AR. Comparison of radiation exposure in lumbar pedicle screw placement with fluoroscopy vs computer-assisted image guidance with intraoperative three-dimensional imaging. J Spinal Cord Med. 2008;31(5):532-7.
24. Kochanski RB, Lombardi JM, Laratta JL, Lehman RA, O'Toole JE. Image-guided navigation and robotics in spine surgery. Neurosurgery. 2019;84(6):1179-89.
25. Tabaraee E, Gibson AG, Karahalios DG, Potts EA, Mobasser JP, Burch S. Intraoperative cone beam-computed tomography with navigation (O-ARM) versus conventional fluoroscopy (C-ARM): a cadaveric study comparing accuracy, efficiency, and safety for spinal instrumentation. Spine (Phila Pa 1976). 2013;38(22):1953-8.
26. Mendelsohn D, Strelzow J, Dea N, Ford NL, Batke J, Pennington A, et al. Patient and surgeon radiation exposure during spinal instrumentation using intraoperative computed tomography-based navigation. Spine J. 2016;16(3):343-54.
27. Van de Kelft E, Costa F, Van der Planken D, Schils F. A prospective multicenter registry on the accuracy of pedicle screw placement in the thoracic, lumbar, and sacral levels with the use of the O-arm imaging system and StealthStation Navigation. Spine (Phila Pa 1976). 2012;37(25):E1580-7.
28. Freedman BA, Nassr A, Currier BL. Stereotactic navigation in complex spinal surgery: tips and tricks. In: Operative Techniques in Orthopaedics, Volume 27. Netherlands: Elsevier; 2017. pp. 260-8.
29. Agarwal A, Freedman RA, Goicuria F, Rhinehart C, Murphy K, Kelly E, et al. Prior authorization for medications in a breast oncology practice: Navigation of a complex process. J Oncol Pract. 2017;13(4):e273-82.
30. Quinones-Hinojosa A, Robert Kolen E, Jun P, Rosenberg WS, Weinstein PR. Accuracy over space and time of computer-assisted fluoroscopic navigation in the lumbar spine in vivo. J Spinal Disord Tech. 2006;19(2):109-13.
31. Rahmathulla G, Nottmeier EW, Pirris SM, Deen HG, Pichelmann MA. Intraoperative image-guided spinal navigation: technical pitfalls and their avoidance. Neurosurg Focus. 2014;36(3):E3.

CHAPTER 29

Technical Pearls in the Management of Spinal Cord Injury

Daniel Franco, Aria Mahtabfar, Glenn Gonzalez, James Harrop

■ INTRODUCTION

Spinal cord injury (SCI) is a life-changing, disruptive event. This entity puts significant strain on the United States public health system; it can cost anywhere from $368,000 up to $1,110,000 in the first year postinjury to care for each of these patients, followed by an average of $110,000 each subsequent year, though there is great variability depending of level and extent of neurological injury.[1] Incomplete tetraplegia is the most common type of injury, and typically results in longstanding neurological defects as <1% of persons experienced complete recovery before discharge.[1] Moreover, SCI is an increasingly common pathology, with a recent estimate showing that the annual incidence of SCI is approximately 54 cases per 1 million people in the United States, or about 17,730 new SCI cases each year.[1,2] These estimates do not include those who die at the location of the incident that caused the SCI. The most common causes for SCI are motor vehicle accidents (31.4%), falls (19.0%), and violent crimes, and gunshots (18.3%), while the remaining 31.3% are attributed to a variety of additional causes.[4]

Federally backed Spinal Cord Injury Model Systems (SCIMS) were conceptualized and brought to fruition in 1971, with a goal of standardizing comprehensive care and reducing morbidity and mortality after SCI.[3] The SCIMS have, by design, five key components of care: Prevention, emergency care/resuscitation/transport, acute care, rehabilitation, and follow-up.[4] Concurrently, nationwide Emergency Medical Services (EMS) were developed, creating a new streamlined process which attempted to immediately identify SCIs, properly retrieve injured victims, and deliver these patients to specialized centers in both acute trauma and SCI.[3,4] The architecture of this structure was based on two primary goals: Saving lives and preventing additional progressive neurologic injury.

In this chapter, the authors will focus on the management of the acute care phase. Depending on the etiology of the SCI, management strategies can vary, with the two main strategies being operative and medical management. In patients who have suffered a motor vehicle accident, it is likely that the cause of the SCI is associated with unstable fractures, therefore, this population usually is managed surgically with decompression and instrumented fusion[5] **(Figs. 1A and B)**. In contrast, patients who have had penetrating injuries, which tend to cause complete neurological injury below the affected level[1] **(Fig. 2)**, are predominantly treated nonoperatively.[5]

■ INITIAL ASSESSMENT AND DIAGNOSIS

Any traumatic injury should initially be managed following the steps outlined on the Advanced Trauma Life Support (ATLS) from the American College of Surgeons (ACS).[6] Upon arrival at the care facility, primary survey should be performed following the ABCDEs (airway, breathing, circulation, disability, exposure), which will allow clinicians to identify any other potentially life-threatening injuries that need to be addressed immediately. Once the patient has been stabilized and issues identified during the primary survey have been addressed, initial neurological assessment should be performed in a very careful and detailed manner. This should include a complete cranial nerve examination, examination of isolated muscle groups, dermatomal sensory testing, and rectal sensation, tone, and volition evaluation.[8] After this evaluation has been completed, a baseline American Spinal Injury Association (ASIA) Impairment Scale (AIS) designation is given[7] **(Table 1)**.

Diagnostic Imaging

Patients with clinical findings concerning for SCI should undergo diagnostic imaging immediately. Historically, the patient would get three-view plain radiographs of the different sections of the spine, however, presently, the computerized tomography (CT) scan has essentially replaced

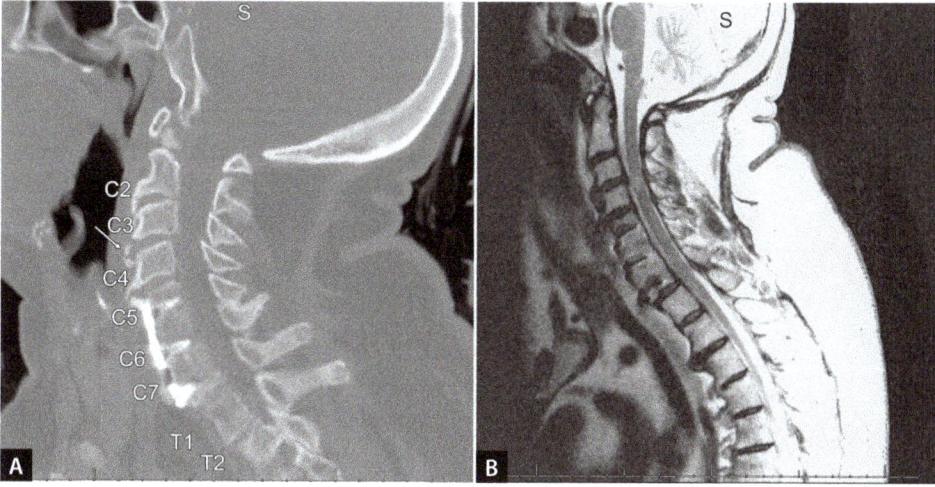

Figs. 1A and B: Computerized tomography scan reveals C3–C4 anterior osteophyte fracture after and extension-distraction injury. Magnetic resonance image C-spine, T2-weighted images show hyperintensity at the level of C3–C4, indicating injury to the spinal cord. Noted below is a previous C5–C7 anterior cervical discectomies and fusion.

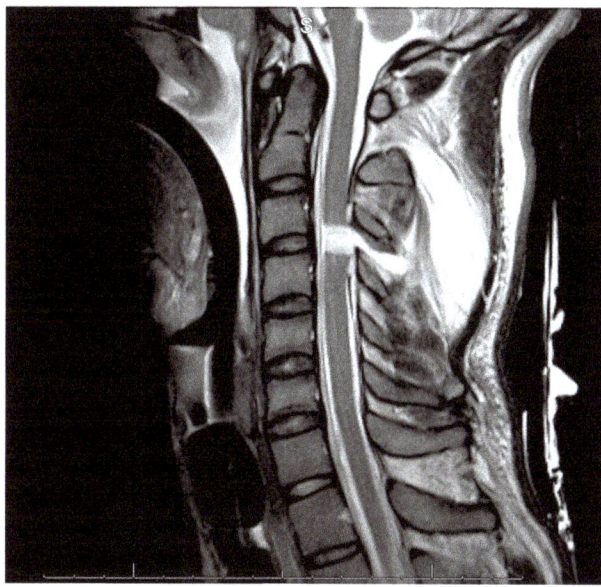

Fig. 2: T2-weigthed sagittal C-spine magnetic resonance image showing complete transection of the spinal cord at the C3–C4 level, caused by direct stabbing of posterior neck. There were no associated bony element disruptions in this case. Patient was a C4 American Spinal Injury Association (ASIA).

TABLE 1: American Spinal Injury Association (ASIA) impairment scale.

ASIA Impairment Scale (AIS) designations	
A = Complete	No sensory or motor function in the S4–S5 segments
B = Sensory incomplete	Sensory but not motor function is preserved below the neurological level and includes S4–S5, and no motor function is preserved more than three levels below the motor level on either side of the body
C = Motor incomplete	Motor function is preserved below the neurological level, and more than half of key muscle functions below the single neurological level of injury (NLI) have a muscle grade <3 (Grades 0–2)
D = Motor incomplete	Motor function is preserved below the neurological level, and at least half of key muscle functions below the NLI have a muscle grade >3
E = Normal	If sensation and motor function are graded as normal in all segments, and the patient had prior deficits, then AIS grade is E. Patients without an initial spinal cord injury do not receive an AIS grade

these radiographs as the initial modality of choice.[9,10] In our institution, transferred spinal cord injured patients undergo a full body CT scan by the trauma team. This is to be sure that there is no other concurrent body injuries. This CT scan is then reformatted to show the entire spine in order to rule out fractures. There can be an up to 40% chance of a simultaneous, noncontiguous injury.[10] At our institution, an imaging protocol is in place for any patient for whom there is suspicion of an SCI, in which CTs of the cervical, thoracic, and lumbar spine are performed. A detailed neurologic examination helps define the area of further imaging. After all initial images are completed and reviewed, magnetic resonance images (MRIs) are tailored to the patient's neurological condition and CT scan findings.

In some cases, CT scans can be negative for fractures or gross bony misalignment, yet the patient still presents with significant neurological impairment. Subsequent MRI should still be considered and possibly obtained under these circumstances. MRIs have been shown to play a protagonist role in the identification of occult injuries, as well as SCIs that might be obscured due to alteration of mental status at the moment of the initial insult.[11] This

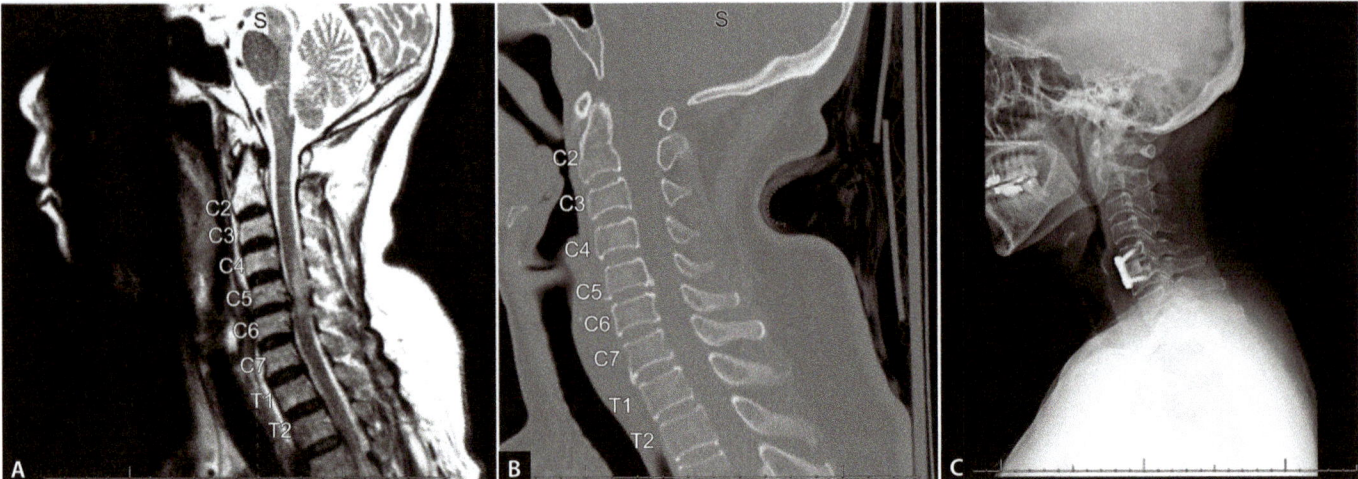

Figs. 3A to C: A 57-year-old female who presented with acute central cord syndrome after a motor vehicle accident. Computerized tomography scan revealed no abnormalities, magnetic resonance image however showed a large C5–C6 disk herniation, causing injury to the spinal cord with increased signal at that level. Patient was treated with a C5–C6 anterior cervical discectomies and fusion.

imaging study is also of particular benefit when attempting to predict prognosis; severe edema, hemorrhage, and cord discontinuity are some of the indicators of poor prognosis[12] (**Figs. 3A to C**).

SURGICAL MANAGEMENT OF SPINAL CORD INJURY

Depending on the etiology of the injury, some patients will benefit from surgical intervention after an SCI. Regardless of the neurological level of injury (NLI), the goals of surgical management are to provide structural stabilization, ensure adequate decompression of the level of interest, and to prevent secondary injury during the recovery process.[13,14] In 2012, the Surgical Timing in Acute Spinal Cord Injury Study (STASCIS) concluded that surgical intervention performed within the first 24 hours postinjury was associated with better neurologic outcomes.[14] Laboratory evidence also supports this hypothesis. Animal models show attenuation of secondary injury mechanisms and improved outcomes when persistent spinal cord compression is relieved. Moreover, the degree to which these results were noted was inversely related to time to surgery.[14-22] Although data is not conclusive on the timing of surgery, we tend to take a more aggressive approach and decompressing the spinal cord, weighing the risks of concomitant medical conditions against the potential benefits of improving the patient's neurological status.

Cervical and High Thoracic Spinal Cord Injury

If a patient is deemed a surgical candidate, surgery is typically performed as soon as possible. Although the literature has not defined the optimal timing of surgery particularly and central cord injury, we tend to take to believe that decompression potentially improves neurologic recovery. Although this is weight on each patient's general medical risks, operative risks as well as neurologic deficits. One benefit of early surgical decompression is that it provides the patient to progress to the next stage of care, involving early mobilization and aggressive rehabilitation, especially with cervical SCIs and with an incomplete neurological injury as defined by AIS designation.[16] High thoracic SCIs also carry a high level of morbidity and significantly impact a person's way of life. Thus, surgical needs for this patient population should be addressed in a similar, urgent fashion as are cervical injuries.

Central cord syndrome is defined by Schneider in 1954[23] as greater weakness in the upper versus lower extremities with variable sensory loss, bladder, bowel, and sexual dysfunction. This type of injury often times presents with no evidence of gross instability or compression and has expected neurological recovery in the long term.[25] Although recent studies suggest that early surgery (within 24 hours) can certainly be performed in an effective and safe manner, there is insufficient evidence to formulate a clear indication.[24] In our practice, patients with central cord syndrome are almost uniformly taken to the operating room for decompression and fusion within 24 hours of injury. Postoperatively, these patients are transferred to an intensive care unit (ICU), where mean arterial pressures (MAPs) are kept above 85 mm Hg for 5–7 days, and aggressive physical therapy is started as early as possible. Steroids are not routinely used, although this practice is under evaluation in light of recent recommendations of AO Spine.[26] Addressing the level of injury requires close attention to the imaging studies performed, decompression of the segment involved is necessary when obvious compression is noted; however, there are other times where there is no significant stenosis but T2 cord signal is seen. In these cases, decompression of the levels spanning said signal is preferred.

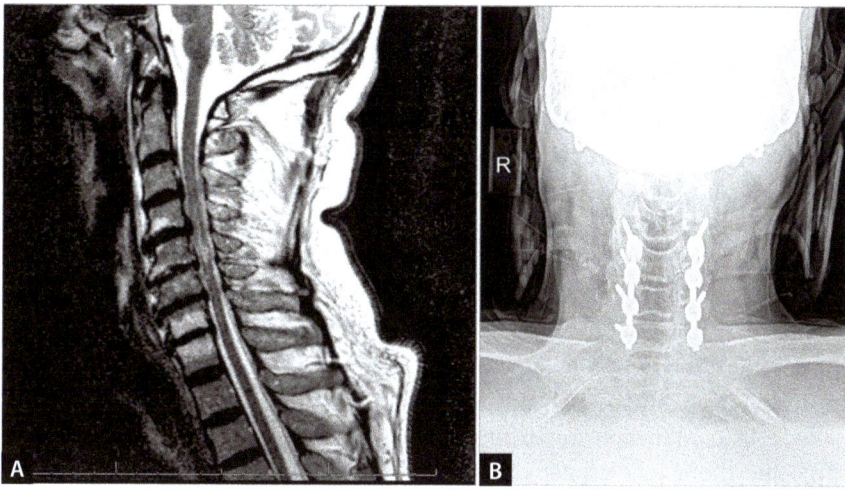

Figs. 4A and B: T2-weighted sagittal C-spine magnetic resonance image showing increased cord signal spanning C4–C6 with severe stenosis at the same levels, patient was a 48-year-old male who presented acutely quadriparetic after slipping on ice. Underwent emergent posterior cervical decompression and instrumented fusion.

Since there is no single optimal surgical technique to address SCI, an operative plan should be individually formulated in order to maximize achievement of the aforementioned goals **(Figs. 4A and B)**.

Low Thoracic and Lumbar Injuries

The most common areas for spinal fractures occur in the thoracolumbar region;[29-31] however, there is significant debate in determining management, timing, and surgical approach in this region. This is due to a multitude of reasons, such as the wide spectrum of injuries (from simple fractures to large complex ligamentous and osseous disruptions), the unique transitional anatomy of the thoracolumbar region, where the spine biomechanical properties change dramatically (thoracic spine being rigid and protected anteriorly with rib cage and lumbar spine being much more dynamic).[28,29] Neurological deficit is more likely to occur following injury to the thoracic versus lumbar spine. This is due to the relatively narrow spinal canal as compared to the lumbar spine, as well as the greater resilience of the cauda equina nerve roots in contrast with the spinal cord or conus medullaris.

In an effort to standardize categorization to injury to this area, there have been many different classification systems that have attempted to categorize the different types of fracture morphology, mechanisms of injury, and neurologic status on arrival. Some of the better known classification systems are the three-column system, described by Denis[32] in 1983; the AO Spine Classification, first described by Magerl[33] in 1994 with more recent validations in 2016,[34,35] which focused more on mechanism of injury and morphology; and the "Thoracolumbar Injury Classification System, TLICS" by The Spine Trauma Study Group[27] in 2005 **(Table 2)**, which also provided the surgeon with a score to aid with surgical decision-making.

TABLE 2: Thoracolumbar injury classification system (TLICS) score.

TLICS score			
Morphology immediate stability	• Compression • Burst • Translation/ rotation • Distraction	1 2 3 4	• X-rays • CT
Integrity of posterior ligamentous complex long-term stability	• Intact • Suspected • Injured	0 2 3	MRI
Neurological status	• Intact • Nerve root • Complete cord • Incomplete cord • Cauda equina	0 2 2 3 3	Physical examination
Recommendation	Need for surgery	0–3 4 >4	• Nonsurgical • Surgeon's choice • Surgical

(CT: computerized tomography; MRI: magnetic resonance image)

In the absence of neurologic injury and evidence of Frank instability, most thoracolumbar spine fractures may be managed nonoperatively. Patients in this setting are typically given thoracolumbar orthoses and/or hyperextension casts with the goal of allowing for early ambulation.[28,36,37] At the institution at which the authors practice, the preference is to brace initially, with follow-up at 1–2 months with repeat X-rays, after which the physician will reassess if a modification of management should be made. Although there is evidence that bracing does not improve outcomes for patients (Bally and Fischer). If considering a surgical correction, careful evaluation of potential morbidity must be weighed against the expected benefits. Surgical decompression of compressing bone fragments over the spinal cord also reliably provides a better environment for restoration of neurologic function.[28] There are certain situations that are better managed with early surgical intervention in our opinion, some of these include severe pain making the patient severely handicapped, large body habitus where bracing would not be effective, fracture morphology known to have poor healing chance down the line.

As is the case with cervical SCI, there are multiple ways of addressing thoracolumbar injuries and there is no scientific evidence to support one technique over others. Surgical plan should be individualized to each patient. Important factors that come into plan are concomitant injuries, baseline morbidity, anesthetic use, expected blood loss, and surgeon's expertise.[28] The thoracolumbar region offers great versatility in surgical approaches, essentially this region can be surgically accessed in all of its circumference.

The posterior approach remains the most popular way of addressing thoracolumbar fractures; posterior decompression and pedicle screw fixation and arthrodesis have been shown to effectively reduce fractures and relieve neurologic compression; all with a reasonably low complication profile.[28,38-40] However, late complications may occur, such as instrumentation failure and kyphotic deformity. Some authors[41,42] have suggested transpedicular intracorporeal bone grafting and vertebroplasty, but this has not been shown to have a significant impact in outcomes. Others have described the addition of "intermediate screws" at the fracture level, which have had more promising results on biomechanical studies.[43-46] The authors of this chapter tend evaluate these patients on a case-by-case basis, and have found that a majority of these can be satisfactorily addressed from a posterior approach. Additionally, the authors favor the use of intermediate screws when possible. It is always kept in mind what the goals of the surgical procedure are: (1) decompression, (2) stabilization/arthrodesis, (3) fusion, and (4) restoration of alignment. To that end, there are some instances in which a combination of anterior and posterior approaches is preferred; primarily cases that present with significant deformity which cannot be corrected from a posterior approach alone (i.e., hyperkyphosis, lateral listhesis, etc.).

Anterior, stand-alone approach for thoracolumbar fractures plays a role mainly when the anterior column is substantially injured, there is absence of posterior element disruption, and neural element compression could not be otherwise adequately decompressed from a posterior approach. Spinal stability and alignment seem to also be better restored from an anterior approach.[30]

Combined anterior-posterior techniques may also be used in select cases. Indications for combined approach would include burst fractures with significant kyphosis (>40°), >50% canal compromise, and neurological deficit in the presence of spinal cord compression.[28] Combined approaches offer the benefits of anterior approaches, they afford direct ventral canal decompression and anterior structural grafting, improving height and sagittal alignment, with also the added benefits of posterior approach allowing directly addressing posterior canal stenosis, and posterior bony or ligamentous injury with three-column fixation from pedicle screws and rods.

Overall, in the setting of spinal trauma, surgical management provides the means of adequate spinal stabilization and neural element decompression with a reasonably low risk profile. However, there are complications that can be associated to surgical correction, which are to be taken into account when selecting and tailoring management. Posterior pedicle screw fixation is a safe way to provide rigid stabilization of the spine, as the most common complication that arises from this method is screw malposition, which is typically asymptomatic. Injury to surrounding visceral or vascular structures is much less common.[28,47,48,50] In an anterior approach, complication is uncommon but has the potential to be devastating. Vascular injury is the most common complication. If small, like a segmental vein injury, it can be treated with compression of the structure, bipolar cauterization, or clip ligation; if large, such as an inferior vena cava or aortic injury, this may require immediate pressure to be held, either manually or with a sponge stick, as well as massive transfusion protocol to be activated and complex repair by vascular surgeon.[49]

MEDICAL MANAGEMENT OF SPINAL CORD INJURY

Contrary to the common opinion that surgical stabilization and decompression will provide the most ideal environment for recovery, a number of clinical studies have found no significant difference in outcomes between early (<3 days) and late (>3 days) surgical intervention.[13,15] However, this cannot directly repair or correct the neurologic injury. After the initial injury, as discussed before, one of the main goals of management is to prevent secondary insults and complications. In the acute setting, patient should be carefully monitored in an ICU setting, as they are at a high risk of cardiac and respiratory dysfunction, particularly in patients with cervical SCI.[10,51] At our institution, depending on the presence and extent of other injuries, the patient is kept in the ICU for at least 5-7 days. Deep vein thrombosis (DVT) prophylaxis is started immediately, the patient's blood pressure is closely monitored (MAP > 85), and ventilator liberation is attempted every day (if applicable). Additionally, physical medicine and rehabilitation (PM&R) clinicians, physical therapists, and occupational therapists are promptly brought in for assessment, and continue to re-evaluate and work with the patient on a daily basis.

Data suggest that an aggressive pulmonary-recovery focused protocol early after SCI is associated with reduced need of long-term ventilator support.[51,52] Patients with high cervical injury are at a high likelihood of requiring tracheostomy to ensure adequate airway protection, and although the timing of placement of tracheostomy has not been firmly determined, there have been some general critical care studies that demonstrated reduction in ICU length of stay, as well as reduced amount of time requiring active mechanical ventilation down the line.[53-55] Patients with cervical cord injury might present with altered respiratory patterns. High cervical lesions might affect the bulbospinal fibers integrity, thus affecting transmission of the respiratory signals arising from the brainstem to the phrenic motor neurons. These descending fibers will reach the ventral-lateral region of the cervical spinal cord before reaching the gray matter where the phrenic nucleus will be placed. Disconnection of this circuitry is what eventually leads to respiratory instability due to the predominance of accessory respiratory muscles.[57] Therefore, in patients whose injury involves high cervical levels (i.e., C1-C3) where ventilator dysfunction is to be expected, early tracheostomy in conjunction with all other pulmonary protective measures might be of benefit.

Sympathetic preganglionic neurons are commonly located in the intermediolateral cell column (IML) of the first thoracic to the second lumbar spinal cord segment (T1-L2). Based on this anatomic correlation, lesions involving lower cervical and high thoracic regions might disrupt the normal activity of the sympathetic nervous system. This leads to decreased systemic vascular resistance, which includes arteriolar vasodilation, pooling of venous blood, bradycardia, and decreased myocardial activity signifying the cause of hypotension in patients with SCI.[58,59] Hemodynamic control is essential in the immediate period after SCI. Depending on where the injury focus lies, patients can present with cardiovascular collapse. Hypotension is thought to cause a reduction in spinal cord perfusion and has been associated with poorer neurologic outcomes.[51,55] Current recommendations are to keep MAP between 85 and 95 mm Hg for 7 days following acute SCI.[10,51,52] Initially, perform volume resuscitation with crystalloids, then followed with vasopressors. There is no single recommended agent, preference is the use of an agent with α- and β-adrenergic properties.[10] At our institution, we keep MAP goals above 85 mm Hg for at least 5-7 days.

Steroids were previously thought to improve neurologic outcomes; thus they were widely used in the acute setting postinjury. This practice has mostly been abandoned. In 2013, the revised guidelines for management of acute cervical spine and spinal cord injuries recommend against administering methylprednisolone[56] as no clear benefit was identified and the practice was associated with significant side effects, such as uncontrolled hyperglycemia, gastrointestinal bleeding, and infections. We do not routinely use steroids in the setting of SCI.

Once the patient has been stabilized and no longer has intensive care needs, focus should shift to promoting aggressive mobilization and rehabilitation. Inpatient PM&R specialist consultation is strongly recommended, as well as twice daily SCI-focused physical and occupational therapy.

■ PROGNOSTICATION

Every SCI diagnosis is life-changing, and providing accurate, sensitive, and reliable prognostic counseling is an essential part of the patient's healing process. Questions regarding expected neurological recovery and prognostication in SCI are complex and multifaceted. During counseling, it is particularly important to emphasize the significant variability observed from patient to patient.

The physiologic basis for interventions and recovery in SCI is preserving functional neural tissue and facilitating axonal repair, and patients must be counseled as such during their clinical course. Aside from MRI, many modalities may be used to assess the extent of injury, which some clinicians use for prognostic value. Various molecular markers, diffusion tensor imaging, and evoked potentials can provide valuable physiologic data regarding the extent of injury.[60] However, despite its ubiquitous use in assessing and classifying SCI, the ASIA classification should not be used as a prognostic tool for counseling patients. As described by Flett et al., an estimated 10-20% of complete spinal cord injuries convert to incomplete injuries 1 year following the injury, with many showing significant functional recovery.[61] Despite anecdotal concerns of poor reliability and precision on initial assessment, the potential functional recovery many complete injury patients have shown should dissuade clinicians from using the ASIA scale as a prognostic tool when counseling patients.

At our institution, we incorporate pastoral care, rehabilitation medicine, and the operative team into the discussion. We emphasize to patients and families that a severe injury has occurred and that ample resources being provided to create the best opportunity for functional recovery, but that true prognostication should be put on hold for about two weeks after injury. We believe the delay allows for better clinical evaluation of the extent of injury, as it allows all the necessary surgical interventions to take place and neuronal edema to decrease prior to assessment. Most importantly, we ensure patients and families recognize that improvement is incredibly variable, and the recovery period is extended, with most functional recovery taking place within the first year and a majority of recovery seen by 2 years postinjury.

REFERENCES

1. National Spinal Cord Injury Statistical Center, Facts and Figures at a Glance. Birmingham, AL: University of Alabama at Birmingham; 2019.
2. Jain NB, Ayers GD, Peterson EN, Harris MB, Morse L, O'Connor KC, et al. Traumatic spinal cord injury in the United States, 1993-2012. JAMA. 2015;313(22):2236-43.
3. Chen Y, Devivo MJ, Richards JS, SanAgustin TB. Spinal cord injury model systems: review of program and national database from 1970 to 2015. Arch Phys Med Rehabil. 2016;97(10):1797-804.
4. Nobunaga A, Go B, Karunas R. Recent demographic and injury trends in people served by the Model Spinal Cord Injury Care Systems. Arch Phys Med Rehabil. 1999;80(11):1372-82.
5. Waters R, Meyer P, Adkins R, Felton D. Emergency, acute, and surgical management of spine trauma. Arch Phys Med Rehabil. 1999;80(11):1383-90.
6. American College of Surgeons. ATLS Advanced Trauma Life Support Program for Doctors. 7th edition. Chicago, IL: American College of Surgeons; 2004.
7. American Spinal Injury Association. International Standards for Neurological Classification of Spinal Cord Injury. Atlanta, GA: American Spinal Injury Association; 2008.
8. Hadley MN, Walters BC, Aarabi B, Dhall SS, Gelb DE, Hurlbert RJ, et al. Clinical assessment following acute cervical spinal cord injury. Neurosurgery. 2013;72(suppl 2):40-53.
9. Ryken TC, Hadley MN, Walters BC, Aarabi B, Dhall SS, Gelb DE, et al. Radiographic assessment. Neurosurgery. 2013;72(suppl 2):54-72.
10. Consortium for Spinal Cord Medicine. Early acute management in adults with spinal cord injury: clinical practice guideline for health-care professionals. J Spinal Cord Med. 2008;31(4):403-79.
11. Bozzo A, Marcoux J, Radhakrishna M, Pelletier J, Goulet B. The role of magnetic resonance imaging in the management of acute spinal cord injury. J Neurotrauma. 2011;28(8):1401-11.
12. Yucesoy K, Yuksel KZ. SCIWORA in MRI era. Clin Neurol Neurosurg. 2008;110(5):429-33.
13. Vaccaro AR, Daugherty RJ, Sheehan TP, Dante SJ, Cotler JM, Balderston RA, et al. Neurologic outcome of early versus late surgery for cervical spinal cord injury. Spine (Phila Pa 1976). 1997;22(22):2609-13.
14. Fehlings MG, Vaccaro A, Wilson JR, Singh A, W Cadotte D, Harrop JS, et al. Early versus delayed decompression for traumatic cervical spinal cord injury: results of the Surgical Timing in Acute Spinal Cord Injury Study (STASCIS). PLoS One. 2012;7(2):e32037.
15. Mirza SK, Krengel WF 3rd, Chapman JR, Anderson PA, Bailey JC, Grady MS, et al. Early versus delayed surgery for acute cervical spinal cord injury. Clin Orthop Relat Res. 1999;(359):104-14.
16. Gelb DE, Aarabi B, Dhall SS, Hurlbert RJ, Rozzelle CJ, Ryken TC, et al. Treatment of subaxial cervical spinal injuries. Neurosurgery. 2013;72(suppl 2):187-94.
17. Brodkey J, Richards D, Blasingame J, Nulsen F. Reversible spinal cord trauma in cats. Additive effects of direct pressure and ischemia. J Neurosurgery. 1972;37:591-3.
18. Carlson G, Minato Y, Okada A, Gorden C, Warden K, Barbeau JM, et al. Early time-dependent decompression for spinal cord injury: Vascular mechanisms of recovery. J Neurotrauma. 1997;14(12):951-62.
19. Delamarter R, Sherman J, Carr J. Pathophysiology of spinal cord injury. Recovery after immediate and delayed decompression. J Bone Joint Surg Am. 1995;77(7):1042-9.
20. Dimar J, Glassman S, Raque G, Zhang Y, Shields C. The influence of spinal canal narrowing and timing of decompression on neurologic recovery after spinal cord contusion in a rat model. Spine. 1999;24(16):1623-33.
21. Carlson G, Gorden C, Oliff H, Pillai J, LaManna J. Sustained spinal cord compression: Part I: Time-dependent effect on long-term pathophysiology. J Bone Joint Surg Am. 2003;85(1):86-94.
22. Fehlings MG, Tetreault LA, Wilson JR, Kwon BK, Burns AS, Martin AR, et al. A Clinical Practice Guideline for the management of acute spinal cord injury: Introduction, rationale, and scope. Global Spine J. 2017;7(3 Suppl):84S-94S.
23. Schneider RC, Cherry G, Pantek H. The syndrome of acute central cervical spinal cord injury; with special reference to the mechanisms involved in hyperextension injuries of cervical spine. J Neurosurg. 1954;11(6):546-77.
24. Anderson KK, Tetreault L, Shamji MF, Singh A, Vukas RR, Harrop JS, et al. Optimal timing of surgical decompression for acute traumatic central cord syndrome: a systematic review of the literature. Neurosurgery. 2015;77(suppl 4):S15-32.
25. Kepler CK, Kong C, Schroeder GD, Hjelm N, Sayadipour A, Vaccaro AR, et al. Early outcome and predictors of early outcome in patients treated surgically for central cord syndrome. J Neurosurg Spine. 2015;23(4):490-4.
26. Fehlings MG, Wilson JR, Tetreault LA, Aarabi B, Anderson P, Arnold PM, et al. A Clinical practice guideline for the management of patients with acute spinal cord injury: Recommendations on the use of methylprednisolone sodium succinate. Global Spine J. 2017;7(3 Suppl):203S-11S.
27. Vaccaro AR, Lehman RA Jr, Hurlbert RJ, Anderson PA, Harris M, Hedlund R, et al. A new classification of thoracolumbar injuries: The importance of injury morphology, the integrity of the posterior ligamentous complex, and neurologic status. Spine (Phila Pa 1976). 2005;30(20):2325-33.
28. Rajasekaran S, Kanna RM, Shetty AP. Management of thoracolumbar spine trauma: An overview. Indian J Orthop. 2015;49(1):72-82.
29. Wood KB, Li W, Lebl DR, Ploumis A. Management of thoracolumbar spine fractures. Spine J. 2014;14(1):145-64.
30. Gertzbein SD. Scoliosis Research Society. Multicenter spine fracture study. Spine (Phila Pa 1976). 1992;17(5):528-40.
31. Gertzbein SD, Khoury D, Bullington A, St John TA, Larson AI. Thoracic and lumbar fractures associated with skiing and snowboarding injuries according to the AO Comprehensive Classification. Am J Sports Med. 2012;40(8):1750-4.
32. Denis F. The three column spine and its significance in the classification of acute thoracolumbar spinal injuries. Spine (Phila Pa 1976). 1983;8(8):817-31.
33. Magerl F, Aebi M, Gertzbein SD, Harms J, Nazarian S. A comprehensive classification of thoracic and lumbar injuries. Eur Spine J. 1994;3(4):184-201.
34. Vaccaro AR, Oner C, Kepler CK, Dvorak M, Schnake K, Bellabarba C, et al. AO Spine thoracolumbar spine injury classification system: fracture description, neurological status, and key modifiers. Spine (Philla PA 1976). 2013;38(23):2028-37.

35. Kepler CK, Vaccaro AR, Koerner JD, Dvorak MF, Kandziora F, Rajasekaran S, et al. Reliability analysis of the AOSpine thoracolumbar spine injury classification system by a worldwide group of naïve spinal surgeons. Eur Spine J. 2016;25(4):1082-6.
36. Weinstein JN, Collalto P, Lehmann TR. Thoracolumbar "burst" fractures treated conservatively: A long term follow-up. Spine (Phila Pa 1976). 1988;13:33-8.
37. Mumford J, Weinstein JN, Spratt KF, Goel VK. Thoracolumbar burst fractures. The clinical efficacy and outcome of nonoperative management. Spine (Phila Pa 1976). 1993;18(8):955-70.
38. Alanay A, Acaroglu E, Yazici M, Oznur A, Surat A. Short-segment pedicle instrumentation of thoracolumbar burst fractures: Does transpedicular intracorporeal grafting prevent early failure? Spine (Phila Pa 1976). 2001;26(2):213-7.
39. Shin TS, Kim HW, Park KS, Kim JM, Jung CK. Short-segment pedicle instrumentation of thoracolumbar burst-compression fractures; short term follow-up results. J Korean Neurosurg Soc. 2007;42(4):265-70.
40. Xu BS, Tang TS, Yang HL. Long term results of thoracolumbar and lumbar burst fractures after short-segment pedicle instrumentation, with special reference to implant failure and correction loss. Orthop Surg. 2009;1(2):85-93.
41. Cho DY, Lee WY, Sheu PC. Treatment of thoracolumbar burst fractures with polymethyl methacrylate vertebroplasty and short-segment pedicle screw fixation. Neurosurgery. 2003;53(6):1354-60.
42. Marco RA, Kushwaha VP. Thoracolumbar burst fractures treated with posterior decompression and pedicle screw instrumentation supplemented with balloon-assisted vertebroplasty and calcium phosphate reconstruction. J Bone Joint Surg Am. 2009;91:20-8.
43. Dick JC, Jones MP, Zdeblick TA, Kunz DN, Horton WC. A biomechanical comparison evaluating the use of intermediate screws and cross-linkage in lumbar pedicle fixation. J Spinal Disord. 1994;7(5):402-7.
44. Guven O, Kocaoglu B, Bezer M, Aydin N, Nalbantoglu U. The use of screw at the fracture level in the treatment of thoracolumbar burst fractures. J Spinal Disord Tech. 2009;22(6):417-21.
45. Mahar A, Kim C, Wedemeyer M, Mitsunaga L, Odell T, Johnson B, et al. Short-segment fixation of lumbar burst fractures using pedicle fixation at the level of the fracture. Spine (Phila Pa 1976). 2007;32(14):1503-7.
46. Farrokhi MR, Razmkon A, Maghami Z, Nikoo Z. Inclusion of the fracture level in short segment fixation of thoracolumbar fractures. Eur Spine J. 2010;19(10):1651-6.
47. Lonstein JE, Denis F, Perra JH, Pinto MR, Smith MD, Winter RB. Complications associated with pedicle screws. J Bone Joint Surg Am. 1999;81(11):1519-28.
48. Matsuzaki H, Tokuhashi Y, Matsumoto F, Hoshino M, Kiuchi T, Toriyama S. Problems and solutions of pedicle screw plate fixation of lumbar spine. Spine (Phila Pa 1976). 1990;15(11):1159-65.
49. Foxx KC, Kwak RC, Latzman JM, Samadani U. A retrospective analysis of pedicle screws in contact with the great vessels. J Neurosurg Spine. 2010;13(3):403-6.
50. Inamasu J, Guiot BH. Vascular injury and complication in neurosurgical spine surgery. Acta Neurochir (Wien). 2006;148:375-87.
51. Ryken T, Hurlbert RJ, Hadley MN, Aarabi B, Dhall SS, Gelb DE, et al. The acute cardiopulmonary management of patients with cervical spinal cord injuries. Neurosurgery. 2013;72(suppl 2):84-92.
52. Vale F, Burns J, Jackson A, Hadley M. Combined medical and surgical treatment after acute spinal cord injury: results of a prospective pilot study to assess the merits of aggressive medical resuscitation and blood pressure management. J Neurosurg. 1997;87(2):239-46.
53. Menaker J, Kufera JA, Glaser J, Stein DM, Scalea TM. Admission ASIA motor score predicting need for tracheostomy in adults patients undergoing artificial ventilation. BMJ 2005;330(7502):1243.
54. Posluszny JA Jr, Onders R, Kerwin AJ, Weinstein MS, Stein DM, Knight J, et al. Multicenter review of diaphragm pacing in spinal cord injury: successful not only in weaning from ventilators but also in bridging to independent ventilation. J Trauma Acute Care Surg. 2014;76(2):303-9.
55. Tator CH. Experimental and clinical studies of the pathophysiology and management of acute spinal cord injury. J Spinal Cord Med. 1996;19(4):206-14.
56. Hurlbert RJ, Hadley MN, Walters BC, Aarabi B, Dhall SS, Gelb DE, et al. Pharmacological therapy for acute spinal cord injury. Neurosurgery. 2013;72(suppl 2):93-105.
57. Zimmer MB, Nantwi K, Goshgarian HG. Effect of spinal cord injury on the respiratory system: basic research and current clinical treatment options. 2007;30(4):319-30.
58. Hadley MN, Walters BC, Grabb PA, Oyesiku NM, Przybylski GJ, Resnick DK, et al. Blood pressure management after acute spinal cord injury. Neurosurgery. 2002;50(3 Suppl):S58-62.
59. Deuchars SA. How sympathetic are your spinal cord circuits? Exper Physiol. 2015;100(4):365-71.
60. Krishna V, Andrews H, Varma A, Mintzer J, Kindy MS, Guest J. Spinal cord injury: how can we improve the classification and quantification of its severity and prognosis? J Neurotrauma. 2014;31(3):215-27.
61. Burns AS, Marino RJ, Flanders AE, Flett H. Clinical diagnosis and prognosis following spinal cord injury. Handb Clin Neurol. 2012;109:47-62.

Dural Repair Strategies

Fadi Al-Saiegh, Anthony Stefanelli, Srinivas Prasad

■ INTRODUCTION

Incidental durotomies during spinal procedures occur with a reported incidence of 14%[1] and can be as high 15.9%[2] in revision lumbar surgery. The risk of durotomies is higher with increasing patient age, lumbar spine surgery, revision spine surgery, degenerative disease, instrumentation, and increasing operative duration.[3] They are associated with substantial morbidity and often complicate the post-operative course of patients leading to postural headaches, pseudomeningocele formation, or persistent wound drainage. If left untreated, large cerebrospinal fluid (CSF) collections (CSFomas) may form over time and some patients may even develop cranial subdural hematomas. However, having a reliable strategy achieving dural repair can prevent persistent CSF leakage and limit postoperative complications. In this chapter, we discuss various strategies and techniques for dural repair after incidental durotomies.

■ PRIMARY DUROTOMY CLOSURE

Once an accidental durotomy occurs and CSF is encountered, it is important to remain calm and to ensure that suctioning CSF is limited and done over cottonoids to avoid injury to the spinal cord or cauda equina fibers.

In order to be able to repair the dural defect, it is paramount to obtain adequate exposure and visualization of the defect, which may necessitate additional removal of bone along the perimeter of the durotomy cranially, caudally and/or laterally. This can involve extension of the laminectomy or facetectomy until the dural edges are clearly visualized.

Instruments, Suture, and Needle Choices

Additional microsurgical instruments that are not routinely included in spinal fusion sets are necessary to perform a satisfactory primary dural closure. These instruments should be requested when a durotomy is encountered. They include a Castroviejo needle driver, which allows better maneuvering of the needle in narrow corridors, as well as small cottonoids or Merocel neurosurgical patties (Medtronic, Minneapolis, MN), which can be helpful if nerve rootlets have herniated through the dural defect.

There is a variety of suture options for the dural repair. An important consideration is the use of tapered instead of cutting needles as the latter make larger holes as they traverse the dura, which can lead to egress of CSF. A commonly used suture is Nurolon 4-0 (Ethicon, Somerville, NJ), which is a nonabsorbable synthetic braided suture with good tensile strength and a controlled-release needle. An alternative is Gore-Tex 5-0 (Gore, Flagstaff, AZ), which is a nonabsorbable monofilament with a cutting needle whose diameter is nearly equal to the suture it carries, thus, reducing the risk of CSF leakage from the needle holes.

The dura should be closed in a running fashion starting at the apex of the dural defect. It is important that an assistant maintains tension on the suture while the operator is performing the closure. A knot pusher can be useful in tight corridors. Before the last stitch is placed and the final knot is made, the turgor of the thecal sac should be reinstituted with normal saline using a syringe and a blunt catheter.

After the closure is completed, it is important to confirm its integrity by performing a Valsalva maneuver. An additional stitch may be necessary if CSF is encountered.

■ DURAPLASTY

In cases of a large dural defect or when the dural edges are irregular, primary dural closure may not be attainable. In such cases, a patch graft can be sutured in place to achieve closure. There are a variety of patch graft materials including synthetic dural substitutes such as DuraGen (Integra, Plainsboro, NJ), decellularized biological materials such as bovine pericardium, or autograft, such as local lumbodorsal fascia. The optimal choice depends on the size of the dural defect and the availability of the material. Fat or muscle autograft can be used in small dural defects typically as an onlay graft. In addition to providing coverage of the defect, it provokes a local inflammatory reaction which augments the healing process of the dura.

The patch graft should be shaped to match the dural defect it is going to cover. Once that is achieved, it is advisable to start suturing the apices to hold the graft in place and proceed with a continuous stitch. Once the dural patch is sutured satisfactorily, a Valsalva maneuver should be performed to confirm that a watertight closure was achieved and there is no egress of CSF.

SEALANT ADJUNCTS

Once a durotomy has been primarily repaired or a patch graft duraplasty has been applied, many surgeons will opt to use an adjunct sealant over the suture line or graft edges to help ensure a watertight closure and to help reduce continuous leakage of CSF through the defect as the durotomy heals. An ideal sealant should be able to rapidly conform to the applied surface, remain flexible, and produce no inflammatory reaction to the underlying neural structures.[4]

There are many different types of sealants used in clinical practice today. These are composed of a range of materials including fibrin glue, polymer hydrogel, collagen matrix, and cyanoacrylate. The choice as to which sealant to use can be complicated as the data varies about efficacy of each sealant. Preferred dural sealants are DuraSeal (Integra, Plainsboro, NJ), which is a polymer composed of two components that cross-link when mixed together.

Another dural sealant is TISSEEL (Baxter Medical), which is a fibrin sealant that is less toxic and is favored whenever there is concern it may come in contact with neural tissue.

The application of each sealant is relatively similar amongst products and involves the application of a light coat of sealant over the suture line and edges of the patch graft duraplasty. Most sealants are either applied directly from a syringe or sprayed from a gas- or pressure-assisted applicator. During the application process, it is important to avoid overapplication of the sealants as many of them can exert mass effect on the subjacent neural tissue. There are many reports in the literature of patients who developed postoperative neurological dysfunction, including paralysis, from expanding dural sealants.[5] In the case of durotomy repair, more is not always better.

LUMBAR SUBARACHNOID DRAIN PLACEMENT AND MANAGEMENT

Often times, the surgeon cannot get a true watertight closure on the durotomy either due to its location (e.g., ventral thecal sac) or its size and morphology. When this occurs, many surgeons will elect to place drains in different anatomical locations to divert CSF away from the healing durotomy to allow the tissue to remain dry and prevent the egress of CSF through the wound, which is a risk factor for developing local infection and meningitis.

Several options for drain placement exist. Many surgeons will elect to place a subfascial epidural drain to closed suction to prevent the epidural space from filling up with CSF and developing into a pseudomeningocele.[6] The length of time that these drains remain in place is traditionally decided based on output and surgeon preference.

Another adjunct that can be used to reduce CSF pressure is the placement of a traditional subarachnoid lumbar drain. As opposed to subfascial drains which drain only what leaks through the healing durotomy, a lumbar drain directly diverts flow of CSF out of the thecal sac to reduce the overall pressure that is placed internally on the repaired dura. Lumbar subarachnoid drains are most often used when primary closure is incomplete or unachievable or when durotomies are exposed to negative intrathoracic pressure as seen with thoracic durotomies. Postoperative management of a lumbar drain typically involves removing 5–15 cc of CSF per hour for several days as the durotomy heals. As a general rule, the average person produces about 20 cc of CSF per hour and typical target drainage from a lumbar drain is between 5 and 10 cc per hour with rare need to go beyond this. It is of particular importance to avoid overdrainage from a lumbar drain, especially in elderly patients, as the negative pressure created in the cranial vault can lead to the development of a subdural hematoma which could be fatal.[7-9] Great caution should be exercised when a lumbar drain is in place with a patient who is being mobilized as inadvertent drainage can be catastrophic.

REFERENCES

1. Wang JC, Bohlman HH, Riew KD. Dural tears secondary to operations on the lumbar spine. Management and results after a two-year-minimum follow-up of eighty-eight patients. J Bone Joint Surg Am. 1998;80(12):1728-32.
2. Khan MH, Rihn J, Steele G, Davis R, Donaldson WF 3rd, Kang JD, et al. Postoperative management protocol for incidental dural tears during degenerative lumbar spine surgery: a review of 3,183 consecutive degenerative lumbar cases. Spine. 2006;31(22):2609-13.
3. Baker GA, Cizik AM, Bransford RJ, Bellabarba C, Konodi MA, Chapman J, et al. Risk factors for unintended durotomy during spine surgery: a multivariate analysis. Spine J. 2012;12(2):121-6.
4. Preul MC, Bichard WD, Spetzler RF. Toward optimal tissue sealants for neurosurgery: use of a novel hydrogel sealant in a canine durotomy repair model. Neurosurgery. 2003;53(5):1189-98; discussion 1198-89.
5. Epstein NE. Dural repair with four spinal sealants: focused review of the manufacturers' inserts and the current literature. Spine J. 2010;10(12):1065-8.
6. Niu T, Lu DS, Yew A, Lau D, Hoffman H, McArthur D, et al. Postoperative cerebrospinal fluid leak rates with subfascial epidural drain placement after intentional durotomy in spine surgery. Global Spine J. 2016;6(8):780-5.
7. McHardy FE, Bayly PJ, Wyatt MG. Fatal subdural haemorrhage following lumbar spinal drainage during repair of thoraco-abdominal aneurysm. Anaesthesia. 2001;56(2):168-70.
8. Rosario LE, Rajan GR. Repeat subdural hematoma after uncomplicated lumbar drain discontinuation: A case report. A A Pract. 2019;13(3):107-9.
9. Tan VE, Liew D. A case of chronic subdural hematoma following lumbar drainage for the management of iatrogenic cerebrospinal fluid rhinorrhea: pitfalls and lessons. Ear Nose Throat J. 2013;92(10-11):513-5.

Minimally Invasive Sacroiliac Joint Fusion

Matthew J Sabatino, Glenn S Russo, Peter G Whang

INTRODUCTION

- For patients with a diagnosis of sacroiliac joint (SIJ) dysfunction or disruption, studies have shown that minimally invasive fusion of the SIJ is associated with superior outcomes in terms of pain, function, and quality of life when compared to nonsurgical treatment.[1-3]
- Over the past decade, multiple SIJ fusion systems have been developed which have been shown to give rise to notable improvements in clinical outcomes. **Table 1** lists recent publications assessing these various SIJ fusion systems.[4]
- Minimally invasive techniques utilizing a lateral-to-medial trajectory have less morbidity than open approaches[5,6] and currently account for about 90% of all SIJ fusions.[7]
- Minimally invasive SIJ fusion can generally be performed in the outpatient setting with the patient being discharged a few hours after the completion of the operation.
- The use of stereotactic navigation in conjunction with minimally invasive SIJ fusion techniques has been described with patient outcomes comparable to minimally invasive techniques without navigation. Use of stereotactic navigation does tend to increase the procedure time, particularly during a surgeon's initial application of the technique, owing to a learning curve.[8,9]
- In the treatment of pelvic fractures and fracture-dislocations, use of three-dimensional navigation for minimally invasive SIJ fusion has been demonstrated to significantly improve implant placement over traditional two-dimensional fluoroscopic navigation. This improvement in implant placement is magnified in patients with dysmorphic sacrum.[10,11]

PREOPERATIVE DIAGNOSIS

- Establishing the diagnosis of SIJ-mediated pain involves obtaining an accurate history from patients who will typically report pain in the lower back and buttock which will frequently radiate into the groin, thigh, or leg. These symptoms may commonly have been precipitated by a traumatic incident, previous lumbar fusion, or childbirth.
- Physical examination findings indicative of SIJ dysfunction include a positive Fortin finger test, where individuals will point to their posterior superior iliac spine as being the primary location of their pain. In addition, there are also a number of provocative maneuvers that have been described to identify the SIJ as being a pain generator (**Figs. 1A to E**).[2]
- A positive response (i.e., at least >50% pain relief) to image-guided local anesthetic injections into the symptomatic SIJ is considered to be the "gold standard" method for confirming the diagnosis of SIJ dysfunction prior to considering SIJ fusion.
- Obtaining a preoperative computerized tomography (CT) scan for accurate surgical planning is recommended. CT scan provides the surgeon with a three-dimensional visualization of the SIJ and the presence of any sacral dysmorphism that will impact the placement and effectiveness of fusion implants.[12,13]

INSTRUMENTS

- Jackson table
- Intraoperative imaging modality—fluoroscopy versus navigation
- SIJ fusion instrumentation—multiple systems are commercially available which generally include a guide pin, tissue protection sleeve, cannulated drill/tap/broach, and cannulated implants.

SETUP

- The patient is positioned prone on a Jackson table.
- Prior to draping, the fluoroscopy unit should be brought into the field to ensure that clear lateral, inlet, and outlet radiographic images of the pelvis may be obtained;

TABLE 1: Published studies on sacroiliac joint instrumented arthrodesis.[4]

Study and year	Year	Study type	Number of patients	Implant system	Clinical outcome	Patient satisfaction	Reoperation Rate, n (%)	Follow-up (months)
Wise and Dall	2008	Prospective	13	Titanium cages (Medtronic, Memphis, Tennessee, USA)	VAS	77% overall	1/13 (7.7)	29.5
Khurana et al.	2009	Consecutive case study	15	Hollow Anchorage screws (Aesculap Ltd., Tuttlingen, Germany)	SE-36, Majeed scoring system	–	0	17
Cummings and Capabianco	2013	Retrospective	18	iFuse Implant System (SI-BONE Inc., San Jose, California, USA)	VAS, ODI, SF-12	56% very satisfied: 83% consider surgery again	1/18 (5.6)	12
Gaetani et al.	2013	Retrospective	12	iFuse Implant System (SI-BONE Inc., San Jose, California, USA)	NRS, ODI and RDQ	100%	2/12 (0.17)	3
Rudolf and Capobianco	2014	Retrospective	50	iFuse Implant System (SI-BONE Inc., San Jose, California, USA)	QOL questionnaire, NRS 0–10	91% satisfied	4/50 (8)	40
Ledonio et al.	2014	Retrospective	22	iFuse Implant System (SI-BONE Inc., San Jose, California, USA)	ODI	–	2/22 (9)	13
Duhon et al.	2016	Prospective (26 centers)	172	iFuse Implant System (SI-BONE Inc., San Jose, California, USA)	VAS, ODI, EQ-5D	78.1% very satisfied: 74.7% consider surgery again	8 (4.7)	24
Rapapport et al.	2017	Prospective	32	SI-LOK (Globus Medical, Inc., Audubon, Pennsylvania, USA)	VAS, ODI, Odom's criteria	97% consider surgery again	2/32 (6.3)	12
Bornemann et al.	2017	Prospective	24	iFuse Implant System (SI-BONE Inc., San Jose, California, USA)	VAS, ODI	–	0	24
Darr et al.	2018	Prospective (12 centers)	103	iFuse Implant System (SI-BONE Inc., San Jose, California, USA)	VAS, ODI, EQ-5D	82% Improved with the pain	1/103 (0.009)	36
Cross et al.	2018	Prospective	18	–	NPS (MCID)	17/18 (94%) met the MCID	0	24

(EQ-5D: EuroQol-5D health survey; MCID: minimum clinically important difference; NPS: numerical pain scale; NRS: numerical rating scale; ODI: Oswestry disability index; QOL: quality of life; VAS: visual analog scale; RDQ: Roland-Morris disability questionnaire)

it may be helpful to make appropriate marks on the floor and the C-arm to facilitate moving efficiently between these different views during the procedure.
- It is critical to obtain a "true" lateral view with confluence of the left and right iliac cortical densities (i.e., alar lines). It may be necessary to change the angle of the C-arm gantry or even readjust the position of the patient until the lines are superimposed.
- Using a pin, mark the following lines on the skin: (1) Iliac cortical densities; (2) anterior sacral wall; and (3) posterior sacral wall. These lines should form a triangle approximating the shape of the sacrum, with the iliac cortical density line serving as a short ventral base of the triangle.
- Mark the proposed incision measuring approximately 2–3 cm starting approximately 1 cm dorsal to the iliac cortical density which bisects the anterior and posterior sacral lines **(Fig. 2)**.
- This incision, 1 cm away from the alar line between the anterior and posterior sacral body lines **(Fig. 2)**, allows for appropriate implant spacing to accommodate three implants across the SIJ.

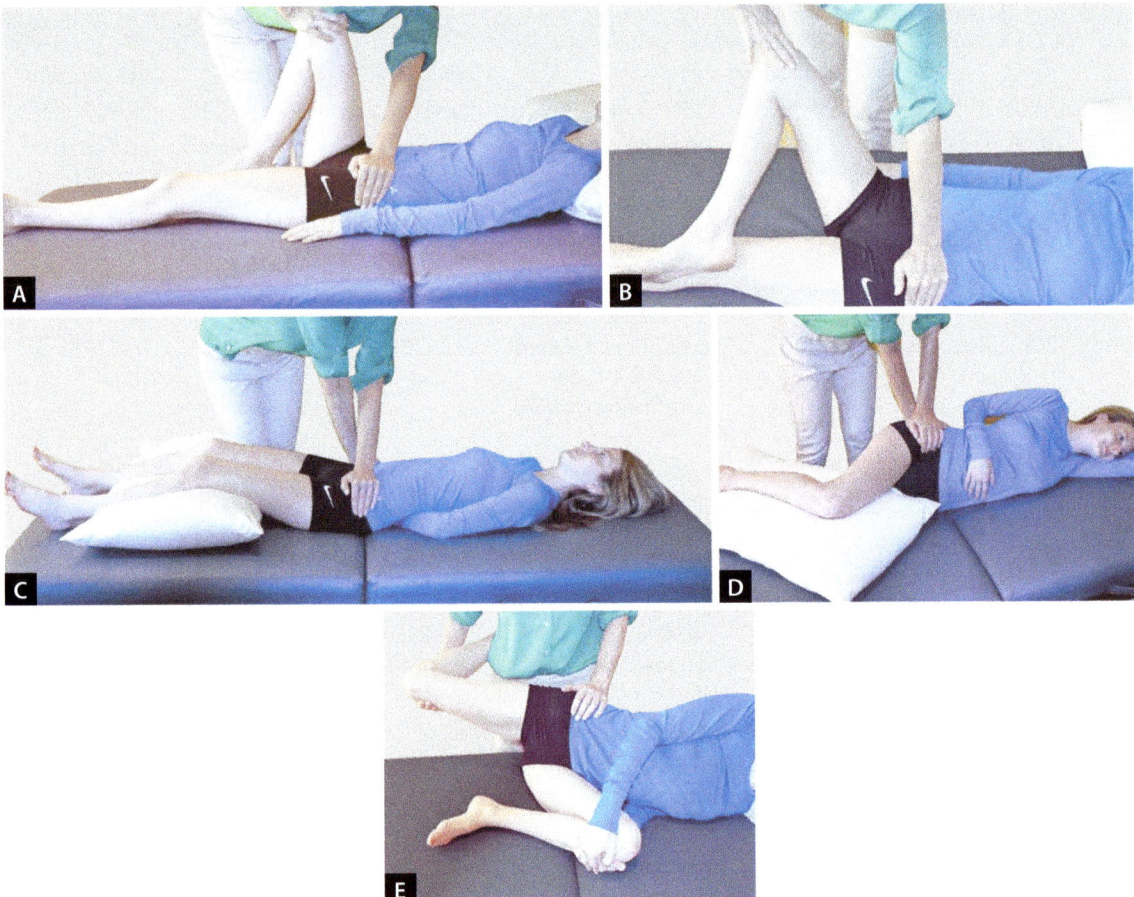

Figs. 1A to E: Physical examination tests for sacroiliac joint dysfunction. (A) Thigh thrust; (B) Flexion, abduction, and external rotation (FABER); (C) Pelvic distraction (gapping); (D) Compression; (E) Gaenslen test.[2]

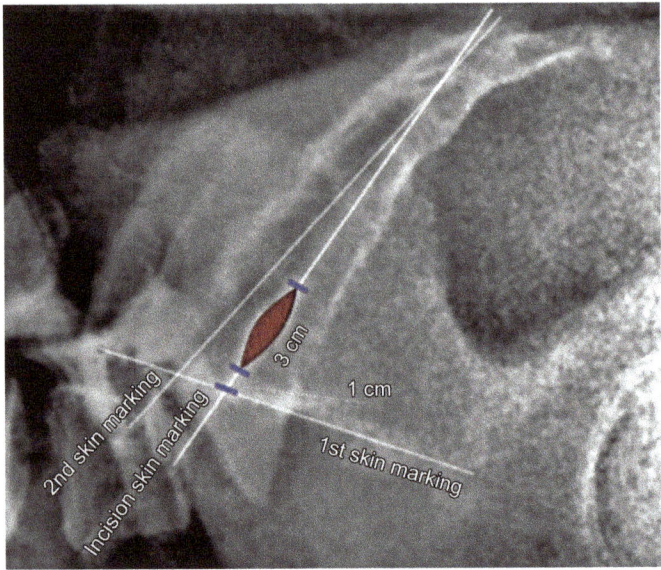

Fig. 2: Markings for the skin incision including the first line along the iliac cortical density (i.e., alar line) and a second skin overlying the posterior sacral wall.
Courtesy: SI-Bone iFuse technique guide

PROCEDURE

- The skin is incised and a finger may be used to bluntly dissect down to the fascial layer. It is generally feasible to preserve the majority of the fascial layer by simply inserting the instrumentation through it rather than sharply dividing it to minimize the risk of a superior gluteal artery injury.
- On the lateral fluoroscopic view, the first guidewire is docked on a starting point between the anterior and posterior sacral lines just dorsal to the iliac cortical density **(Figs. 3A to C)**; it is helpful to use a Kocher clamp so that the position of the wire may be observed while minimizing the radiation exposure of the surgeon.
- Once a suitable start point is identified, the wire is gently tapped with a mallet to dock it in the lateral cortex of the ilium and advanced further under fluoroscopic guidance.
- After the first wire has been introduced into the ilium, it is visualized on the inlet view to ensure that its trajectory will remain in bone and not pass through the anterior portion of the sacrum. The wire is inserted to its final position on the outlet view to ensure that the tip is outside of the S1 foramen (i.e., either superior or lateral). An oblique fluoroscopic image may be used to confirm that the wire has not violated the lateral wall of the foramen.
- The length of implant is determined once the wire is advanced to the appropriate depth into sacrum.

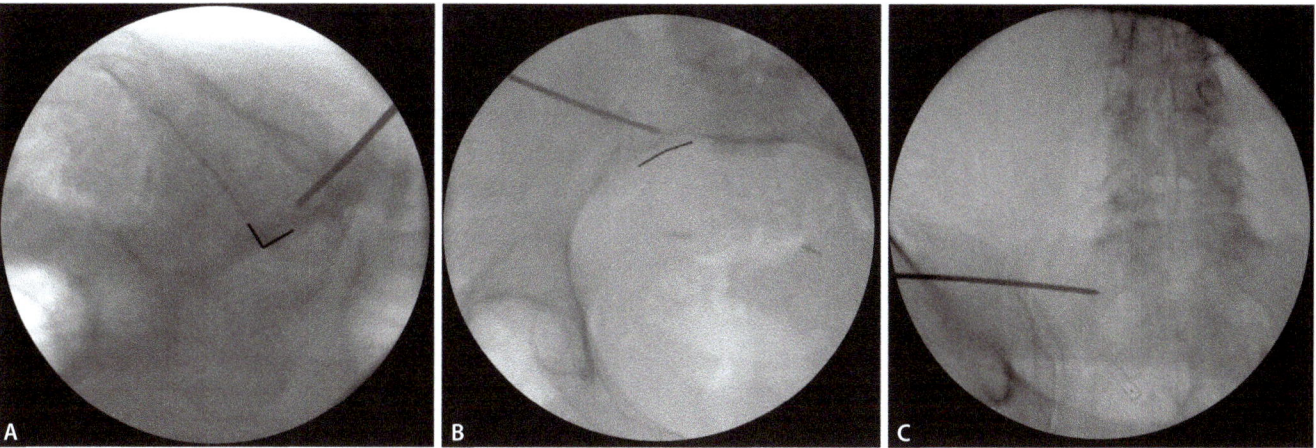

Figs. 3A to C: (A) The initial pin placement on the lateral fluoroscopic view should be dorsal to the sacral ala, between anterior and posterior sacral walls, and below the alar line; (B) On the inlet view, the pin should be within the ventral portion of the bony sacrum (thin curved line); (C) On the outlet view, the pin is placed outside of the S1 foramen.[4]

- Tactile feedback can be useful for informing the surgeon of the location of the instrumentation. Greater resistance is encountered when crossing the dense subchondral bone of the SIJ, and then it should advance more easily once it is in the cancellous bone of the sacrum at which time the surgeon should use less force.
- Once the first wire is in place and confirmed on all three fluoroscopic views, a drill with a cannulated bit is passed over the first guidewire to prepare the tract for the implant; this step will be dependent upon the size and type of implant specific to each SIJ fusion system.
- If the sharp pin enters the foramen, it may be prudent to exchange it with a blunt-tipped wire to minimize any trauma to the S1 nerve root.
- Insert the cannulated implant over the wire and confirm its final position using multiplanar fluoroscopic images—it should be below the alar line on the lateral view, within the bony pelvis on the inlet view, and outside of the sacral foramen on the outlet view.
- Once the first implant is fully seated, keep the wire in place because it may be used as a reference for a guide to assist with placement of the subsequent pins.
  - *Important note:* Attention to "pin management" is critical to the safety and workflow of this procedure. If the wire is ever withdrawn out of the bone (particularly during the removal of the cannulated drill), a considerable amount of time may be needed to find the correct trajectory and replace it within the tract. Thus, every effort should be made to keep the pin in the proper position during insertion and removal of all of the instruments.
- Using an alignment guide, the first pin is used to find an appropriate starting point for the second wire, slightly caudal and anterior to the initial implant.
- Once the starting point is confirmed on all three fluoroscopic views, the pin is advanced using the same steps. At this point, the first wire may be removed and the second one will be used as a reference for the third implant.
- While theoretically, a greater degree of biomechanical stability is obtained with the use of three implants instead of two, current evidence does not demonstrate an increased fusion rate or increase in SIJ bone bridging based on number of implants.[14] This author's recommendation is to place three implants across the SIJ when technically feasible in order to provide greatest stability.
- After all of the implants are in place, the final construct should be visualized to make sure that they are in appropriate position (i.e., below the alar line on the lateral view, within the sacrum on the inlet and view, and outside of the foramina on the outlet view).
- **Figures 4 to 8** show fluoroscopic images and radiographs of SIJ fusion procedures performed with different systems.

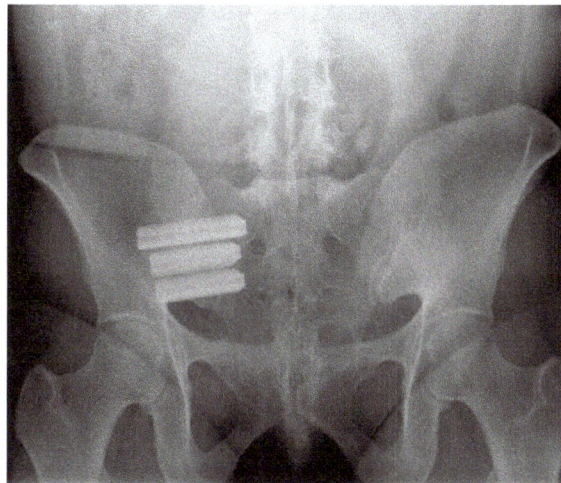

Fig. 4: Anteroposterior radiograph of a sacroiliac joint fusion using triangular implants.

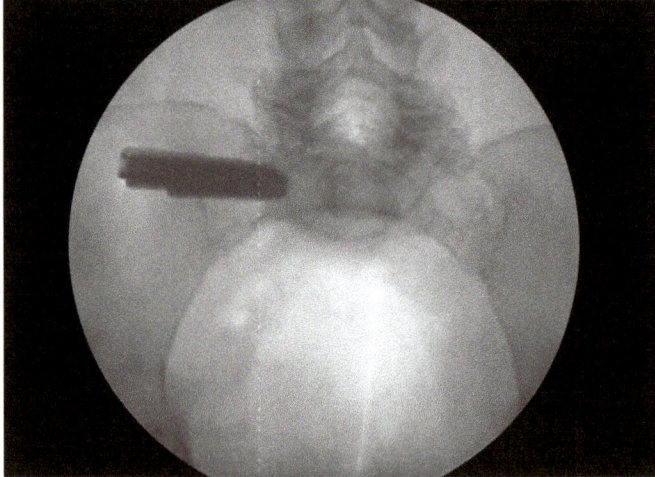

Fig. 5: Inlet fluoroscopic image of a sacroiliac joint fusion using triangular implants.

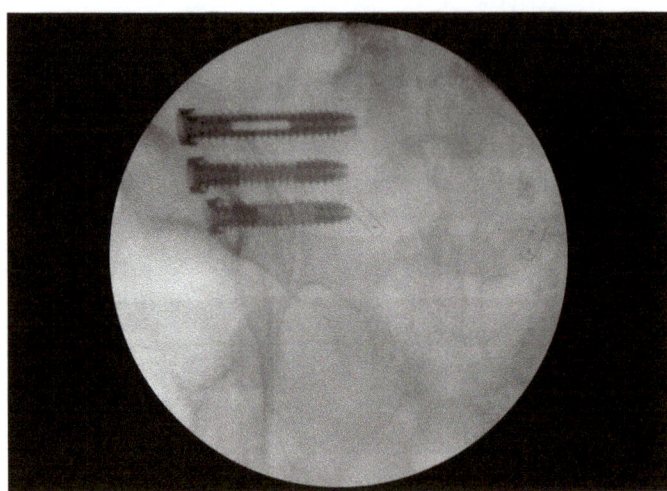

Fig. 7: Outlet fluoroscopic image of a sacroiliac joint fusion using cannulated screws.

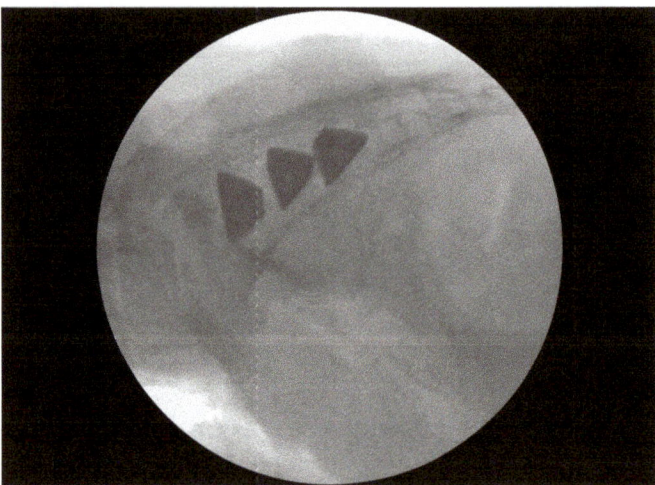

Fig. 6: Lateral fluoroscopic image of a sacroiliac joint fusion using triangular implants.

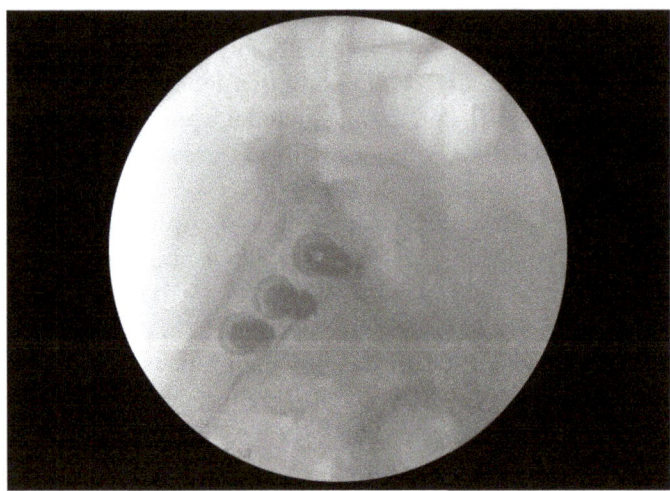

Fig. 8: Lateral fluoroscopic image of a sacroiliac joint fusion using cannulated screws.

CLOSURE AND POSTOPERATIVE CARE

- The wound should be thoroughly irrigated prior to closure.
- If possible, the fascial defect may be approximated and the incision is closed in a layered fashion.
- Patients should be restricted to partial weight-bearing on the extremity with crutches or a walker for at least 7–10 days after surgery at which the point their activity level may be increased as tolerated.
- Postoperative improvements in SIJ dysfunction symptoms are generally observed within the first 6 months as the fusion matures.[3]

REFERENCES

1. Dengler J, Duhon B, Whang P, Frank C, Glaser J, Sturesson B, et al. Predictors of outcome in conservative and minimally invasive surgical management of pain originating from the sacroiliac joint: A pooled analysis. Spine. 2017;42(21):1664-73.
2. Polly DW, Cher DJ, Wine KD, Whang PG, Frank CJ, Harvey CF, et al. Randomized controlled trial of minimally invasive sacroiliac joint fusion using triangular titanium implants vs nonsurgical management for sacroiliac joint dysfunction: 12-month outcomes. Neurosurgery. 2015;77(5):674-90; discussion 690-71.
3. Whang P, Cher D, Polly D, Frank C, Lockstadt H, Glaser J, et al. Sacroiliac joint fusion using triangular titanium implants vs. non-surgical management: six-month outcomes from a prospective randomized controlled trial. Int J Spine Surg. 2015;9:6.
4. Janjua MB, Ozturk A, Piazza M, Passias P, Arlet V, Welch WC. Technical nuances of percutaneous sacroiliac joint fixation: A cadaveric study. J Clin Neurosci. 2019;61:315-21.
5. Waisbrod H, Krainick JU, Gerbershagen HU. Sacroiliac joint arthrodesis for chronic lower back pain. Arch Orthop Trauma Surg. 1987;106(4):238-40.
6. Ashman B, Norvell DC, Hermsmeyer JT. Chronic sacroiliac joint pain: fusion versus denervation as treatment options. Evid Based Spine Care J. 2010;1(3):35-44.

7. Lorio MP, Polly DW Jr, Ninkovic I, Ledonio CG, Hallas K, Andersson G. Utilization of minimally invasive surgical approach for sacroiliac joint fusion in surgeon population of ISASS and SMISS membership. Open Orthop J. 2014;8:1-6.
8. Rajpal S, Burneikiene S. Minimally invasive sacroiliac joint fusion with cylindrical threaded implants using intraoperative stereotactic navigation. World Neurosurg. 2019;122:e1588-e1591.
9. Lee DJ, Kim SB, Rosenthal P, Panchal RR, Kim KD. Stereotactic guidance for navigated percutaneous sacroiliac joint fusion. J Biomed Res. 2016;30(2):162-7.
10. Matityahu A, Kahler D, Krettek C, Stöckle U, Grutzner PA, Messmer P, et al. Three-dimensional navigation is more accurate than two-dimensional navigation or conventional fluoroscopy for percutaneous sacroiliac screw fixation in the dysmorphic sacrum: a randomized multicenter study. J Orthop Trauma. 2014;28(12):707-10.
11. Yu T, Zheng S, Zhang X, Wang D, Kang M, Dong R, et al. A novel computer navigation method for accurate percutaneous sacroiliac screw implantation: A technical note and literature review. Medicine (Baltimore). 2019;98(7):e14548.
12. Miller AN, Routt ML Jr. Variations in sacral morphology and implications for iliosacral screw fixation. J Am Acad Orthop Surg. 2012;20(1):8-16.
13. Kaiser SP, Gardner MJ, Liu J, Routt ML Jr, Morshed S. Anatomic determinants of sacral dysmorphism and implications for safe iliosacral screw placement. J Bone Joint Surg Am. 2014;96(14):e120.
14. Zaidi HA, Montoure AJ, Dickman CA. Surgical and clinical efficacy of sacroiliac joint fusion: a systematic review of the literature. J Neurosurg Spine. 2015;23(1):59-66.

Index

Page numbers followed by *b* refer to box, *f* refer to figure, *fc* refer to flowchart, and *t* refer to table.

A

Abaloparatide 164
Abduction 192*f*
Absorbable monofilament suture 148
Acute central cord syndrome 182*f*
Adequate decompression 37
Adequate hemostasis 172
Adequate sagittal trajectory 51
Adequate scapular retraction 75
Adhesions, lysis of 67
AdiS classification 118
Adjacent level disease 21
Adjacent segment disease 17, 34, 39
Adson clamp 25
Adult degenerative scoliosis 118, 119
Adult idiopathic scoliosis 118, 121*f*
Adult scoliosis, management of 118
Advanced trauma life support 180
Airway management 43
Alar ligament avulsion, unilateral 42
Alar line 191, 193
Alexander elevator 75
Alignment changes 62
Allen medical systems 58
Allen table 149
Allis clamps 177*f*
Allograft 77, 104
    disk 33*f*
    preparations 78
American Board of Orthopaedic Surgery 127
American College of Surgeons 180
Anesthesia 21, 57
    team 59
Aneurysmal bone cysts 84
Angled curettes 21, 166
Ankylosing spine 134
    conditions 57
Ankylosing spondylitis 50, 57, 62*f*
Annulotomy 31, 32*f*, 33
    inferior level 33
    middle level 33
Anomalous vertebral artery anatomy 28
Ansa cervicalis 29, 30*f*, 31
Ante-psoas interbody fusion 164, 165*f*, 169
Anterior central herniations 72
Anterior cervical
    corpectomy and fusion 35
    decompression and fusion 126
    discectomy 6*f*, 39, 153
        and fusion 17, 28, 39, 51, 57*f*
    landmarks 28*f*
Anterior column
    reconstruction techniques 88, 101
    support options 101
Anterior compressive lesions 72
Anterior cortex 94
Anterior decompression 67
Anterior odontoid
    osteosynthesis 51
    screws 8
    systems 51
Anterior osteosynthesis 51
    screw 50, 50*f*
Anterior sacral
    body lines 191
    wall 191
Anterior spinal
    columns 61
    cord 51
Anterior thoracic
    discectomy 72
    plate 79*f*
Antibiotic 35, 119
    perioperative 4, 103
    powder 7
    prophylaxis 15
Antifibrinolytic medication 129
AOSpine classification 55
    system 61
AOSpine Knowledge Forums 62
AOSpine Subaxial Cervical Spine Classification
    system 55, 56*f*
AOSpine's Research Department 62
Apex pointed caudally 97
Apical soft tissue 97, 98
Appendiceal retractor 31, 35
Arcuate foramen 48
Arm rests 73
Arterial pressure 21
Arthrodesis 122
Articular facet fragment, medial superior 19
Articular process
    composed of inferior 17
    composed of superior 17
    inferior 98, 116
Asymptomatic patients 47
Atlanto-dens interval 45, 45*f*, 47
    posterior 47
Atlanto-occipital articulation 43
Atlas fractures 44, 45*t*, 47
Auditory canal, external 18
Avascular midline raphe 22
Awake fiberoptic intubation 57
Awl-tip tap 177
Axial computed tomography 53*f*
Axillary roll 73
Azygous vein 73, 77, 102

B

B1 and B2 fractures 60
Bacteriostatic properties 78
Bail-out 8
Ball-tipped
    pedicle 107
    probe 11, 66
    sounder 103
Barrel-chested patients 51
Baseline neuromonitoring 12, 30
Basic instruments 119
Basion-axis interval 42, 43*f*
Basion-dens interval 42
Bayoneted instruments 149
Beam radiation therapy, external 81, 87
Beneath platysma, neck immediately 29
Bicortical fixation 79
Bicortical purchase 80
Bicortical screw 4
    fixation 4
    purchase 79, 79*f*
Bicycling accident 10*f*
Bifid spinous processes 13
Biopsy 81
    confirmed metastasis 82
    pearls 82
    technique 82
Biopsy-proven metastatic disease, history
    of 82
Biplanar fluoroscopy 51, 131
Bipolar cautery 25, 26, 37, 98, 153
Bipolar electrocautery 31, 38, 58, 138, 139,
    158
    combination of 20
Bivector traction 18
    set up 18
Bleeding, reduce 22
Blood loss
    decrease 97
    increased 96
Blood pressure 13
    inflatable 57
    monitoring, continuous 21
Bluntly palpated 36
Body resection, partial 96*f*
Bone
    direct anatomic reduction of 60
    fragments 20, 72
    hinge 23
    injury, acute 49
    landmarks, intraoperative 23
    longest corridor of 11
    matrix, demineralized 164

mineral density 119
morphogenetic protein 9, 122
scan 73
wax 20, 23, 38, 40, 103, 141, 159
Bone graft 77
  fragments, limit 70
  placement 70
  posterolateral 117
Bone quality 88, 118
  poor 70
Bone-instrumentation interface 78
Bony corridor 14
Bony element disruptions 181f
Bony osteophytes 161
Bony sacrum 193f
Bony structure 60
Bony tunnel, abnormal 48
Bovie electrocautery 58, 138, 141
Bovie tip 138
Box cutters 160
Brachial plexopathy 13
Brachial plexus 73
Bracing, orthopedic principle of 43
Bradycardia 185
Breast cancer 84
Bridging osteophytes 97
Bryan disk 39
B-type injuries 60
Burr
  down 32
  side-cutting 14
  technique 23f
  tip 23
Burst fracture 42, 72, 133f, 134f

C

C1 lateral mass fixation, techniques of 46
C1-C2
  alignment 9
  instability, acute 47
  screws, transarticular 48
Cage
  insertion 78
  placement 70
  shapes 77
  sizing 78
  types 78
Calcified disk, excision of 76
Canal expanding 52
Cancellous allograft 135
  chips 70
Cancellous bone 19, 23, 193
Cancellous cavity 67
Cannulated drill 190
Cannulated systems 52
Cannulated tap 94
Cantilever bending 100
Cantilever reduction 135
Capsular tissue 24
Capsuloligamentous complex, posterior 55, 60
C-arm 123, 126, 156, 165, 169
  aligned 93
  drape, lateral 40
  extreme obliquity of 91
  fluoroscopy 9, 110
  images, frequent 51

Carotid artery 37
  internal 29, 29f, 31
Carotid sheath 29, 29f
Carotid tubercle estimate C6 28
Caspar disk retractors 39
Caspar pin 28, 32, 37
  distractor 35
Caspar-type
  distracting pins 40
  retaining pins 40
Castroviejo needle 188
Catastrophic neurologic
  deficit 75
  injury 13
Cauda equine
  fibers 188
  nerve roots 183
  syndrome 159
Caudad pedicle 151
Caudad vertebral body 61
Caudal directions 131
Caudal extent 4
Caudal facet superior articular process 61
Caudal nerve roots 98
Caudal orientation 11
Caudal vertebra medially 14
Caudal-to-cephalad direction 15
Cell saver 58
Cement augmentation 132
  role of 86
Central compression 132f
Central disk herniations 28
Central stenosis 140, 145f
  decompression of 145f
Cephalad and caudal
  direction 32
  disk 69
  ribs 68
  starting location 11
Cephalad angulation 14, 103
Cephalad boarder 9
Cephalad body 61
Cephalad extent 4
Cephalad pars interarticularis 138
Cephalad pedicle 140
Cephalad segment 61
Cephalad vertebral body 37
Cephalocaudal starting point 104
Cerebellar retractor 12, 149
  angled self-retaining 22
Cerebrospinal fluid 4, 58, 69, 132, 188
Cervical 1, 182
  ball hook 18
  closure of posterior 15
  cobb 32
  corpectomy cage 70
  deformity 10f
  disk herniation 35
  facet joints 18
  fascial layer, superficial 38
  flexion 22f
  foramen 17
  foramina 17
  foraminotomy 17
  incisions, closing posterior 26
  instability 39
  kerrison rongeurs 18
  level 17

midline posterior 21, 22
morphology 17
neoplasm 35
osteomyelitis 35
pedicles 19f
radiculopathy 28
rods 4
spondylotic myelopathy 35
sympathetic plexus runs superficial 29
Cervical collar 38
  well-fitted rigid 46
  well-padded rigid 46
Cervical disk arthroplasty 39, 40f
  contraindications for 39b
  implantation 40
  indications for 39b
Cervical nerve
  hook 18, 19
  roots 17
Cervical spine 3, 12, 22f, 26, 28-30, 35
  alignment, influences 57
  postop 25
  precautions 3
  research society 127
  trauma, surgical management of 55
Cervicothoracic approach 87
Cervicothoracic junction 55, 66
C-flex apparatus 58
Chemosensitive tumors, highly 87
Chest
  radiographs, upright 68
  tubes 73
Chlorhexidine scrub brush 13
Chronic pain 50
Clamp, appropriate type of 25
Clear visual landmarks 67
Clydesdale trials 166
Coagulating veins 25f
Cobalt chromium rods 103
Cobb angle 164
Cobb elevator 75, 170f
  series of 68
Codman microcurette set 18
Collagen matrix 189
Comb malalign 118
Commencing surgery 13
Comminuted lateral masses 46
Communicating vein 29, 30
  courses 29
  reside superficial 28
Communication systems 79
Comorbidities 65
Complete blood count 81
Complete relaxation 137
Completed instrumentation 26f
Complex hemodynamic monitoring 96, 97
Compression 192f
Compressive disk herniation 57
Compressive epidural abscess 35
Compressive lesions, posterior 72
Computed tomography 81, 180, 183
  guided biopsy, accuracy of 83
  scan, mid-sagittal 10f
Computer-assisted navigation 107
Concomitant injuries 53
Condylar sum 42
Coning down 77
Contemporary spine surgery 127

Contoured rods 155
Contralateral temporary rod 100
Conus medullaris 183
Conventional external beam radiation therapy 87
Copious normal saline 20
Cor malalign 118
Cord signal changes 6*f*
Core needle biopsy 82
Coronal alignment 65
Coronal and sagittal balance 98
Coronal plane deformity 97
Coronal vertical axis 118
Corpectomy 37, 69, 74, 77
    defect 38, 77*f*, 133*f*
    site 59
Correct trajectory 4
Cortex, posterior 37
Cortical attachments 19
Cortical bone 32
    trajectory 106, 106*f*
Cortical trajectory, medial 111
Cortical wall, lateral 98
Corticocancellous autograft 135
Costochondral cartilage tip 76
Costotransverse joint 130
Costotransversectomy 65, 68, 87
Costovertebral junction 68
Cotton patties 129
Counter-torque force 25
Cover wound 107
Cranial fixation 44
Cranial nerve root 97, 98
Cranial orientation 11
Cranialcaudal axis 32
Craniocaudal direction 25
Craniocervical junction 87
C-reactive protein 81
Cricoid cartilage 28
Cross-table radiograph 21, 22
Cryoablation 86
    role of 86
Cubital and carpal tunnels 18
Curved pedicle probe 103
Cyanoacrylate 189

D

Dark blue blade 165
Dead space 15
Decompression 14, 98
    window 70
Decompressive trajectory 92
Deep cervical fascia 28-30
Deep dermal vicryl sutures 136
Deep dissection 31*f*
Deep fascial incision 31
Deep Gelpi retractors 66, 149
Deformity correction 122
Deformity magnitude and flexibility, evaluation of 96
Deformity parameters 164
Degenerative conditions 115
Degenerative disk disease 50, 140
Degenerative spondylolisthesis 110
Depuy synthes 127
Dermal layer 38
Dermatomal sensory testing 180

De-rotation 122
Diagnostic yield, lower 83
Dickman's classification 45*t*
Direct osteosynthesis screws 54
Discectomy 31, 36, 76, 125, 139, 153, 158, 162, 171*f*
    instruments, long-handled 164
    preliminary 33
Disk
    annulotomy, box-shaped 162
    arthroplasty 39
    fragments 37
    height, posterior 167*f*
    location 72
    material 32
    nature of 72
    posterior intervertebral 100
Disk herniation 39, 55
    calcified 76
Disk space 32
    adequate visualization of 36
    collapse 140
    one-third of 169*f*
Dislocation 42
    anterior 42
    bilateral 57
    indicative of 42
    unilateral 57
Displaced fracture 50
Displaced lamina fracture 133
Displaced type C injuries 57
Dissection 128, 150
    plane 29
    remains medial 31
Distal thoracic upper instrumented vertebra 118
Distinct fascial layers 28
Distort intraoperative anatomy 48
Dome laminectomy 21
Dorsal cortex 23
Dorsal root ganglion 17, 69
Down pushing curettes 69
Doyen rib dissector 75
Drains 73, 136
Dressing 7
Du and Chao method 105
Dual-rod
    constructs 79
    systems 79
Dura, midline anterior 65
Dural adhesions 15
Dural repair strategies 188
Duraplasty 188
Durotomy 189
    closure, primary 188
Dust 20
Dysphagia, high rate of 54
Dysplastic pedicles 91

E

Edema 38
Elbow flexion 146
Electrocautery 18, 35, 37, 103, 159
Electromyograph 107
Elevators, combination of 97
Emergency medical services 180
Emergency room 43, 60

Empty disk space 69
Enbloc excision, undergoing 87
Enbloc resection, role for 88
Endotracheal tube 36
    double-lumen 73
Endplate 171
    distraction 35
    preparation techniques 40
    prepare 33
    superior 32, 92
        and inferior 92*f*
Epidural fat 97
Epidural hematoma 132*f*, 159
Epidural spinal cord compression scale 85*f*, 85*t*
Epidural veins 24, 25*f*, 158*f*
Epinephrine 22
Eponymous Hangman's fracture 42
Epstein curette 69
Erector spinae muscles 93, 150
Errant screw placement 92
Erythrocyte
    salvage technology 58
    sedimentation rate 81
Esophagus 102
Ethylene vinyl alcohol copolymer 84
Evaluate decompression 153
Excessive cervical extension 13
Excessive kyphosis 72
Expandable cage 35, 38
    placement 133*f*
Expandable tube 149
Expose quadratus lumborum 130
Extension injury 62*f*
Extension-distraction injury 181*f*
Extensor muscle tendons 22
External beam radiation therapy 83
Extracavitary approaches, lateral 87
Extracavitary corpectomy 132
Extraforaminal disk herniations 149, 153
    treatment of 149
Extraforaminal space 153
Extraforaminal stenosis 141

F

Facet capsule 96, 96*f*
Facet complex 17
    and lamina 17
Facet dislocations, unilateral 61
Facet fracture 110
    dislocation, bilateral 38
Facet joint 18
Facet perch 57
Facet resection, medial 19
Facet rule, superior 104
Facetectomy 103, 115, 119, 158
Facial fractures 42
Facilitate adequate laminar excursion 21
Facilitate rod placement 14
Fascial incision 137, 152
Fascial layer 172, 192
    closure 26
Fashion bone graft 35
Feeler probe 103
Femoral ring allograft 123
Femoral shaft 77
Fiber 169*f*

Fiber-wire spanning 101
Fibrin glue 189
Fibular strut allograft 35
Figure-8 stitches, interrupted 7
Final fixation increases, time of 44
Final fluoroscopic imaging 95
Final four-rod satellite construct 99
Fine needle aspiration biopsy 82
Finochietto rib 130
Fishhook 95, 95f
    upside-down 111
Fixation
    anterior 126
    caudal level of 44
    posterior 38
Fixed head screws 79
Flat Jackson table 57, 123, 124f
Flat-plate digital radiograph 44
Flexion 34, 192f
Flexion-distraction
    injuries 35
    type mechanism 57
Flexion-extension studies 52
Floseal™ 77, 152, 153, 163, 166
Fluoroscopic guidance 11, 38, 146
Fluoroscopic guided 130
Fluoroscopic localization 161
Fluoroscopic technique 66
Fluoroscopic visualization 40
Fluoroscopy 5, 12, 18, 39, 115, 126, 138, 145, 156, 165, 170f, 171, 174, 190
    arm 155
    based navigation 107
    facilitate intraoperative 57
    guided technique 131
    image 58, 161
    intraoperative 36, 65, 67, 133f, 137, 145, 149, 155, 160, 164
    lateral 3, 11
    similar 152
    unit 157
Food and Drug Administration 39
Footprint interbody placement, large 160
Foraminal stenosis 137, 140, 149, 153
Foraminotomy
    bilateral 37
    kerrisons curve 141
Forearm fractures 42
Fortin finger test 190
Four-post Jackson frame 155
Fracture 9, 80
    bone, displacement of 58
    diagnosis of 66
    displacement 52
        high risk of 52
    distracted 50
    fragment 55
        posterior 53f
    morphology 52f
    pedicle-based 54
    reduction 10f
    type 2 49, 54
    unstable 79
Frazier suction tip 140, 153
Free-hand technique 59, 131
Freer elevator 97, 98
Fungal disease 72
Fusion 33f, 135, 184
    augmentation materials 164
    consider 40
    mass 120f
    posterior 60
    procedure 18

G

Gaenslen test 192f
Gardner-wells tong 18, 35, 57, 61
    routine 97
    traction 59
Gear shift probing 106
Gel head pad 39
Gelatin hemostatic matrix 20
Gelfoam 77, 166
    thrombin 138, 152, 153
Gelpi retractor 12, 152
General anesthesia, induction of 18
Generous flaps 36
Gentle exposure techniques 44
Gentle extension 54
Gerald forceps 30
Geriatric odontoid fractures, surgical management of 49
Global alignment modifier 118
Gluteal artery injury, superior 192
Glycocalyx, formation of 78
Graft
    inferior level 33
    insert inferior 33
    insert superior 33
    middle level 33
    placement 69
        and instrumentation 38
    subsidence 32
Grafton putty 172
Granulomatous disease 72
Guide pin 190
Guidewire 156, 159
    damage 52
    placement 156
    systems 52
    within pedicle, center placement of 157f
Gunshots 180

H

Half-inch straight osteotome 97
Halo immobilization 46
Halo vest immobilization 48
Handheld Cloward retractor 31, 35, 36
Handheld retractors 169
Hangman's fracture 52, 53f, 53t
Hard collar 16
Hardware complications 62
Hardware failure 52
Harmonic bone scalpel 137
Harvested tricortical iliac crest autograft 38
Hawk-beak 72
Head clamp, three-pronged 66
Hemangiomas 84
Hematologic malignancy 87
Hemilaminotomy 149
Hemoglobin 84
Hemostasis 20, 25f, 71, 103, 129, 139, 141, 147, 148, 150, 152
Hemostatic agents 38, 98, 138, 159

Hemostatic technologies 58
Herniated nucleus pulposus 141
Heterotopic ossification, higher rates of 39
Hibbs retractor 152
High standalone failure rate 80
High-speed burr 9, 18, 35, 38, 59, 98, 100, 103, 137, 155
High-speed drill 9
High-speed side cutting burr 19
Hinge trough 24f
Historical treatment method 44
Hoarseness, postoperative 31
Hollow anchorage screws 191
Human bone morphogenetic protein 163, 164
Humeral shaft 77
Hybrid procedures 40
Hydroxyapatite 9
Hyoid bone 28, 29
Hypervascular tumors, embolization of 84
Hypoglossal nerve 29, 31
Hypointense signal 46

I

Iatrogenic dural injury 139
Iatrogenic flatback deformity 99f
Iatrogenic spinal cord injury, risk of 58
Iatrogenic upper extremity nerve injury 13
Iatrogenic vascular injury 112f
Ideal spinal column alignment 77
Identify trajectory 104, 106
Idiopathic scoliosis 120
    adolescent 79
Idiopathic skeletal hyperostosis, diffuse 50, 57
Iliac bolt system 110
Iliac cortical density 191, 192, 192f
Iliac crest 9, 77f, 131, 161f
    autograft 135
    bone 5
        graft 7, 77, 135
    caudally 74
    posterior 8
    structural 88
Iliac screws 113, 113f
Iliac spine
    anterior superior 119
    posterior superior 114, 135, 175f
Iliac trajectories 112f
Iliac vein and artery
    left common 166f
    right common 166f
Iliohypogastric nerve fibers 163
Impairment scale 180
Implant
    cannulated 190
    handle 167f
    placement 125
Implantation, general principles of 40
Incision 30, 128-130, 156
    and exposure 103
    midline-based 149
    toward costochondral junction 75
Incisional negative pressure dressing 7
Index surgery 44
Infection
    increased risk of 96
    risk, minimize 26

Index

Inferior disk, annulotomy of 32
Inflatable pressure infusion bag 30
Infolded ligamentum flavum 133
Infrared camera 176f
Injuring tissue 30
Injury
    displacement of 44
    distraction across zone of 135
    morphology, guide identification of 47
    occurs, unintentional 75
    spinous processes, caudad level of 61
    zone of 135
Innominate artery 76
Instrumentation 14
    final 5
    final posterior 70
    inaccurate placement of 92
    placement 38
Instrumented fusion 12
Instruments 188
Intact ligamentous structures 54
Intact postintubation neurologic function 57
Intensive care unit 16, 136, 182
Interbody cage 115, 155, 159
    placement 158
Interbody curettes and pituitaries 115
Interbody fusion
    anterior 76
    direct lateral 165
    incision 165f
Interbody grafts 59, 61
Interbody implant 69
Interbody placement 162
Interbody segments, bony fusion of 164
Interbody shavers and dilators 115
Interbody spacer 77
Interbody trial and spacers 155, 164
Intercostal muscle
    external 80
    fibers 75
Intercostal vessels, superior 102
Interlaminar space 18, 137
    cephalad 21
Interlaminar window 138
Intermediolateral cell column 185
Internal instrumentation, type of 49
Interscapular bump 57
Interspinales muscles 22
Interspinous ligament 96, 97
Intertransverse membrane 153
Interventional radiology 81, 82
Intervertebral disk 17, 60, 65, 77, 127
    neighboring 96f
    space 158f
Intervertebral space 115, 146
Intra-arterial
    catheter 21
    pressure monitor 21
Intradural disk herniation 72
Intraoperative computed tomography 44, 107, 110, 174
    navigation guide 174
    scan 73, 74, 177f
Intraoperative imaging 174, 176
    modality 190
    type of 173, 174
Intra-substance transverse ligament tears 48
Intrawound antibiotics 119

Intubation 155
Invasive spine pedicle screw systems 95
Ioban strips 30
Ipsilateral facet joint 158
Ipsilateral intervertebral segment autofusion 170
Isolated atlas fractures, surgical management of 46
Isolated muscle groups, examination of 180
Isthmic spondylolisthesis 110, 126
    high-grade 91

J

Jackson frame 110
Jackson table 3, 18, 65, 103, 145, 146, 164, 175, 190
Jamshidi needle 93, 111, 155, 156
Jamshidi tip 156
Jugular vein
    anterior 29
    external 28, 29
    internal 29, 29f
Jumped facet 57, 60
Juxtapedicular screw technique 120

K

Kambin's triangle 116, 117
Karlin curettes 32
Karnofsky performance status 83, 83t
Keel cuts 40
Keel fixation 40
Kerrison cephalad 141
Kerrison cranially 18
Kerrison punch 59, 158
Kerrison rongeur 5, 15, 23, 37, 67, 68, 97, 100, 116, 125, 139-141, 145, 147, 153, 157
Kickstand screw 121
Kidney
    cancer 84
    rests 73
Kirschner guidewire 156
Kirschner wires 155, 159
Kittner dissection 75
Kocher clamp 67, 115, 192
Koros rotating rongeur 32
K-wire 88, 92
Kyphoplasty 86, 132
Kyphosis 84, 88
    assess flexibility of 96
    cases of 99
    correction 28
Kyphotic alignment 10f, 12
    correction of 77
Kyphotic cervical spines 51

L

Lactate dehydrogenase 81
Lag-by-design 51
Lag-by-technique 51
Lamina
    spreader 115
    superior 146f
Lamina-lateral mass junction 21, 23
Lamina-ligamentum interface 15

Laminar screw 11, 25, 48
    trajectory 4
Laminectomy 12, 14, 132, 137-140, 145, 147, 157
    interspace partial 12
    partial 21
    plus fusion 17
    posterior 21
Laminoplasty 21, 24, 25f
    opening 25f
    plate 21
Laminotomy 138, 145
Landell's classification 45t, 46
Landells atlas fracture classification 45
Large curettes, basic instruments of 119
Large disk space 97
Largest diameter mesh cage 38
Laryngeal nerves 31
    superior 29
Laryngoscopy 30
Laser interstitial thermal therapy 86
Lateral disk
    annulus fibrosus 76
    herniations 28
Lateral mass 9, 14
    cannulation 14
    combination of 12
    displacement 45
    instrumentation 15
    portion 26
    screw 12, 15, 54
        and insert 25
        technique 4
Latissimus dorsi 129
Leg length discrepancy 119
Leksell rongeur 14, 37, 66, 68, 97
    basic instruments of 119
    down 97
Levin and Edwards
    classification 53t, 54
    method 105
Life-threatening condition 42
Ligament
    anterior longitudinal 36, 53, 60, 77, 162, 170
    posterior longitudinal 32, 37, 40, 53, 59, 72, 97, 133, 153, 166
Ligamentotaxis 134
Ligamentous complex, posterior 53, 55, 127
Ligamentous injury 43, 45, 184
    acute 46
    partial 46
Ligamentum flavum 15, 19, 24, 25f, 96, 96f, 116, 120, 138-140, 146f, 147, 157, 158
    facilitate removal of 21
    layer of 120
    removing 25f
    resection of 158
Light blue retractor 166f
Listhesis, lateral 110
Liver function test 81
Local ablative techniques 86
Local autograft 70, 77
Longus colli
    flap of 36
    muscles 29, 36
Loose areolar tissue 30

Loose spinous processes 58
Lordosis 88
  restoration 35
  trial 166
Lordotic angle 169
Lordotic malalignment 122
Lordotic rod, high degree of 44
Lower lumbar area 91
Lower thoracic
  lesions 73
  pathology 65
  spine 70
Lumbar curve 122
Lumbar decompression 120
Lumbar injury 183
Lumbar interbody fusion
  lateral 160
  technique, anterior 123
Lumbar lordosis
  facilitate 97
  high degrees of 111
Lumbar pedicle
  fixation principles 105
  starting point 105*f*
Lumbar plexus 162*f*
Lumbar spine 12, 99, 161*f*
Lumbar subarachnoid drains 189
Lumbar vertebra, number of 66
Lumbodorsal fascia, thicker 93
Lumbopelvic dissociation 113*f*
Lumbosacral curve 122
Lumbosacral dysmorphism 91
Lumbosacral junction 92
  anatomy 91
Lumbosacral modifier 118
Lumbosacral plexus 160, 161
Lumbosacral spine, hyperlordosis of 91
Lymphatic plexus 29
Lymphoma 87
Lytic lesions, particularly 86

M

Machine vision image 174
Magnetic resonance imaging 62*f*, 81
Mandible, inferior border of 28
Mandible-cervical distance 3
Manual manipulation 100
Marcaine 22
Margel's technique 105
Match stick 23
Maximal flexion, position of 19
Maximal insertional arc 104
Mayfield attachment 21, 58
Mayfield clamp 60
Mayfield extension 12
Mayfield head
  attachment 8
  clamp 48, 51
  holder 8, 12, 13, 15, 39
  positioner 3, 60
Mayfield horseshoe 57
Mayfield position 3
Mayfield tongs 3, 15, 21
Mayfield type tongs 44
Mayfield vice 60
  head holder 58
Mayo table 40

McCullough retractor 149
  set 18
McRae's line 3
Mean arterial pressure 13, 69, 97, 182
Medial pedicle wall 100, 102, 104*f*
Medication, perioperative 119
Medtronic Clydesdale
  system 164
  trials 171
Medtronic divergence
  system 164, 166
  trials 166
Medtronic StealthStation™ 174
Medtronic Thompson retractor 169
  system 164, 165
Merocel neurosurgical patties 188
Metastasis, history of 81
Metastatic disease 81, 83, 86
Metastatic epidural spinal cord compression 86
Metastatic group 89
Metastatic spine disease 83
Metastatic tumors, treatment of 86
Meticulous hemostasis 37, 38, 40, 44
  first ensure 26
Meticulous periosteal dissection 18
Meticulous subperiosteal dissection 97
Metzenbaum scissors 30, 36
  pair of 30
Micro Kerrison rongeur 35, 37
Microdiscectomy 137, 138, 145, 145*f*, 146
  case of 141
Microwave ablation 86
Military tuck position 15
Minimally invasive spine 92
  surgery 127
Minimally invasive surgical
  approaches 149, 150
  discectomy 145
  laminectomy 145
  lateral approach 160
Minimally invasive techniques 87
Minimally invasive thoracoscopic approach 87
Minneapolis 173, 174
Mono- and bipolar electrocautery,
  combination of 22
Motion-sparing operation 26
Motor and sensory function 10*f*
Motor evoked potential 3, 18, 35, 57, 73, 97, 128
Motor vehicle accident 62*f*, 180
Multilevel cervical
  myelopathy, treatment of 21
  spinal cord compression 35
Multilevel corpectomy 38
Multilevel discectomy 74
Multilevel lumbar access 165*f*
Multimodal neuromonitoring, intraoperative 65
Multimodal pain regimen 16
Multiple myeloma 84, 87
Multiple vertebra, circumferential fusion of 98
Muscle 169
  necrosis 22
  spasms 16
Muscular bands 93

Muscular bleeding 22
Myelopathy 28, 39
  severe 13, 58
  type symptoms 17

N

Navigating pedicle screw placement 178*f*
Navigation 12, 190
  image-guided 131
  intraoperative 51
  system 18, 110, 145, 174
  techniques 173
N-butyl cyanoacrylate 85
Neck
  extension 30
  posterior 181*f*
Needle choices 188
Negative pressure wound therapy 136
  systems 136
Neoplastic disease
  diagnosis of 81
  treatment of 81
Neoplastic spine disease 86
Nerve
  decompression 150*f*, 151*f*
  fibers
    composed of 29
    course 30
  hook 12, 35
  injury, prevent 161*f*
  retractors 149
Nerve root 9, 17, 82
  adjacent 103
  decompress certain 23
  length of 28
  pedicle-inferior 103
  sacrifice 69
  structure 17
Neural elements compromise and
  compression 83
Neural foramen 67
Neural foramina 65
Neural structures, proximity to 102, 103
Neuroforaminal stenosis 97
Neurologic compromise 8, 42
Neurologic deficit 35, 127
Neurologic dysfunction, primary treatment
  for 86
Neurologic function 13, 81
Neurologic injury, potential for 96
Neurologic symptoms 65, 83
Neurological decline secondary,
  postoperative 16
Neurological injury 35, 55, 66, 132*f*, 181, 182
Neuromonitoring 3, 8, 18, 12, 30, 35, 65, 97,
  107, 145, 153, 155
  intraoperative 21, 119, 149, 160, 164
Neuropathic pain 154
Neuropathy, median 13
Neurophysiologic monitoring 135
  intraoperative 57, 145
Neurovascular structures 31
  higher risk of 163
  number of 31
New spinal lesions 81*fc*
Noncannulated systems 52
Noncontiguous linear collagen fibers 46

Nonexpandable tubular retractors 155
Nonself-tapping screws 131
Nonsmall-cell lung carcinoma 88
Nonsteroidal anti-inflammatory drugs 41, 136
Nonunion with conservative management, risk factors for 50*b*
Normal anatomy, distortion of 55
Nuchal line risk, superior 4
Numerical pain scale 191
Numerical rating scale 191

O

O-arm™ 173, 176, 177
    spin 176
    system 174
Oblique muscles
    external 169*f*
    internal 169*f*
Occipital bone 5*f*, 6*f*
Occipital condyle 44
    C1 interval 42
Occipital fusion 3
Occipital plate 3, 4
Occipital protuberance, external 4, 43, 44
Occipitocervical angle 3, 44*f*
Occipitocervical dislocation 42, 48
Occipitocervical distance 3
Occipitocervical fusion 3, 44, 46
Occipitocervical injuries 43*f*
Occipitocervical junction 5
Occult bleeding points 22
Occult occipital-cervical injury 57
Occult pneumothorax 70
Odontoid fracture 9, 10*f*, 51, 48
    transverse 50*f*
    type 2 8
    type 3 49*f*
Omohyoid muscle 36
Open door laminoplasty 23
Open Jackson frame 8, 119
Open-mouth odontoid 45, 47
Operating microscope 145
Operating room 3, 8, 13, 157, 178
    set-up 145
    specific 73
Operative technique 30, 87
Optimal screw positions 4
Os odontoideum 49*f*
Osseous fixation, posterior 58
Osteomyelitis 72
Osteopenia 51
Osteophyte 151
    anterior 37, 38
    fracture 181*f*
Osteoporosis 51, 80
Osteoporotic bone 94
Osteosynthesis 46
Osteotomes 115
    basic instruments of 119
Osteotomy 119
    closure 97
    posterior 118
    techniques 96
    three-column 118
Oswestry disability index 86, 191
Overgrown degenerative facets 152
Overhang 15

Owl eye 157
    technique 131

P

Pack allograft bone 5
Packed red blood cell 119
Paddle distractors 155, 166
Painful spinal metastases 86
Palliative embolization 86
Paracentral thoracic disk herniations 65
Paracentral-subarticular disk herniation 145*f*
Paraspinal muscles 13
Paraspinal musculature 157
Parietal pleura 74*f*, 75, 100
Pars fracture 53
Pars interarticularis 105, 105*f*
Pars screws 11
Partial thromboplastin time 81
Patellar wedges 77
Pedicle 17, 67, 110
    breech, lateral 91
    cannulation 67
    diameter 102
    fixation 104
    length 102
    path, tapping of 94*f*
    preparation 93
    subtraction osteotomy 97, 98, 99*f*
    taps 155
    tract taps 103
    zone 17
Pedicle screw 8, 11, 48, 93*f*, 95*f*, 110, 118, 131, 157
    cannulated 95, 159
    fixation 8
    placement 11, 14, 66, 93, 173, 177
    trajectory 92*f*
    value of 91
Peek and titanium mesh 77
Pelvic distraction 192*f*
Penfield
    basic instruments of 119
    dissectors 97
Percutaneous cryoablation 86
Percutaneous pedicle screw 111, 155, 172
    placement 157, 159
        complications of 95
Percutaneous technique 131
Percutaneous thoracolumbar pedicle screw fixation 91
Percutaneous transpedicular biopsy 82
Philadelphia cervical collar 33
Phlegmon, cavity of 75
Physical and neurologic examination 81
Physical medicine 184
Physical therapist, supervision of 27
Physical therapy 34, 122
Pin management 193
Pituitary rongeur 37, 97, 116, 137, 155, 166
Place instrumentation 58
Place neural structures 70
Place pedicle screws 135
Place plate 33
Place rods bilaterally 11
Plain radiograph 3, 5
    evaluation, acute 42
    thoracic 73

Planned vertebra coronal 79
Plasmacytoma 87
Plate 79
    anterior 61, 79
    application of 38
    holder 25
    insertion 26*f*
    positioning 26*f*
Platysma 29*f*, 30
Pleural scarring 72
Pleural tears, inadvertent 80
Polyaxial pedicle screws 103
Polyetheretherketone 35, 73, 115, 167
Polymer hydrogel 189
Polymethyl methacrylate 86, 104
    bone cement 88
Polyvinyl alcohol 84
Ponticulus posticus 48
Pop-off vicryl sutures 15
Postanesthesia care unit 52
Posterior cervical
    C1-2 fusion 8
    decompression 12
    foraminotomy 17
    fusion 12, 22*f*, 46, 48
    laminoplasty 21
    lateral mass screws 3
    musculature 14
    procedure 12, 18*f*
    screws 8
Posterior column
    osteotomy 97, 119, 120, 120*f*
    resection, amount of 97
Posterior element 22, 131
    resection, extent of 67
Posterior extent of Basion 43*f*
Posterior instrumentation techniques 51
Posterior instrumented fusion 48
Posterior lumbar 87
    interbody fusion 123
    pedicle screws 115
Posterior sacral
    lines 191
    wall 191
Posterior spinal
    columns 61
    fusion 99*f*, 100*f*
Posterior subaxial instrumentation, technical pearls for 58
Postfinal hardware placement 35
Postflip baseline signals 73
Potential kyphotic deformity 59
Potential ligamentous avulsions 45
Potential spinal cord ischemia 75
Potentially catastrophic complications 37
Preprocedural fluoroscopy 160
Pre-psoas space 170
Pressure bag 35
Presurgical planning 57
Pretracheal fascia 29, 31
Prevertebral edema 52
Prevertebral fascia 29, 31, 36
    lies directly 29
Primary tumor
    groups 85
    histology 83
    treatment of 86
Proaxis table 98

Progenitor cells 9
Proper pedicle screw 92
Prostate
    cancer 84
        specific antigen 81
Prosthetic cage 123
Provisional fixation 33
Provisionally tighten endcaps 11
Pseudoarthrosis 17, 159
Pseudohernia 163
Psoas muscle 100, 160, 161, 169, 170
    major 130
Psoas tendon 169, 169*f*
Pulled back 54
Pulmonary compromise, significant 72
Pulmonary embolus 72
Pulmonary function testing 73
Pyogenic osteomyelitis 72

R

Radiation exposure 174
Radiation therapy 87
    delivery systems, image-guided 88
    history of 88
    options 88*fc*
Radiation-resistant tumors 89
Radiculopathy, bilateral 17
Radiofrequency ablation 86
    role of 86
Radiofrequency, role of 86
Radiograph
    extension lateral 34
    facilitate 58
    intraoperative 98, 101
    visualization 65
Radiolucent bed 39
Radiolucent bite block 51
Radiolucent Jackson table 73
Radiolucent table 65, 150
Radioresistant tumors 88
Radiosensitive tumors, highly 87
Radiotherapy 84
Range of motion exercise, active 27
Rapid-sequence intubation 57
Raytec sponge 30
Rectal sensation 180
Rectangular prism shape 32
Rectus abdominis 124*f*
Recurrent laryngeal nerve 17, 29
Reduce venous pressure 21
Reduction techniques 54, 60
Reference frame insertion 175*f*
Regional lumbar hypolordosis 98
Regular surgical operating room 30
Rehabilitation 26, 184
Remnant nerve root 69
Renal cell carcinoma 85
Residual bony bridges 15
Residual ligamentum flavum 67
Retractor
    blades 22, 166*f*
    placement 22, 128, 146, 161
    position 151, 162
    removal 163
Retroperitoneal corridor 161
Retroperitoneal lumbar resections 87

Retropharyngeal hematoma 38
Retropharyngeal space 17
Retropharyngeal tissues 45
Retrovertebral stenosis 35
Rheumatoid arthritis 48
Rib
    autograft 78*f*
    bundled resected 78
    disarticulation 68
    heads articulate 76
    number of 73
    resection 130
Right-angle impactor 97
Rigid cervical collar 43
Rigid global kyphotic deformities 98
Rigid occipitocervical fixation 43
Rigid spinal deformity, severe 99
Robotic surgery 107
Robust disk 160
Rod placement 95, 131
    and fusion 11
Rod system 79
Roland-Morris disability questionnaire 191
Room set-up 8
Rotational stability 7
Roy-Camille method 105
Rule out spondylolysis 164

S

S1 pedicle screws 111*f*
Sacral and pelvic instrumentation 110
Sacral artery, middle 124*f*, 125*f*
Sacral body lines, posterior 191
Sacral screws 110
Sacroiliac joint 190
    dysfunction 192*f*
        symptoms 194
    fusion 193*f*, 194*f*
        instrumentation 190
    instrumented arthrodesis 191*t*
    pain 190
Safe pelvic screw placement 112*f*
Scheuermann's kyphosis 72
Schwab grade 96
Sclerotic lesions 83
Scoliosis
    lateral 100*f*
    Research Society 118
    severe 72
Screw
    construct 4
    designs 104
    heads 15
    intermediate 184
    placement 11, 91, 107, 117, 177*f*
    trajectory, medial-lateral 10*f*
Scrub solution, iodine-based 18
Seal bleeding points 23
Sealant adjuncts 189
Segmental fixation 5
Self-retaining retraction system 35
Self-retaining retractors 40
Sensitivity breast cancer prostate cancer 87
Sensory incomplete 181
Serum protein electrophoresis 81
Sharp rib tip fragments 75

Shoe-horn 162
Short tau inversion recovery 46, 65
Short-segment temporary rod 99
Single cervical nerve root 17
Single laminar screw 25
Single radiolucent line 92
Single-rod constructs 79
Sinus, transverse 4
Skeletal screening for cancer 73
Skeletal survey 81
Skin 13, 75
    glue 38
    incision 93*f*, 192*f*
    staples, spaced superficial 71
Skull base fractures 42
Skytron table 164
Smith-Robinson approach 36
Smoke evacuator 119
Soft cervical collar 26
Soft disk 65
    herniation, cases of 19
Soft spot 106
Soft tissue 22, 51, 113*f*
    anterior 39
    coverage, adequacy of 88
    disruption 55, 58
    dissection 91
    injury 53, 55, 60, 61
    shadow 45*f*
    significant posterior 55
Solid organ malignancies 88
Solid screw systems 51
Solitary metastatic tumors, cases of 89
Somatosensory evoked potential 35, 65, 73, 97, 130, 164
Sophisticated intraoperative techniques 9
Space disk 160
Spinal canal
    compromise 132*f*
    lateral 65
    roof of 104*f*
    stenosis 23
Spinal cord 14, 17, 66, 82, 127, 183, 188
    complete transection of 181*f*
    compression 21, 23, 50, 83
    infarction 21
    perfusion 35
    tolerance varies 88
Spinal cord injury 13, 35, 55, 88, 180
    acute 182
    management of 180
    medical management of 184
    model systems 180
    secondary 55
    surgical management of 182
Spinal deformity, significant 91
Spinal instability
    increase 91
    neoplastic score 83, 84, 85*t*
Spinal instrumentation 77, 78
Spinal metastases, treatment of 88
Spinal navigation 178*b*
Spinal needle 18
    placed 92
Spinal nerve root lateral 17
Spinal oncology, management of 81
Spinal osteotomy, classification of 96, 96*f*

Spinal stability 81, 83, 84
Spinal stenosis 97
Spinal tumor
    ablation, image-guided 86
    hypervascular 86*t*
    primary 81
    unresectable 85
Spine
    exposure, technical pearls for 58
    navigation systems 174*t*
    surgery, techniques of 155
Spinolaminar junction 52
Spinolaminar line 14
Spinopelvic parameters 164
Spinous process 22, 44, 115, 131
Splayed lateral masses 46
Spontaneous electromyography 160
Stable craniocervical injuries 42
Standard fluoroscopy 174
Standard orthopedic table 57
Standard sterile dressings 7
Starr-Eismont variant 53
Static supine imaging scan 47
Static tube 149
Stenosis 12
Stereotactic body radiotherapy 87, 88
    high-dose 88
    integration of 88
Stereotactic navigation 173
    computer-based 173
Stereotactic placement technique 131
Stereotactic radiosurgery 87, 88
Steri strips 38
Sterile fashion 18
Sternal notch 36, 92
Sternocleidomastoid muscles 36
Sternum 92
Straight screw trajectory 51
Strap muscles 28-31, 36
Structural allograft 35, 88
Structural coronal plane 118
Structural graft 38
Subarticular lateral recess 137
    stenosis 140
Subaxial burst fractures, surgical
    management of 59
Subaxial cervical
    approach, anterior 87
    trauma, management of 55
Subaxial flexion-compression injuries,
    surgical management of 60
Subaxial injury
    classification system 55
    pattern 55
Subaxial spine 13
Subaxial spinolaminar junction 44
Subaxial subluxations and dislocations,
    surgical management of 60
Subaxial trauma 58
Subchondral juxta-endplate bone 105
Subclavian artery 29
Subcutaneous tissues 15, 75, 129
Subfascial drain 7, 26
Subluxation 55
    dislocation 57
Subperiosteal dissection minimizes
    blood loss 66
    damage 31

Superior articular facet 17, 19, 61, 104, 106*f*, 119
    resection 19
Superior articular process 17, 97, 116, 140
Superior disk, annulotomy of 32
Superman position 65
Supplemental foraminotomies 23
Surgeon pass instruments 95
Surgery
    anterior 55, 57
    image-guided 174
    posterior 55
Surgical anatomy 28
Surgical approach 85
Surgical field adequate 21
Surgical indications 55
Surgical navigation system 174
Surgical power drill 145
Suture 188
Sympathetic chain 77, 102
Sympathetic trunk 69
Synovial capsule 18
Systemic disease 83
Systemic therapy 87

T

T score 164
T1 transverse process 14
Table-mounted
    retractor system, placement of 166*f*, 170*f*
    tubular retractor system 145, 164
Tamponade 103
T-cut 157
Tear drop 112
    type fractures 35
Temporary pins 38
Teriparatide 164
Terminal management 43, 46, 47, 49, 54
Thecal sac 97
Theoretical claim 8
Thick fascial layer, first 31
Thickest bone 4
Thoracic and lumbar trauma, surgical
    management of 127
Thoracic approach
    left 73*f*, 74*f*
    right 74*f*
Thoracic cavity 75
Thoracic curve 122
Thoracic disk herniation 72
Thoracic duct 77, 102
    injury 74*f*
Thoracic durotomy 189
Thoracic injury, low 183
Thoracic level 100
Thoracic myelogram 72
Thoracic nerve, long 76
Thoracic pedicle
    anatomical considerations 102
    fixation principles 104
    trajectory 105*f*
Thoracic probe, straight 66
Thoracic spinal cord injury 182
Thoracic spine 66, 72, 97, 99
    mid 70
Thoracic stenosis, primary 72

Thoracic transpedicular approach 65
Thoracic upper instrumented vertebra 118, 119
Thoracolumbar approach
    left 74*f*
    right 76*f*
Thoracolumbar injury classification 127, 127*t*, 134, 183, 183*t*
Thoracolumbar instrumentation 102
Thoracolumbar junction 61, 66, 76, 97
Thoracolumbar kyphosis 100*f*
Thoracolumbar osteotomy 96
Thoracolumbar spine 87, 135
    trauma 127
Thoracotomy 129
    instruments 73
    posterolateral 87
Three fluoroscopic views 193
Thrombin 20
Thrombin-soaked
    gelfoam 129
    hemostatic matrix 147
Thumb, rule of 97, 122
Thyroid
    arteries 29, 31
    drape 30
    panel 81
Tidal volume 74
Tip of Basion, posterior 43*f*
Tissue
    burden 91
    protection sleeve 190
    tension, maintain 128
Titanium 103
    alloy 87
    cages 191
    mesh cage 78*f*
    rod 3
Toggling 26*f*
Tokuhashi score 83, 84*t*
    system 84*fc*
Tomita grading scales 83
Tomita score 83, 84*t*
Tonsil clamp 70
Tonsillar hemostats 161
Towel clip 12
    technique 61
Tracheoesophageal groove 29
Tracheoesophageal structures 36
Tracheostomy 43
Traditional fluoroscopically-assisted
    techniques 108
Traditional subarachnoid lumbar drain 189
Traditionally radioresistant tumors 88
Tranexamic acid 4, 119, 129
Transarticular fixation 50
Transarticular screw 48
Transcervical craniocervical approach 87
Transforaminal lumbar interbody fusion 110, 115, 118, 123, 155
Translaminar screw 48
Transoral odontoid resection 48
Transpedicular decompression 66, 132
Transpedicular fixation points 98, 99
Transpleural approach, case of 80

Transpsoas 164
Transversalis fascia 161, 165, 168, 169*f*
Transverse foramen 37
Transverse ligament injuries 45*t*
    classification system of 47
Transverse pedicle angulation 102
Transverse skin markings 93*f*
Transversus abdominis 161
Trap door 76
Trapezius muscle posteriorly 28
Trauma bay 43
Traumatic injury 58, 60
Trendelenburg position 13
Tricalcium phosphate 9
Tricortical graft 38
Tri-cortical structural autograft 77*f*
Troughs 140
Tuberculosis 72
Tubular dilators 155
Tubular retractor 160
    placement 157
Tumor 38, 72, 75, 80
    diagnosis of 66
    histology, favorable 89
    location 85

U

Ulnar neuropathy 13
Uncovertebral joint 17, 31, 32, 37, 59
    bilateral 36
    medial 40
Unicortical screws 4
Unintended migration, risk of 94
Unknown isolated spine lesion, management of 82*fc*
Upper cervical spine 47
    injuries 42
    trauma management 42
Upper chest traveling dorsally 65
Upper instrumented vertebra 107, 118, 172
Upper lumbar instrumentation 92
Upper thoracic spine 21, 70, 75

Urine protein electrophoresis 81
Urological anatomy 160

V

Vagus nerve 29, 29*f*
Valsalva maneuver 68, 70, 188, 189
Vancomycin 7
    powder 26
Vascular access, increased 43
Vein
    retractor 36
    thrombosis, deep 184
Vena cava 77, 165
    inferior 73, 102, 123, 129
Ventral and dorsal rootlets, bundles of 17
Ventral bundles 17
Ventral corpectomy 37
Ventral cortex 23
Ventral lamina 104, 104*f*
Ventral spine 28
Ventral thecal sac 189
Vertebra
    aiming slightly medial 38
    lower instrumented 107, 118
    multiple adjacent 96*f*
    prominens 13
    second 96*f*
    superior 33, 93
Vertebral artery 4, 14, 28, 30, 32, 37
    anatomy 48
    injury 11, 28
    location 28
    posterior to 17
    runs 30
Vertebral body 30, 35, 36, 53, 69, 100
    anterior 36, 98
    decancellated 98
    depth 38
    fracture, risk of 39
    inferior 70
    junction 94
    length 28

    multiple 38
    posterior 100
    posterolateral 65
    sixth 36
    staple, current systems 79
    tumors 72
Vertebral burst fracture 35
Vertebral column resection 97, 99, 100*f*
Vertebral endplates 40
Vertebral fracture 126
Vertebral levels 36
Vertebroplasty 86
Viable osteoblasts, presence of 9
Vicryl 38
Violent crimes 180
Visceral injury 94
Visceral neck injuries 55
Visual analog scale 86, 191
Vocal cords 30
Volition evaluation 180

W

Weitlaner retractor 12
    self-retaining 66
White blood cell 84
Wilson frame 103, 145, 146, 149
Wiltse approach 150, 152
Wiltse incision placement 92*f*
Wiltse plane 111
Woodson elevator 15, 67, 97, 98, 120*f*, 137, 139, 140, 149, 152, 153
Woodson probe, basic instruments of 119
Worsen cervical stenosis 13
Wound closure and dressing 136

X

X-ray 58, 154, 169
    lateral view 170
    extension 48
    postpositioning 44
    preoperative 91

EU GSPR Authorised Reprsentative
Logos Europe, 9 rue Nicolas Poussin
1700, La Rochelle, France
Phone: +33 (0) 6 67 93 73 78
E-mail: contact@logoseurope.eu

www.ingramcontent.com/pod-product-compliance
Ingram Content Group UK Ltd.
Pitfield, Milton Keynes, MK11 3LW, UK
UKHW051846210426
5322IPUK00005B/184